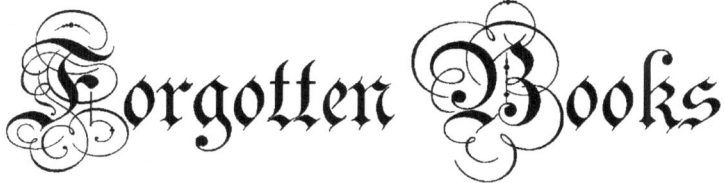
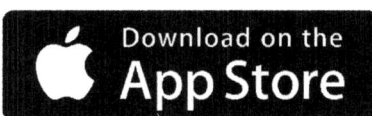
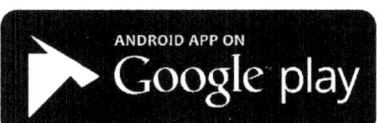

ISBN 978-1-334-64659-1
PIBN 10670780

This book is a reproduction of an important historical work. Forgotten Books uses state-of-the-art technology to digitally reconstruct the work, preserving the original format whilst repairing imperfections present in the aged copy. In rare cases, an imperfection in the original, such as a blemish or missing page, may be replicated in our edition. We do, however, repair the vast majority of imperfections successfully; any imperfections that remain are intentionally left to preserve the state of such historical works.

1 MONTH OF
FREE
READING

at

www.ForgottenBooks.com

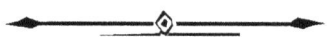

By purchasing this book you are eligible for one month membership to ForgottenBooks.com, giving you unlimited access to our entire collection of over 700,000 titles via our web site and mobile apps.

To claim your free month visit:

www.forgottenbooks.com/free670780

English
Français
Deutsche
Italiano
Español
Português

www.forgottenbooks.com

Mythology Photography **Fiction**
Fishing Christianity **Art** Cooking
Essays Buddhism Freemasonry
Medicine **Biology** Music **Ancient
Egypt** Evolution Carpentry Physics
Dance Geology **Mathematics** Fitness
Shakespeare **Folklore** Yoga Marketing
Confidence Immortality Biographies
Poetry **Psychology** Witchcraft
Electronics Chemistry History **Law**
Accounting **Philosophy** Anthropology
Alchemy Drama Quantum Mechanics
Atheism Sexual Health **Ancient History**
Entrepreneurship Languages Sport
Paleontology Needlework Islam
Metaphysics Investment Archaeology
Parenting Statistics Criminology
Motivational

REPORT

ON THE

CAUSE AND MODE OF DIFFUSION

OF

EPIDEMIC CHOLERA,

BY

WILLIAM BALY, M.D., F.R.S.,

PHYSICIAN TO MILLBANK PRISON.

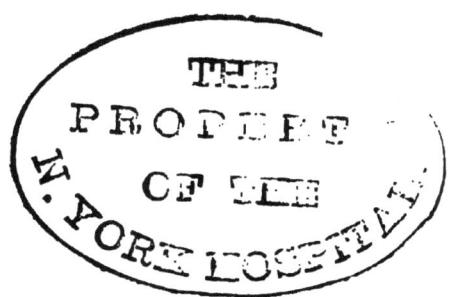

IN AYRTON PARIS, M.D., D.C.L., F.R.S.,

PRESIDENT OF THE ROYAL COLLEGE OF PHYSICIANS OF LONDON.

IR,

  I have the honour to place in your hands the
ort on the " Cause and Mode of Diffusion of Epidemic
era," which was undertaken by me in compliance with
resolution of the Cholera Committee in the summer of
rear 1849. It is due to the College, and also to myself,
the circumstances which have so long delayed its com-
su should now be explained.

he replies of Members of the Profession in all parts of
country to the circular letters and series of questions
ared by Dr. Gull and myself, and issued in the name
e Cholera Committee, were not received until the end
se year 1849 and the beginning of the year 1850.
r were more than four hundred in number, and were
any instances of considerable length. It was necessary
ttract from them the statements relating to the several
s which were to be treated of, and subsequently, as
extracts would have been far too voluminous for pub-
on, to abstract and tabulate, for the sake of more easy
ance, the facts detailed in them. In this work, of
le, much time was consumed.

any of the communications bore proof of having
prepared with great care and after searching inquiry.
afforded very valuable evidence with regard to several

questions of high interest and importance, and entitle the
Gentlemen who so readily and zealously lent their aid in
promoting the objects of the Cholera Committee to the best
thanks of the College. These communications were, however, necessarily defective in that kind of information from
which alone the course of the epidemic in England in the
years 1848 and 1849, could be safely deduced, namely,
statistical facts. I had, therefore, to seek for further materials from different public offices; and consulted many
publications on the subject of Cholera. The Reports
of Dr. Sutherland and Mr. Grainger to the General Board
of Health, which were issued, the one in 1850, the other
in 1851, were, in particular, found replete with valuable matter, more especially in relation to sanitary questions. But my hopes of gathering from these different
sources the statistics of the epidemic were wholly disappointed. It had, however, in the meantime become
known to me, that the data at the command of the Registrar-General would be published under the superintendence of Mr. Farr; and being now sure that no satisfactory
report on Cholera, such as I believed to be desired by the
Cholera Committee, could be prepared without reference to
those data, I determined to wait until they should be made
available.

Mr. Farr's most able and elaborate "Report on the Mortality of Cholera in England in 1848-49," was not published
until the spring of last year. My attention was then immediately given to the facts and generalisations it contained;
and the preparation of the Report I had undertaken was
proceeded with. It was, even, in part printed during the
months of November and December, 1852; and the maps
and diagrams intended to illustrate it were also then, in
part, designed and drawn. I still felt, however, that much
additional light might be thrown on the progress of the
epidemic from place to place in England, and on the
causes of its extension, by the original Registration Returns.

These Returns, giving the dates and other particulars of 55,149 deaths, had not been printed, on account of their great extent. But they were preserved at the General Register Office; and, at the commencement of the present year, they were, with the sanction of the Registrar-General, placed, for a time, at my disposal. The analysis of them, which, without the aid of clerks, was a labour of no little magnitude, furnished the materials for Tables showing the progress of Cholera and Diarrhœa in all the towns and sub-districts of England and Wales; and Tables of this kind were drawn up for every county. A few of them only have been printed; but the statistical history of the epidemic of 1849, extending from page 53 to page 110 of the Report, is almost entirely founded on the results which they afforded.

Since this task was brought to a conclusion every effort has been made to complete the Report, and no obstacle that could be avoided has been permitted to interfere with its progress.

Such, Sir, is the explanation I have to offer of the delay which, I know, has caused surprise to yourself and many Fellows of the College. A perusal of the Report will, I trust, show that the postponement of its publication has been attended with some compensatory advantage,—that the matter it has enabled me to add is not devoid of value and interest. An opposite judgment, I must own, would disappoint and pain me. But even then I should have the satisfaction of knowing that my error had arisen from an anxious desire to fulfil the trust committed to me in a manner not altogether unworthy of the College.

I have the honour to be,
Sir,
Your obedient humble Servant,
WILLIAM BALY.

London, December, 1853.

TABLE OF CONTENTS.

CONTENTS OF THE APPENDIX.

MAPS AND DIAGRAMS.

CORRIGENDUM.

Page 38, line 22, *for* Chilton *read* Clutton.

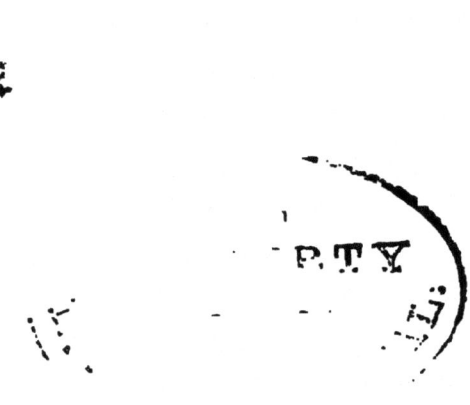

REPORT

ON

THE CAUSE OF ASIATIC CHOLERA,

AND ITS

MODES OF INCREASE AND DIFFUSION.

In the first circular letter addressed by the Cholera Committee to Hospital Physicians and to members of the College generally, two questions were proposed in relation to this subject.

The first was :—

"Can you communicate any facts observed or investigated by yourself which appear to you demonstrative of the contagious or infectious nature of Cholera, or of its communicability in any way?"

The second question related to the character of the localities in which Cholera manifested itself most frequently and with most intensity.

Can you detail any facts illustrative of the influence of deficient ventilation, damp, foul air, and bad water, respectively, or of other external circumstances in determining or favouring the production of Cholera?"

These questions did not procure that distinct statement of facts, especially with regard to the former subject of inquiry, which the Committee desired. A second series of questions was, therefore, prepared, and, with the sanction of the President, distributed very widely through the profession; the

B

chief objects of this more detailed
determine the mode of origin
towns, villages, or large publi
it was spontaneous or the
duction of infection from
value of the theory that the
or aggravated by the water
persons exposed to frequent
clothes which they had worn,
and others, are attacked by
viduals of the same rank
posed; and fourth, to learn
particular part of the town,
in which the first case the

* Roy

Sir,—We are instructed by
the accompanying copies of
to request that you will dist
Profession in your neighbou
had the largest experience
which those gentlemen may
objects indicated, would be r

The Committee are also
special inquiry respecting th
They believe that much mig
important question, by collec
first cases of the disease in t
tutions throughout England
submit to you the subjoined
obtaining for them as detailed

1. Had the person first attacked
   recently been in an infected p
   house clothes or other articles
   or had he been in contact with
   locality?

2. If the disease appears not to have
   these ways, is it possible that the drink
   conveying the infection, by its being co
   passage (as a river or canal) through infecte

3. What was the character of the part of

nded by Dr. Snow—gives a
e of contagion. It supposes
llowed, and acts directly on
estines, is at the same time
il, and passes out, much in-
that these discharges after-
fly by becoming mixed with
wells, reach the alimentary
roduce the like disease in

es that the cause of Cholera
ut supposes that it is repro-
the bodies of those whom it
s due to the agency of the

fication of the fourth. It
r is increased by a species
of reproduction in impure,
aintains that it nevertheless
cans of human intercourse;
her vehicles, and even in the
foul clothes of vagrants, and
ties.
the second and fourth, as-
of the disease may be in-
by impure air, as well as in

object of this Report is to
hich of these theories is

tious, or evidently lean to the adoption of that view, and seven in which the contagious or infectious nature of the disease is asserted in an unqualified manner. On the other hand, in fifteen of the replies received by the Committee, the writers advocate, or, at least, admit, the probability, that Cholera is propagated in more than one way; in twenty-four no opinion is expressed, although in several of these the facts communicated are so stated as to show that the writers would not altogether exclude infection of some kind from the modes of diffusion, yet clearly regard it as only of partial influence; and in six other papers, it is simply stated that the disease is communicable under some circumstances, or that instances of infection have been observed by the writers.

The varieties of opinion as to the remote cause of Asiatic Cholera and the cause of its spreading are very numerous, but all that need be referred to may be reduced to six principal theories which must be briefly stated here, since it is only by reference to them that the value and import of the facts to be examined in this Report can be estimated.

The *first* theory is, that the disease spreads by an "atmospheric influence or epidemic constitution," its progress consisting of a succession of local outbreaks, and that the particular localities affected are determined by certain "localizing conditions," which are, first, all those well-known circumstances which render places insalubrious; and, second, a susceptibility of the disease in the inhabitants of such places, produced by the habitual respiration of an impure atmosphere*.

The *second* theory following the analogy of diseases known to be due to morbid poisons regards the cause of Cholera as a morbific matter which undergoes increase only within the human body, and is propagated by means of emanations from the bodies of the sick, in other words, by contagion†.

* See Report of the General Board of Health on the Epidemic Cholera of 1848 and 1849, pp. 36 and 146. Report on Quarantine, p. 14.

† In the succeeding pages of this Report the terms "contagion" and

The *third* theory—that propounded by Dr. Snow—gives a more specific form to the doctrine of contagion. It supposes that the poison of Cholera is swallowed, and acts directly on the mucous membrane of the intestines, is at the same time reproduced in the intestinal canal, and passes out, much increased, with the discharges; and that these discharges afterwards, in various ways, but chiefly by becoming mixed with the drinking water in rivers or wells, reach the alimentary canals of other persons, and produce the like disease in them.

The *fourth* theory also assumes that the cause of Cholera is a morbific matter or poison, but supposes that it is reproduced only in the air, not within the bodies of those whom it affects, and that its diffusion is due to the agency of the atmosphere.

The *fifth* theory is a modification of the fourth. It admits that the cholera matter is increased by a species of fermentation or other mode of reproduction in impure, damp, and stagnant air, but maintains that it nevertheless is distributed and diffused by means of human intercourse; it being carried in ships and other vehicles, and even in the clothes of men, especially the foul clothes of vagrants, and the accumulated baggage of armies.

The *sixth* theory combines the second and fourth, assuming that the material causes of the disease may be increased and propagated in and by impure air, as well as in and by the human body.

Such are the theories. The object of this Report is to inquire into the facts, and to learn which of these theories is most in accordance with them. But, in the first place, reference will be chiefly made only to the most general views that may be taken of the cause and mode of pro-

"contagious" are alone restricted to the sense here indicated; the words "infection" and "infected" are used in their most general significations of pollution and polluted, without any inference as to the source of the polluting cause or poison.

pagation of the disease; those, namely, which respectively regard it—1, as dependent on a general state of the atmosphere or an atmospheric influence; 2, as due to a poisonous matter partially distributed through the atmosphere and conveyed from place to place by atmospheric currents; and 3, as communicable in some way or other by human intercourse.

The facts which will be submitted to examination do not consist merely of those furnished by members of the profession in answer to the letters addressed to them by the Cholera Committee of the College: documentary evidence of much value has been obtained from other sources. And special acknowledgment must here be made of the aid in this way rendered to the College by the Registrar-General, by Sir William Burnett, Director-General of the Medical Department of the Navy, by the Commissioners in Lunacy, and by Sir Charles Hastings, President of the Provincial Medical and Surgical Association *.

Certain general characters observed in a cholera epidemic are too well established to be disputed. These must, in the first place, be carefully considered; since no theory which is inconsistent with them can be the true one; and since from them alone some conclusions may perhaps be drawn regarding the nature of the cause on which the epidemic depends, and the mode of its propagation.

I. Of the characters here referred to, the most obvious one is *the unequal and very partial distribution of the epidemic,* which in this respect presents a remarkable contrast

* From the sources above indicated, together with the statistical " Report on the Mortality of Cholera in England, in 1848, 1849," prepared by Mr. Farr, by direction of the Registrar-General, the information relating to the distribution and propagation of the epidemic in this country has been almost exclusively derived. The published works of individual writers, and the communications contained in periodicals, have rarely been referred to; for, in the use of such materials, it seemed scarcely possible to avoid the risk of partial selection.

to epidemic influenza. For while the latter disease, in its visitations, has pervaded within a very short period the whole of Europe, and at one and the same time has involved every part of this island, affecting four-fifths of its inhabitants, Cholera has left whole districts unvisited, and has fallen severely on comparatively few localities.

The unequal and partial distribution of the cholera epidemic is manifest, whether Europe is regarded as a whole, or the attention is confined to this country alone, or even to a single town, or a single public institution.

With regard to England, the fact is demonstrated from statistical data in the Report prepared by Mr. Farr, by direction of the Registrar-General. It is shown that four-fifths of the deaths from Cholera in England and Wales during the year 1849 (namely 46,592 out of 53,293 deaths) occurred in 134 registration districts, the total number of districts being 623, and that on the other hand, there are 85 districts in which no death was caused by Cholera. The partial distribution of the epidemic is further illustrated by the maps Nos. I. and II., which show the spots in which deaths from Cholera were registered in the two periods of the epidemic, extending respectively from the 1st of October, 1848, to the end of April, 1849, and from the 1st of May, 1849, to the close of the year. In both maps, but especially in the first, which represents the earlier and less severe portion of the epidemic, it will be observed that the mortality caused by Cholera was considerable in a comparatively small number of places, while over the general surface of the country no deaths were caused by it, or only single deaths. And with regard to these single deaths, it must be borne in mind that some of them must have been due to the common sporadic Cholera, not to the epidemic disease; for deaths from sporadic Cholera occur every year in all parts of the country*, and in the returns made to the

* The subjoined Table shows the number of deaths in England and Wales registered as due to Cholera in the several years 1838, 1839, 1840, 1841, 1842, 1848, 1849.

Registrar-General * from which the data for these maps are derived, the deaths caused by it are not, and could not, with

Years.	No. of Deaths from Cholera.
1838	339
1839	394
1840	702
1841	443
1842	1,620
1848	1,057
1849	53,293

The distribution of the deaths from sporadic Cholera over the different quarters of the year, is shown, in the case of the metropolis, in the next Table, constructed, like the last, from data derived from the Reports of the Registrar-General; and if the numbers of the deaths are distributed in similar proportions through the different quarters of the year, in the whole country, the average number occurring in England and Wales, in the six winter months of the year 1848–1849, will have been (calculating from the mean of the two years 1841 1842) about 150.

	Quarters ending				
Year.	March.	June.	September.	December.	The Year.
1840	3	4	53	6	66
1841	1	1	23	3	28
1842	0	7	106	13	126
1843	6	8	60	14	88
1844	4	9	47	5	65
1845	4	2	26	11	43
1846	7	9	197	15	228
1847	3	4	98	12	117
Total in 8 years	28	44	610	79	761
Annual Average	3·5	5·5	76·25	9·86	94·62
1848	9	17	158	468	662

* The Registrar-General entrusted the Cholera Committee with the manuscript documents, from which the data referred to were extracted.

ny accuracy, be distinguished from those due to the super-
dded epidemic.

It must be remembered, too, that these maps represent
he aggregate of the local visitations during several months,
nd that in any given month of either period, the distribution
f the epidemic was even more partial than it here appears.

Again, if the attention be fixed on single towns, single
treets, or public institutions, the same character is ob-
erved. One part of a town suffers most severely; others
scape altogether. In a few houses in a street half the inha-
itants are carried off by the disease; in the remainder not
single death occurs. In a large public establishment, such
s a barrack, a lunatic asylum, or a prison, it often happens
at the disease is, at least, for a time, confined to one wing
f the building, one ward, or one series of rooms. (See
stances in the Appendix.)

11. The second general character of a Cholera epidemic
, that *the localities, especially, and most severely, visited by
, have certain features by which they are distinguished
om those other places which entirely escape, or suffer only
a slight degree.* In the first place, it may be observed,
at the *parts of England* in which the rate of mortality was
ighest in 1849, as well as in 1832, are, with few exceptions,
e more densely-populated regions lying around great rivers,
on the sea-coast, or in the neighbourhood of mines, espe-
ally coal-mines. The districts having the relations last
scribed have sometimes a high level, and lie in the central
gions of the country where the rivers take their rise; such,
r example, are the districts about Wolverhampton, and New-
stle-under-Lyne. But those lying on the coast or about
vers, which are the more numerous, have almost always a low
vel, and an alluvial soil, as in the instances of the borders
f the Thames and the Humber, and the district of South-
mpton and Portsmouth. The preference of Cholera for
ch localities as these is shown by the fact of its having
en three times more fatal in the registration districts on
e coast than it was in the interior of the country.

	Population, March 31, 1851.	Deaths from Cholera in 1849.	Deaths from Cholera to 10,000 persons living in 1849.
England and Wales ...	17,922,768	53,293	30
415 Inland Districts...	10,433,333	17,052	17
208 Coast Districts ...	7,489,435	36,241	50

The districts spared by Cholera are in most cases thinly peopled, have a comparatively high altitude, and more frequently lie far inland, and, when on or near the coast, have usually a very thin population not engaged in active traffic with other places. A large portion of Wales and Herefordshire, and many districts in Norfolk, Suffolk, Westmoreland, Northumberland, and some of the central counties, have these features, and had no deaths from Cholera. (See Maps I. and II.)

The relation of density of population to the mortality from the epidemic is further illustrated by the subjoined Table*.

Districts.	Area in Square Miles.	Population in 1851.	Inhabitants to a square mile.	Deaths from Cholera.	Deaths per 10,000 living.	Deaths per square mile.
The 623 districts of England	57,067	17,922,768	308	52,293	30	·9
134 districts where the mortality was greatest	7,839	7,417,817	915	46,592	65	6·0
404 districts where the mortality was less.	39,824	9,354,172	235	6,701	7	·17
85 districts where no deaths from Cholera occurred	9,404	1,150,779	122	nil.	nil.	nil.

* The data for this Table were in part extracted from Mr. Farr's Report, and in part obtained from the office of the Registrar-General.

Of the *towns* most severely visited, it is a very general character that, like the districts in which they are situated, they lie on the coast or on rivers, especially the parts of rivers near their mouths, where the level is low, and the soil alluvial, and that they have an active traffic,—in many instances with shipping. They have, moreover, usually a large, crowded, and poor population living in ill-constructed and ill-ventilated houses, together with imperfect sewerage, deficient supply of water, and the consequent accumulation of filth of all kinds.

Of these towns in the coast districts the chief seaports suffered most; and the small ports, often inaccessible to ships, least.

Different orders of Coast Districts.	Population in 1851.	Deaths from Cholera, 1849.	Deaths from Cholera to 10,000 living.
17 Districts, including 7 of the Great Ports*	1,047,210	12,636	125
30 Districts, comprising the Secondary Ports	1,106,109	5,067	47
125 other Coast Districts	2,974,476	4,401	15

But several cities and towns far inland suffered a very high mortality from Cholera, for example, Salisbury, Manchester, Durham, Merthyr, Bilston, Wolverhampton, and Newcastle-under-Lyne. Of these several have constant intercourse with seaports, but all alike have the character of containing large and crowded masses of poor, with all the evils that attend crowded dwellings when the provisions necessary for preserving the public health are neglected †.

* Liverpool, Hull, Bristol, Plymouth, Southampton, Portsea, and Tynemouth.

† The foregoing observations on the characters of the districts and towns chiefly visited by Cholera, as well as the Tables, are almost wholly derived from Mr. Farr's Report on Cholera in England in 1848-1849, published by the Registrar-General.

A large population, however, is not a necessary condition. Small towns, and small villages, both on the coast and in the interior of the country, and isolated groups of houses or cottages, and single public institutions, have been devastated by the epidemic. But in these instances the other conditions have rarely, probably never, been wholly wanting; thus Bedford, where thirty-five deaths from Cholera occurred amongst a population of 9,000 or 10,000, has a low marshy site, on the banks of the Ouse; and Hertford, which suffered a mortality of seventy-nine deaths from Cholera amongst 11,000 inhabitants, lies in a low valley close to the junction of three small streams; Noss Mayo, where forty-eight deaths occurred amongst 400 inhabitants, is a village close to the coast, built on the low shores of a creek between high hills, where the air is rendered damp and foul by the exposure of mud at low tide, and of the offal left by fishermen; and the group of six cottages at Long Handboro', in which seven deaths from Cholera occurred in little more than a fortnight, though on a high site, was destitute of drainage, and had heaps of refuse and filth lying around. In the cases of the brickmakers at Southall, of the hop-pickers at East Farleigh, of the pauper children at the Tooting School, of the lunatics in the Wakefield Asylum, and of the convicts in the Wakefield Old Prison (of which the particulars are given in the Appendix), the more important conditions unfavourable to health appear to have existed in the interior of the buildings, and want of adequate ventilation seems to have been the chief of them.

Some or other of the conditions above described as characterizing the towns severely visited by the epidemic seem, then, to have been, at least generally, present wherever a considerable mortality occurred; and a low damp site and a crowded population, with defective ventilation, have been the most rarely wanting.

But it is important to observe that not all the towns, even of considerable size, presenting such conditions have experienced the severe ravages of the epidemic. Three seaports,

Lynn, Deal, and Scarboro' almost entirely escaped, and many large inland towns certainly crowded, and in a more or less defective sanitary condition, had very few deaths. Thus, in Cambridge there were only five deaths—and during the whole of the year 1849 none ; in Colchester four—and only two in 1849 ; in Cheltenham six ; in Stafford three ; in Leicester two, and in Lincoln seven ; the population of these towns ranging from 18,000 to 50,000. And in Hereford with 18,000 inhabitants, and Kendal with 12,000, there was no death from Cholera *. It is impossible, without more local knowledge of these places, to determine with certainty the local causes to which their comparative or complete exemption from the ravages of the epidemic might be ascribed. But it may safely be affirmed, that the characters of the sites and the sanitary condition of several of these towns would afford no reason for their escaping rather than some other towns, which suffered severely.

Of the multitude of smaller towns and villages that escaped altogether from the influence of the epidemic, it cannot be doubted that very many were at least as insalubrious in site and other circumstances as places of the same size which were severely attacked.

Again, if we compare the two periods of the epidemic illustrated by Maps I. and II. respectively, we meet with facts tending in like manner to prove that the epidemic did not operate equally in all places presenting the conditions which apparently fitted them to receive it. Thus it has been mentioned already, that in the districts of mines and potteries in Staffordshire, and the mining district of Merthyr, Cholera prevailed with great intensity during the summer of 1849. It will be seen in Map I. that the disease scarcely showed itself in those districts during the earlier outbreak of the epidemic ; while it may at the same time be noticed that at Carlisle, at Chesham, in the Amersham district in Buckinghamshire,

* In Birmingham and Aston only thirty-five deaths from Cholera were registered, but the deaths recorded as due to Diarrhœa were numerous.

and at several places in Norfolk, where the epidemic prevailed more or less intensely in the earlier period, there were
very few or no deaths in the later period.

The papers forwarded to the Cholera Committee by many
members of the profession, give the means of correcting or
confirming the foregoing statistical results by the testimony
of local observers. They contain descriptions of the sites,
or sanitary condition, and in most cases descriptions of both
the sites and the sanitary condition, of fifty-eight towns, villages, and public institutions. (Table I. in Appendix.)

Of thirty-five of these places which suffered in proportion to their population, much more than the average
mortality from Cholera, nineteen* have low humid sites;
ten† have sites of a mixed or doubtful character, or not
described, but six‡ are described as being situated in decidedly open and elevated situations. The sanitary condition in other respects of the thirty-five places is described
in twenty-one instances, and in thirteen of these appears to
have been very bad, and in all defective, except Boston
Workhouse and Seaham; and both of these places lie
on the coast. Moreover, the town of Boston, adjoining
which the workhouse stands, has a low level, and is in a
bad sanitary condition. But Seaham is described by Dr.

* The following are the nineteen places:—

Ashford Union House	Torton Barracks, Gos-	Croscombe, near Wells
Dreadnought Hospital	port	Tewkesbury
Ship	Stonehouse Marines	Wakefield Old Prison
Woolwich Convict	Barracks	The Lye Waste, near
Hulks	Noss Mayo	Stourbridge
Tooting Pauper School	Newton Torr and Bold-	Cairnbulg
Cottages at Southall	venture	Inveralochy
Chatham and Rochester	Kingsand and Cawsand	Boddam.
Strood		

† Canterbury	Dunston	Wakefield Lunatic
Ilford	Dowlais	Asylum
Southampton	Walsall	Sunderland.
Newton Ferrers	Boston Workhouse	

‡ Margate Infirmary	Brixton, Devon	Walsall Workhouse
Torpoint	Long Handboro'	Seaham Harbour.

Brown as "not damp, having an elevation which secures free ventilation, the lanes and streets not narrow, sewerage and drainage excellent, nuisances few, population well fed;" so that unless, as is probable, the ventilation of the interior of the dwellings is imperfect, the only circumstances in which Seaham appears to resemble other places where the epidemic was severely felt is the constant intercourse with shipping, and, through it, with other infected places.

Twelve of the places described suffered but little, or not at all, from the epidemic; yet three * of these are in low sites, two both in low sites and in a bad sanitary state. Reading, where only seventeen deaths from Cholera occurred out of a population of about 20,000, is described by Dr. Bradshaw as "built on a bog, surrounded by water-meadows, with the Thames on one side, a canal on the other; the atmosphere remarkably humid," and as "by no means in a sanitary state as to drainage and the like." Stafford, where there were only three deaths from Cholera, is said by Dr. Harland to be "very low," "to have numerous stagnant drains in its immediate neighbourhood;" "the river impounded by hills so as to be above the level of the surrounding lands;" "floods frequent and long continued;" while "the most favourable conditions for the attack of Cholera exist within the town, there being no sewers, much filth on the surface, slaughter-houses, pig-styes," &c.

The information furnished by the correspondents of the Cholera Committee, therefore, confirms the rule, that the epidemic rarely prevailed with any severity unless conditions favourable to the development and spread of epidemic diseases were obviously present; but likewise seems to show again, by the examples of Reading and Stafford, that Cholera did not fall severely upon all places presenting such conditions.

The inquiry may be carried further, and it may be learned how far the partial distribution of the epidemic amongst the

* Deptford Dockyard, Reading, and Stafford.

different parts of towns, streets, and even parts of large public establishments, is determined by local differences in respect of elevation and the other circumstances affecting the salubrity of human habitations.

London, from its extent, the various levels of its several districts, their various relations to the great river running through it, and various conditions as to sanitary provisions, and the habits and character of the population, afforded an ample field for observing the influence of these different circumstances. And happily, the opportunity has not been lost: the observations collected and recorded under the directions of the Registrar-General, have been ably analysed by Mr. Farr, who has extracted from them important results.

A very constant inverse relation subsists between the elevation of the different registration districts of the metropolis, and the rate of mortality from Cholera amongst the inhabitants. This is manifest, not merely when the highest districts are compared with the lower districts in groups, but even when the several districts are examined seriatim in respect of these two circumstances. In proportion as the mortality from Cholera rises, the elevation of the soil is, as a general rule, found to be lower. This is shown in the annexed Table, which has been extracted from Mr. Farr's Report.

Districts.	Deaths from Cholera in 1849 to 10,000 Inhabitants.	Estimated elevation above Trinity high-water mark.
1. Rotherhithe	205	0
2. St. Olave	181	2
3. St. George, Southwark	164	0
4. Bermondsey	161	0
5. St. Saviour	153	2
6. Newington	144	2
7. Lambeth	120	3
8. Wandsworth	100*	22
9. Camberwell	97	4
10. West London	96	28
11. Bethnal Green	90	36
12. Shoreditch	76	48
13. Greenwich	75	8
14. Poplar	71	10
15. Westminster	68	2
16. Whitechapel	64	28
17. St. Giles	53	68
18. Stepney	47	16
19. Chelsea	46	12
20. East London	45	42
21. St. George's, East	42	15
22. London, City	38	38
23. St. Martin	37	35
24. Strand	35	50
25. Holborn	35	53
26. St. Luke	34	48
27. Kensington (except Paddington)	33	12
28. Lewisham	30	28
29. Belgrave	28	19
30. Hackney	25	55
31. Islington	22	88
32. Pancras	22	80
33. Clerkenwell	19	63
34. Marylebone	17	100
35. St. James, Westminster	16	43
36. Paddington	8	76
37. Hampstead	8	350
38. Hanover Square and May Fair	8	49

It is obvious that a low level of the soil almost always includes imperfect drainage, and a more stagnant, damp and
impure atmosphere than is met with at a higher level. This

* Excluding the deaths which occurred in Drouet's Asylum for Infant
Paupers, the mortality of the Wandsworth district was at the rate of
72 deaths to 10,000 persons living.

C

is undoubtedly the case in London. In London, too, the lower districts have generally a poorer and more dense population, and, lying for the most part near the river, are more exposed to the vapours rising from it as well as to intercourse with the shipping. The relation borne by lowness of level to the prevalence of Cholera in London may, therefore, show the influence of all these various circumstances, or of one or more of them, on the spreading of the disease. And although no one of these circumstances singly can from statistical data be shown to have so constant a relation to the mortality from Cholera as the level of the surface has, yet several of them, namely, poverty and density of the population, with their attendant evils, filth and foul air, have a manifest connection with the prevalence of Cholera, not dependent on lowness of site *. Thus, Bethnal Green suffered a mortality from Cholera more than double that of the district of St. George's in the East, although it lies further from the Thames, and at a much greater elevation above high-water mark ; and the most obvious conditions with which this exceptional result can be connected is the greater poverty of the inhabitants and the generally worse sanitary condition of the houses in the former district. Again, the far higher mortality from Cholera in St. Giles's than in St. Martin's district, notwithstanding that the latter has a considerably lower level, cannot but be in some way connected with the greater density as well as the greater poverty of the population, and the more defective sanitary provisions in St. Giles's. Instances of this kind, which are found to be very numerous, when the relation between the mortality from Cholera and the elevation of the surface is examined in the cases of the sub-districts of the metropolis, go far to prove that, even in London, the connection between lowness of level and the prevalence of Cholera depends at least in great part on the character of the inhabitants and their dwellings in the lower districts, and on the foulness, as distinguished from mere dampness, of the atmosphere in these localities.

* This was pointed out by Mr. Smith in his paper published in the *Medical Times*, in November, 1849.

The communications received by the Cholera Committee describe the sanitary condition of the chief seats of Cholera in 68 towns, districts, or institutions. The testimony here afforded to the College is complete and convincing as to the very general association of Cholera, where it is rife, with over-crowding and deficient ventilation, imperfect drainage, want of cleanliness, and the effluvia from privies, cesspools, foul drains, &c. Thus, amongst the characters of the chief seat of Cholera in the 68 places described, bad ventilation or overcrowding of the houses is mentioned 54 times; want of cleanliness, 38 times; defective drainage, 28 times; the presence of foul drains, or cesspools, or open sewers, 16 times; and damp, 11 times. The very similar characters ascribed to the parts of towns in which Cholera proved most destructive to human life may be judged of from the abstracts of the communications relating to this part of the subject given in the Appendix (Table II.).

But one or two striking instances in which the limitation of the disease coincided very exactly with the range of the unhealthful influences referred to, may with advantage be here quoted:—

Of Oxford the late Dr. Kidd says,—"Dividing the whole city into two parts, an eastern and a western, by a line of houses nearly a mile in length, which is continued from the Radcliffe Observatory on the north to the bridge called Folly Bridge on the south, only one case of Cholera occurred on the east of that line; all the other cases, amounting to about 70, occurring on the west. The value of this fact is greatly enhanced by the observation that the western side of the line above described is generally a swampy soil, with scarcely any fall for drainage, and is inhabited by a population least attentive either to domestic cleanliness or personal temperance; while the eastern side has as great a proportion of physical and moral advantages as are usually observable under such circumstances." Further particulars of exactly the same import are given in Mr. T. Allen's account of the distribution of the epidemic in Oxford.

Another striking instance of the partial sway of the ep demic, and of its connection with local defects in the sanita conditions, is afforded by the prisons at Wakefield. Thr prisons, known as the Old Prison, the New Prison, and tl Women's Prison, here stand in close proximity, on a plot ground of about 17 acres, along one side of which runs a slu gish brook. The Old Prison stands close to this brook on dead flat. The ground on which the New Prison and tl Women's Prison have been built, gradually rises to the slig elevation of about eight feet above the level of the broo " At the time of the visitation of Cholera, the Old Prison w: not provided with any means for artificially warming ar ventilating it. The outlet of the drains was defective, ar the drains always contained water, which, soaking into tl loose soil on which the prison is built, kept it continual damp. The cells in which the prisoners slept were cold ar damp. The day-rooms were crowded, and the privies, whic opened directly into the day-rooms, were in an objectionab state."

" The New Prison and the Women's Prison are coi structed on the Pentonville plan, and are very efficient drained, ventilated, and warmed. The cells in which tl prisoners both work and sleep are dry and warm, and we supplied with fresh air."

" The drains both of the New and of the Old Prise enter into the brook. But the drains of the Old Prison ru under the building; while those of the New Prison run c the outside of it." Such was the sanitary condition of tl prisons as described by Messrs. Dunn and Milner, the med cal officers. The facts as regards the epidemic, also con municated by those gentlemen, were, that " the Cholera case 31 in number, 19 fatal, were confined to the Old Prison, : not a single case occurred to any prisoner occupying a cel either in the New Prison or in the Women's Prison. Cas of diarrhœa were met with in every part, but the proportic was much higher, and the average duration of the cases muc greater, in the Old Prison."

It is remarkable that in the evidence on this part of the subject received by the Cholera Committee, lowness of site is not very prominently set forth among the unfavourable sanitary conditions. It is, in fact, specifically mentioned only five times. This may be because a difference of level does not strike the attention so much as other points of difference, where one street is compared with another, or one house with another house; and in many instances it may certainly be inferred that the localities visited by Cholera had a low level as well as other features of insalubrity. At the same time it is evident that lowness of level was not more essential as a condition for the prevalence of Cholera in other, smaller places described by the correspondents of the Committee than it was in the metropolis. In Swansea, as Mr. Michael's Report shows, the disease prevailed much more severely in the higher part than in the lower part of the town. In Maidstone, Dr. Plomley remarks,—" There were in no street more than two deaths, and in no house more than one death, *except in the upper part* of Stone Street, the most elevated and the most remote from the river, yet the very worst in its sanitary condition." In Southampton, again, Dr. Oke records that, " Cholera broke out with fearful violence in Charlotte Place, an assemblage of houses in a high situation to the north end of the town, and detached from it; the streets here being wholly formed of small pauper tenements, narrow and dirty, the front built with more respectable houses, but the whole without sewers. And with regard to Leeds, Dr. Castle states that " the disease was least prevalent by the water-side, and most so on the higher ground."

In these instances, where the epidemic fell with such violence upon the more elevated parts of provincial towns, there were found to be present, as in similar instances in London, many of those conditions which are commonly associated with the prevalence of epidemic disease. But it is important that an exaggerated and incorrect view should not be entertained with regard to the relation subsisting between

even these conditions of insalubrity and the spread of Choler
in towns.   It is undoubtedly true that Cholera rarely pre
vailed with great intensity except in badly-drained and fou
spots, or in dirty and badly-ventilated houses, such as are in
habited by the poorest classes.   But it is equally certain tha
in some public institutions, and even in some private house
where, excepting, perhaps, the want of ventilation, the condi
tions of insalubrity did not exist in a marked degree, the dis
ease caused a large mortality in proportion to the numbe
of persons exposed to its ravages; and further, that in th
towns visited by it, some of the localities which presented th
worst features of insalubrity escaped altogether, or suffere
in the slightest degree.   Of the former fact, illustrations wil
be found, if needed, in the Appendix (Tables I. and II.)
and reference will be made to it again in a subsequent part o
this Report.   Of the latter fact,—the escape of parts of town
apparently adapted above most others for the reception o
the epidemic, instance as striking, perhaps, as the followin
will occur to the recollection of every one who has watche
the progress of Cholera in London, or any large town.

After describing the severe ravages of the disease in a par
of Manchester called Gaythorn, Messrs. Leigh and Gardner[*]
give the following as an instance of the seeming capricious
ness of its course :—

On the bank of the Medlock, and lying on the south
east of Gaythorn, but separated from the latter by the Man
chester gas-works, some large manufactories, and a curve o
the river, is the district called ' Little Ireland.'   It is occu
pied almost entirely by the most squalid and indigent Irisł
immigrants; has numerous pigsties, undrained houses anc
cellars, a population crammed to suffocation; has the exha
lations from the river rolled over it by an opposite higł
bank, and has long been known to be one of the most un
healthy localities, and in the worst sanitary condition of any
in Manchester.   In a straight line it is but a few hundred
yards, scarcely more than three hundred, from Gaythorn, and

* History of the Cholera in Manchester in 1849. London : 1850, p. 25

yet a very few cases of Cholera only have occurred in this locality; indeed, but five cases, and four of these happened when the disease was generally declining."

Mr. Simon, in his "Second Annual Report on the Sanitary Condition of the City of London," makes a general statement to the same effect. "It is unquestionably true," he says, "that many habitual seats of fever were visited by Cholera; on the other hand, many of the worst fever-nests in the whole metropolis were unaffected by it;" and the late Dr. Taylor, in his "History of Epidemic Cholera in Huddersfield," observes that "One of the most remarkable singularities of the epidemic is this, that after attacking one, two, or three persons in a bad locality, it will cease there; again, it will altogether pass by other neighbouring spots, as bad or worse than the one visited. One house will be invaded, whilst others, much nearer to the nuisance supposed to be concerned in the production of the disease, will escape."

The foregoing facts have an important bearing on the theories of the epidemic, which may here be briefly noticed. The marked preference of Cholera for low unhealthy sites and crowded dirty dwellings, suggests at once the inference that the morbific cause, whatever its nature, finds the conditions for its increase or for its action, at least in part, in the impure atmosphere of such places. But in the application of that theory of Epidemic Cholera, which attributes it to a "general state of the atmosphere" or "atmospheric influence," brought into action by "localizing causes," a difficulty is already met with. Such a cause would be expected to produce its effects wherever the "localizing conditions" exist. Yet it has been seen that very many places, some towns, and many smaller places and parts of towns, having these conditions, suffered but slightly or wholly escaped. And it is obvious that no supposed want of susceptibility of the disease in the individual inhabitants will explain the absence of the epidemic under such circumstances from entire towns and districts, or indeed from entire groups of the houses of the poor. If, therefore, the cause be one generally present through the atmosphere, there must be some other condition essential for its action besides the known conditions of insalubrity; and this unknown condition must, in some instances, have been absent throughout entire towns,—in others, only in limited spots.

The theory of a "Cholera matter" not equally diffused through the atmosphere, but only partly distributed and transported in some way or other to the places affected, is more easily reconcilable with the facts hitherto examined. The partial distribution of the epidemic, and its absence from some of the places which have the conditions obviously favourable to its development, would be well explained by this theory; and the occurrence of a very small number of cases of the disease in some places having the characters referred to, might be accounted for on the supposition that, although a small portion of the "Cholera matter" reached those places, its increase was prevented by accidental circumstances.

It may further be inferred from the foregoing facts, that if the cause of Cholera be a material poison, it has most probably not a gaseous form, since a gas soon becomes diffused through the air and dissipated, while the cause of Cholera remains many days producing its effects in one limited spot, —even in a part of one building: it must on that assumption be supposed rather to have the form of minute solid or liquid particles, which may become fixed by attaching themselves to the surfaces of other bodies.

Lastly, it may be observed that the close relation in which the intensity of the epidemic seems to stand to density of population and activity of traffic, though not inconsistent with any one theory, especially suggests the probability of the disease being in some way propagated by human intercourse.

III. A third character of an epidemic of Cholera is *its long duration in a country, or even in a town of large size.*

In England the disease persisted through the last three months of the year 1848, and the whole of the year 1849; and in the previous epidemic of 1831 and 1832, its duration was equally protracted. In the individual cities and large towns of England, it continued, in both visitations, uninterruptedly prevalent during several months; and in London itself was persistent through nearly the whole period of its presence in the country.

This character of Cholera distinguishes it from the Epidemic Influenza, the duration of which in one town does not extend beyond a few weeks, and in a whole country does not exceed two or three months; and it is a character which must not be neglected in an inquiry respecting the cause and mode of diffusion of the disease.

The atmosphere of a country, or of a town, is never completely at rest. Perpendicular currents take place in it, when it is not undergoing horizontal movement; and horizontal currents of great rapidity are frequent, and produce in given spots such considerable changes of temperature and of other meteorological conditions, as prove that the air has come from great distances. The very different qualities of the south-west wind and of the north-east wind, respectively, during the winter in London, are, for example, so marked as to leave no doubt that the one has passed over the northern part of the European continent, and the other over the Atlantic Ocean.

Now, marked changes of the atmosphere occurred during the prevalence of Cholera in London in the summer of 1849; and yet there were no corresponding interruptions to the continuance of the epidemic, or variations of its intensity. In illustration of this statement it is only necessary to refer to the annexed Table showing the changes of the wind during the months July, August, and September, as they were noted at Greenwich, and communicated to the Registrar-General by Mr. Glaisher. Among the frequent changes in the direction of the atmospheric currents which took place during these three months, it may be noticed, for instance, that for eight days together, in the middle of July, the wind blew from the north-east and east at the average rate of 55 miles a day; for eleven days together from the south and

STATES OF THE WIND, AND THE MORTALITY FROM CHOLERA, IN LONDON, DURING THE THREE MONTHS JULY, AUGUST, AND SEPTEMBER, 1849.

Months.	Days of Month.	Number of Days.	Prevailing Direction of the Wind.	Average Daily Horizontal Movement of the Air in Miles.	Average Daily Number of Deaths from Cholera.
July...	1st to 5th.	6	Variable	86	25·4
„	6th to 8th.	3	South, South-west, and West	Anemometer broken.	29 3
„	9th to 16th.	7	North-east and East............	55·6	75·5
„	17th to 20th.	4	South-east, South-west, and North-west.	109	96
„	21st to 31st.	11	South and South-west	122·3	122
August	1st and 2nd.	2	North-west and West	87·5	132·5
„	3rd to 6th.	4	North and North-east	39·7	114·7
„	7th to 17th.	11	South-west	116·2	164·2
„	18th to 20th.	3	North-west and West	68·3	179
„	21st to 23rd.	3	West and South-west	30	177
„	24th to 31st.	8	Variable	81·2	232·5
Sept....	1st.	1	East and North-east............	90	250
„	2nd and 3rd.	2	South, South-east, and East...	50	299
„	4th to 8th.	5	North and North-east	73	308·4
„	9th to 16th.	7	South-west	72	203
„	17th to 27th.	11	North and North-east	50·5	81
„	28th to 30th.	3	South-west	73·3	41

south-west at the rate of 122 miles a day; and for eight days at the end of August from various points of the compass at the average rate of 81 miles a day; and that, nevertheless, the number of deaths from Cholera continued to increase almost without check from the beginning of July to the 8th of September.

In other towns in England, and in Paris likewise*, there was the same absence of any fixed relation between the direction of the wind and the degree of prevalence or intensity of the epidemic.

These facts are surely not consistent with the theory which attributes Cholera to a general state of the atmosphere or atmospheric influence, if by this theory it is assumed that the cause of the disease is constantly and exclusively in the air, attached to it and moving with it. It cannot be that the persistence of the epidemic in a town was due to portions of such a pestiferous atmosphere being left within buildings or confined spaces, while the great mass was moved away ; for even supposing that the air within many buildings were fixed instead of constantly changing, as it is, still a great temporary alteration in the force of the epidemic must have attended or followed a change of the wind. Nor is it possible that the continuance of the epidemic for several months in one place was due to successive portions of the morbific atmosphere being brought at intervals : for, in that case, too, there would have been marked remissions and augmentations of the severity of the epidemic according to the direction in which the wind was blowing.

If, then, the epidemic was *primarily* due to a general state of the atmosphere or to an influence moving with the atmosphere, this state or influence must, it would seem, have determined the production of a more fixed morbific agent in various parts of the country and of individual towns, which remained, and was capable of increase after the transient atmospheric influence had long passed by. But this hypothesis has the defect of assuming two causes as necessary, one serving for the transmission of the epidemic from one country to another, and the other being the efficient cause which really produces the disease in the spots where the epidemic reigns.

A more simple explanation of the long continuance of

* See the Table of the states of the wind during the epidemic in Paris given in the Appendix, Table III.

Cholera, in the countries or towns which it visits, is obviously afforded by the theory of its dependence on a morbific *matter*, transportable within limits from place to place by the atmosphere, and capable of increase under favourable conditions in the places to which it is conveyed. For there is no difficulty in supposing that such a matter might attach itself to the surfaces of bodies within these places, so as to remain fixed there and even to increase, as long as the favouring conditions continued, quite independently of subsequent changes in the direction of the wind, or, in other words, of subsequent movements and changes of the great mass of the atmosphere.

The long persistence of the epidemic is equally in accordance with the theory which refers its introduction into a country or a town, and its diffusion there, to human intercourse.

As far as regards that particular character of a Cholera epidemic, which has here been considered, either of these two theories is admissible.

But the facility with which these theories explain the continuance of the epidemic, itself almost suggests an objection to them: namely, the objection that they would not account for its ultimate cessation. This, however, is a difficulty, the discussion of which must for the present be postponed.

IV. It is a fourth character of Cholera, and an important one, which must now be examined, that *the intensity of an epidemic of the disease varies during its continuance in a country or a large city; so that it has periods of little and of great activity, and usually well-marked periods of increase, acme, and decrease.*

The import of this character of the disease, with regard to the principal theories of its cause, cannot be well estimated until something has been learned of the external circumstances or conditions which attend and apparently determine the increase and the decrease of its prevalence in any place where it exists.

And here the first fact to be noticed is, that, although

Cholera may begin and continue to exist in any season of the year, it most frequently appears in summer, and attains its highest degree of intensity in the course of the summer or autumn, namely, in some month between May and October. The period of greatest intensity is the present subject of inquiry, and the annexed Table shows that in a majority of instances this coincides with the month of July, August, or September.

Amongst the thirty-two epidemics, of which particulars are there given, six produced the greatest mortality in the month of July, seven in August, and seven in September; twenty, in all, in one or other of these three months. And amongst thirteen epidemics in the chief cities of the several countries (New Orleans and New York being taken as the capitals of the northern and southern States of America respectively), eleven were most fatal in one or other of the same months, namely, three in July, three in August, and five in September. But the instances in which the greatest mortality occurred in other months and other seasons, are sufficiently numerous to show that season has no *exclusive* influence in determining the time of culmination of the epidemic. Out of the thirty-two instances, three epidemics were most fatal in June, three in October, one in April, two in March, two in January, and one in December. Even in the same city the greatest mortality from the disease has, in different epidemics, occurred in different months. Paris, for example, in 1832 suffered most severely in the month of April, and in 1849 in the month of June.

While, therefore, the more frequent prevalence of Cholera in an intense degree in the later months of summer and the beginning of autumn, taken in conjunction with the known fact that the disease is so much more fatal in hot than in cold climates, would suggest the probability that temperature has a large share in regulating the severity of the epidemic, other facts tend apparently to an opposite conclusion; and further examination of the matter is here evidently needed to determine the connection really subsisting between the epidemic and temperature.

Table of Epidemics of Cholera in Various Cities and Large Mortality Caused by Them During the Several Months

City or Town	London	London	Liverpool	Hull	Sunderland	Belfast[a]	Dublin[a]	Limerick[a]	Glasgow[b]	Paisley[b]	Paris[c]	Paris[c]	Cologne[d]	Berlin[e]	Berlin[e]	Berlin[e]
Year of epidemic	1831-2	1848-9	1849-9	1849	1848-9	1848-9	1849	1849	1848-9	1848-9	1832	1849	1849	1831	1832	1837
October	..	150	..	14	7	..	..	..	..	..	..	..	..	..	..	..
November	..	190	..	..	13	..	..	..	28	..	..	..	..	..	..	..
December	..	133	8	1	15	27	..	345	1	..	..	..	..	..	..	..
January	57	292	5	..	3	65	2	(83)	130	..	..	..	..	..	7	..
February	57	180	7	..	..	110	6	6	149	52	..	..	..	..	..	..
March	830	40	18	1	131	98	8	501	5	..	90	573	..	..	..	..
April	335	9	19	1	11	60	32	143	..	..	12733	1929	..	..	..	..
May	50	24	96	1	..	62	197	4	..	..	811	4500	..	..	..	..
June	194	979	424	2	1	96	477	1	..	..	868	8009	..	..	1	..
July	1953	2555	1005	35	9	265	314	..	..	..	2573	845	99	..	..	..
August	1198	5368	1575	253	55	122	276	..	..	..	969	1302	250	2	5	942
September	670	5031	874	835	109	46	298	1	..	..	357	1142	610	577	29	1167
October	336	337	68	41	32	10	49	..	..	..	62	115	203	502	230	141
November	27	20	2	..	1	6	5	..	..	..	..	..	10	133	114	16
December	..	2	6	..	..	2	..	..	..	..	..	..	..	14	30	..
Total deaths	5275	14610	4181	1184	387	1090	1064	746	1208	103	18463	19184	1174	1306	407	2206
Population	1,424,854 (Census 1831)	2,361,640 (Census 1851)	255,635 (Census 1851)	50,552 (Census 1851)	70,561 (Census 1851)	63,625	238,531	65,296	344,986 (Census 1851)	69,150 (Census 1851)	785,862 (Census 1851)	1,053,857 (Census 1846)	85,449	248,682	246,892 (Census 1851)	333,752
Mortality per 10,000 during the entire epidemic	37	61	163	236	55	154	69	114	35	30	235	182	138	52	16	60
Mortality per 10,000 during the most fatal month	9	22	61	167	18	42	20	90	19	21	162	82	71	23	9	41

[a] Report of the Commissioners of Health, Ireland : Dublin, 1851, p 79.

[b] Report of the General Board of Health on the Epidemic Cholera of 1848 and 1849. Report by Dr. Sutherland, Appendix, pp. 151 and 160.

[c] Rapport sur la Marche et les Effets du Choléra Morbus dans Paris, par la Commission, &c, année 1832, Tableau No. 58; and Rapport sur les Epidemies Chorériques de 1832 et de 1849, &c., par M. Blondel: Paris, 1850, Tableau No. 5.

[d] Die Cholera-Morbus in Köln im Jahre 1849, von Dr. F. Heimann: Köln, 1850, p. 9.

[e] Vergleichende Statistische Uebersicht der in Berlin in den vier Epidemien 1831, 1832, 1837, und 1848, vorgekommenen Cholerafälle, von Dr. W. Schütz: Berlin, 1849, pp. 43-154.

[f] Report on the Epidemic Cholera prevailing in the Kingdom of Poland in 1852, by Romain Tchesyrieur, Inspector-in-Chief of the Service of Health, &c., &c. Printed by the General Board of Health, and communicated by the Board to the Cholera Committee. The data extend only to the first four days of September, but the epidemic was then rapidly declining.

[g] Rapport sur le Choléra-Morbus, par Alex. Moreau de Jonnès : Paris, 1831, p. 297. The data extend only to the 14th of November, but the epidemic was then beginning to decline. On the 18th of December there were only nine deaths. In January, though the epidemic was not extinct, the number of deaths in a day never exceeded eleven, and was as low as one.

.... EUROPE, EGYPT, AND NORTH AMERICA, SHOWING THE ... CH THEY PREVAILED.

Moscow.[a]	Riga.[b]	St. Petersburgh.[b]	Cronstadt.[b]	Stockholm.[b]	Malmö.[b]	Gotheberg.[b]	Alexandria.[b]	Cairo.[b]	New Orleans.[b]	St. Louis.[b]	New York.[b]	New York.[b]	New York.[b]	Philadelphia.[b]	City or Town.
1830.	1848.	1830-31.	1831.	1834.	1850.	1850.	1848.	1848.	1848-49.	1849.	1832.	1834.	1849.	1849.	Year of epidemic.
..	..	1276	..	..	..	..	..	..	..	..	..	..	..	..	October.
..	..	..	..	..	..	..	..	..	853	..	..	..	..	..	November.
..	..	..	..	..	..	..	..	..	710	38	..	..	..	..	December.
..	..	..	..	..	..	..	..	..	187	90	..	..	..	..	January.
..	..	..	..	..	..	..	..	..	710	68	..	..	..	..	February.
..	..	..	..	..	..	..	..	..	332	131	..	..	..	..	March.
..	..	773	..	..	..	..	..	..	420	517	..	..	..	..	April.
..	..	1844	1809	..	..	..	..	..	253	1799	..	..	35	..	May.
7	..	74	..	..	..	243	2207	21	1896	1797	..	775	105	June.
177	..	3	169	103	..	3452	3021	1	69	1909	421	2023	790	July.
101	345	..	3416	131	13	95	160	..	13	451	307	1451	168	August.
240	65	..	52	34	306	..	..	..	2	63	43	161	20	September.
126	17	..	7	111	..	..	..	..	5	..	..	16	..	October.
..	7	..	21	..	9	..	..	..	..	..	..	7	..	November.
..	..	..	..	..	..	..	..	..	..	..	..	..	..	December.
..	2215	..	1146	3003	378	829	3470	6150	3699	4550	3613	971	3070	1022	Total deaths.
350,000 ?	70,000 ?	470,500 ? (Census 1837)	21,000	81,000 (Census 1831)	12,981	21,403	104,339	300,000	85,000 (Census 1850)				450,000	330,000	Population.
	316		546	452	290	251	236	205		826				112	29	Mortality per 10,000 during the entire epidemic.
25	253	15	809	621	149	162	210	117		212				56	90	Mortality per 10,000 during the most fatal month

Cholera in Riga im Jahre 1848, von Dr. C. J. G. Müller: Riga, 1849, p. 112.

Times Paper, July 13, 1848. The epidemic was not at an end. Of the first epide- St. Petersburgh some information is given by Dr. Russell and Barry in their Reports, .. by authority of the Privy Council in 1831. The epidemic began on the 20th of June. the first seven days the deaths were 123; during the next two days, 164; during the .. days, 771; and during the next eleven days, 1006; in all, 2064 deaths from the 20th to the 30th of July. The epidemic of 1848 began in St. Petersburgh about the begin- June, and produced the greatest mortality on the 23th of the month, on which day 576 died. It subsequently declined rapidly, so that on the 7th of August only 34 fresh cases .. ported. See Einige Bemerkungen über die Asiatische Cholera, von Dr. C. Müller: .. 1849.

.... Reports of Drs. Russell and Barry: London, 1832, p. 136.

.... in Sverige ar 1850, Dr. Fr. Th. Berg: Stockholm, 1851, p. 31.

.... Cholera oder Die Polizei der Natur, von Dr. Pruner-Bey: Erlangen, 1851,

.... of General Board of Health. Abstract of Report, by Dr. James Wynne, on Epi- .. olera as it prevailed in the United States in 1849 and 1850: London, 1852, pp. 4, 15,

A comparison of the progress of Cholera in London during the year 1849, with the daily states of the thermometer at the same period, shows that in this instance a very close relation subsisted between the variations in the mortality from the disease and the variations in the atmospheric temperature ; a relation which was not to be traced in the case of any one of the other meteorological conditions *. No great extension or increased intensity of the epidemic took place until the average external temperature during several days had been about 55° Fahr. ; the period of greatest intensity of the epidemic coincided with a temperature constantly above 55° Fahr., and averaging 62° or 63° Fahr., and remaining several days at 66° or 67° Fahr. The rapid decrease of the daily mortality took place during the fall of the mercury in the thermometer first to 51° and, after a temporary rise, to 42° Fahr. ; and throughout the continuance of the epidemic a temporary rise or fall of the temperature, above or below the average of the period, was in several instances followed, in the one case, by a fresh increase of the epidemic, in the other by its decrease, or at least by an arrest of its previous increase of intensity †.

* See the annexed Diagram, No. I., and Plate II., in Mr. Farr's Report, published by the Registrar-General.

† During the seven months, October, 1848, to April 28, 1849, inclusive, the mean daily temperature of the atmosphere never, except during the first week, reached 60° Fahr. From the 8th October to the 13th of December, it ranged from 35° 2' to 59° 1' Fahr., and after the latter date, down to the 28th of April, was always below 51° Fahr. ; ranging for the most part between 32° and 50°, and falling, on the first days of January, as low as 25° Fahr. During this period the mortality from the epidemic never attained a very high rate. The weekly number of deaths during the last three months of 1848 ranged from 18 to 65 in London. During the first six weeks of 1849, the weekly number of deaths ranged from 38 to 90. Subsequently the mortality rapidly decreased, and during the month of April there were only nine deaths from Cholera. Such were the comparatively trifling effects of the epidemic during the cool season.

On the last days of April the temperature suddenly started up to

The inference that the rise and decline of the epidemic were here regulated very much by the temperature of the atmosphere, is strengthened by the fact that the aggregate mortality throughout England corresponded very closely in its increase and decrease with the varying indications of the

54° Fahr., and on the 3rd of May reached 61°. It again fell on the succeeding day, and on the 11th of May was as low as 42°. But it rose again quickly to 54° on the 13th of May, and continued to rise during the succeeding three weeks, until on the 4th of June it attained the height of nearly 69° Fahr. This last rise of temperature was immediately followed by an increased mortality from Cholera.

During the week ending the 2nd of June there were nine deaths from Cholera, and during the four weeks ending the 30th of June, there were 276 deaths.

The high temperature of 69° Fahr. on the 2nd of June was followed by a fall to 52° Fahr. on the 11th. But on the 12th, the temperature again began to rise, and until the 11th of September never was below 55° Fahr., and ranged between that degree of the thermometer and 71° 1'; a remarkably stagnant state of the atmosphere attending the great heat in London, from the 18th of August to the 13th of September. It was during the period here indicated that the great increase of mortality took place. It began during the last week in June. During July 2555 deaths were caused by Cholera in London. During August the number of deaths was 5368. The epidemic attained its greatest intensity on the 4th of September, on which day 336 deaths from Cholera occurred in London.

From the 2nd to the 5th of September the mercury in the thermometer had stood at 67° and 66° Fahr.; on the latter day it began to fall; on the 11th of September it was as low as 51°, on the 26th it had risen to 63°, but it immediately fell again: on the 6th of October it was as low as 48° Fahr., and remained below 48° for a week; namely, till the 15th of October. During this fall of the temperature of the atmosphere the daily mortality from Cholera in London rapidly decreased from 336 to 3.

From the 16th to the 26th October the temperature was between 50° and 60°. But from the 26th October to the end of the year there was but one day on which the temperature was above 55° Fahr., and only a few days on which it was above 53° Fahr., the range of temperature during the last two months of the year, with the exception of these few days, being from 25° to 46°. It was during these two months that the epidemic gradually became extinct; the last death being recorded on the 29th December.

thermometer as recorded at Greenwich*. It is strengthened, too, by the equally close correspondence between the variations in the mortality from Cholera, and the variations in the external temperature, in Berlin, during the decline of the epidemic of 1848, which began during the height of the summer (see Diagram No. 2, and Table IV. in the Appendix), as well as by the general fact, observable in the Table at pages 30-31, that when epidemics of Cholera have begun during the hot season, they have quickly risen to their climax, and have then soon declined and become extinct on the advance of the cold season; whereas, in the instances in which they have commenced at the close of the year, they have, as a rule, not caused any considerable mortality before the following spring or summer.

But no extended inquiry is needed to find abundant proof that the increase of a Cholera epidemic is not necessarily connected with any particular degree of external heat, nor its decline with the loss of that temperature. Thus it is shown in Table IV. in the Appendix, that the Cholera rose to a high degree of intensity in Paris in 1832, and in Stockholm in 1834, in months when the average temperature was below 55° Fahr. And the epidemic reached its height in Glasgow and Paisley, and other towns in Scotland, in the middle of the winter of 1848-49, when the temperature must have been lower than it was at the same time in London.

It is shown, secondly, in Table IV. in the Appendix, that in several instances Cholera having reached its height as an epidemic has rapidly declined, while the temperature continued to rise, or at least remained high; for example, in the instances of London in 1832, and of Paris in 1832 and 1849.

Thirdly, it is shown that great fluctuations in the mortality from Cholera have occurred without any corresponding variation in the temperature of the atmosphere; this fact, as well as the preceding one, being clearly illustrated by the Diagrams No. 3 and 4.

* See the Diagram, Plate II., in Mr. Farr's Report on Cholera in England in 1849.

consists in adding to that impure condition of the atmo.
which so much favours the local development, and pr
also the diffusion, of the disease.

Other meteorological conditions would aid a high
perature in producing the impure state of the atmo
above referred to.   Great stillness of the air would obv
have this effect, especially in cities and towns, wl
would operate in the same way as want of ventilatio
within buildings ; and a certain degree of moisture woul
mote the decomposition of animal matters and tend
same result.   Both these conditions of the air accor
have been present, together with great heat, in some
during the most severe ravages of Cholera*.   In Lon
the time when the epidemic of 1849 was at its heig
air was very dry, but it was remarkably stagnant ; s
even at the level of Greenwich, according to Mr. Gla
observations, the horizontal movement was far bel
average ; and near the banks of the Thames there v
the slightest motion of the air for days together.
the rise of the epidemic, too, in the summer of 1849
stillness, or at most only slight movement of the air pr
a more rapid increase of the epidemic on three occ
namely, from the 6th to the 8th of July, from the 3rd
6th of August, and from the 21st to the 23rd of Augu
the Table at page 26).   These facts strengthen the
bility that a high temperature favours the growth of a C
epidemic by tending to increase the impure condition
atmosphere.

The coincidence—the natural coincidence, it m
termed— of high temperature with the more intense pe
the epidemic being thus accounted for, it remains
seen whether the exceptional   s are consistent wi
belief that the same condit   ch deto   tho
of severity of the discas   er sp   re

* See Mr. Thom's Obser

consists in adding to that impure condition of the atmosphere, which so much favours the local development, and probably also the diffusion, of the disease.

Other meteorological conditions would aid a high temperature in producing the impure state of the atmosphere above referred to. Great stillness of the air would obviously have this effect, especially in cities and towns, where it would operate in the same way as want of ventilation does within buildings; and a certain degree of moisture would promote the decomposition of animal matters and tend to the same result. Both these conditions of the air accordingly have been present, together with great heat, in some places during the most severe ravages of Cholera[*]. In London, at the time when the epidemic of 1849 was at its height, the air was very dry, but it was remarkably stagnant; so that even at the level of Greenwich, according to Mr. Glaisher's observations, the horizontal movement was far below the average; and near the banks of the Thames there was not the slightest motion of the air for days together. During the rise of the epidemic, too, in the summer of 1849, great stillness, or at most only slight movement of the air preceded a more rapid increase of the epidemic on three occasions, namely, from the 6th to the 8th of July, from the 3rd to the 6th of August, and from the 21st to the 23rd of August (see the Table at page 26). These facts strengthen the probability that a high temperature favours the growth of a Cholera epidemic by tending to increase the impure condition of the atmosphere.

The coincidence—the normal coincidence, it may be termed—of high temperature with the more intense period of the epidemic being thus accounted for, it remains to be seen whether the exceptional cases are consistent with the belief that the same conditions which determine the degree of severity of the disease in particular spots, also regulate

* See Mr. Thom's Observations at Kurrachee, quoted in the Report the General Board of Health on Cholera, p. 27.

the variations in its intensity as an epidemic at different periods in the same place.

Here the first question is, whether the prevalence of Cholera with severity during the winter season in certain instances, can with any probability be referred to the existence of those conditions in a high degree ; and some of these instances may at once be dismissed as offering no difficulty. Several of the outbreaks in England during the winter of 1848–49 and the last months of 1849, occurred in large institutions, such as workhouses, lunatic asylums, and prisons; and as the atmosphere of these buildings is artificially warmed, and is as liable to become impure from imperfect ventilation and other causes in winter as in summer, or perhaps more so, it is quite in accordance with the rule as to the influence of temperature, and with the view above taken of the nature of that influence, that Cholera occurring in such institutions should be severe even in the winter season. The large proportion borne by deaths in these public institutions to the total mortality from Cholera in the metropolis, and some other parts of England, during the coldest months of the winter 1848–49, affords, indeed, a strong support to the view in question. Of 472 deaths from Cholera in London, during the months of January and February, 1849, 257 occurred in the Pauper school at Tooting, the Female Refuge in the Hackney Road, Warburton's Lunatic Asylum (Bethnal Green), Millbank Prison, and a few workhouses. Of 10 deaths in the extra-metropolitan part of Middlesex in the same months, 7 occurred in the Edmonton Workhouse; of 29 in Hertfordshire, 12 occurred in the County Gaol and Union Workhouse; of 17 in the East Riding of Yorkshire, 12 occurred in the workhouse at Howden; and of 61 in the West Riding, 16 occurred in the Wakefield House of Correction, and 7 in the Union Workhouse at Selby.

At the end of the year 1849, again, the deaths in large institutions preponderated at many places. Thus in November, the only deaths in Taunton were 58 in the Union

Workhouse, there being only 168 deaths in the whole county of Somerset; and the only deaths in Hertford were 7 in the County Gaol, the whole number in the county being only 23.

But there are other instances in which the disease was certainly diffused over a village or town, or, at least, over many distinct dwellings, and in these instances it is necessary to seek for conditions favourable to the disease in the general character of the town or village, or, at least, in circumstances external to the dwellings. In the majority of the places most severely visited in England during the winter of 1848-49, and during the last two months of 1849, as well as in the Scotch towns, which suffered severely between November, 1848, and February, 1849, the low site on rivers or sea-coasts, the dense and poor population, in great part employed as workers in factories, miners, or as sailors, and intemperate and uncleanly in their habits, and the general want of sanitary provisions, furnish conditions amply accounting for the diffusion of the disease widely through these places, even in the absence of a high temperature. The places referred to are Sunderland, Newcastle, and Chesham in Buckinghamshire, all visited in the winter of 1848-49; Chilton and Bridgewater in Somersetshire, and Bedlington in Northumberland, severely affected in November and December, 1849; and Paisley and Glasgow, where the mortality was very high in January, 1849*. That the height to which the epidemic rose in these places, even in cold weather, depended largely on the conditions specified above, seems to be proved by the fact that it showed then and there the same preference, as it has done in other places in summer, for the localities in which those conditions chiefly abounded†.

It cannot, however, be affirmed that all the places thus

* Particulars of the visitations of these places will be found in the Maps I. and II., and in the Appendix.

† See, for example, the description of the parts of Glasgow and Paisley visited by Cholera, quoted from Dr. Sutherland's Report, in the Appendix.

severely visited in the cold season present obviously, and in
an extraordinary degree, the known conditions of insalubrity.
It does not appear easy to explain, for example, the outbreaks in the villages of Rudham and Mileham, in Norfolk,
in the winter of 1848-49. It would seem, therefore, that in
these and similar instances, some other cause must have
been at work, either increasing the effect of the local conditions, or, perhaps, acting in some totally different manner.

In the cases, too, where the local conditions which generally
favour the increase of Cholera, were abundant, it is difficult
to explain why the epidemic, which had been severe during
the cold season, should have afterwards quickly declined,
unless under the influence of some other agency than those
hitherto considered.

Stronger reasons will presently be adduced for believing
that some unknown cause exerts an important influence over
the degree of prevalence of Cholera. But, before proceeding to the consideration of them, it is well to remark that,
although the existence of this unknown influence must be
assumed, the importance of the obvious conditions of
unhealthiness ought not to be overlooked. London, of all
the large cities of Europe, is the one in which the removal
of them has been most strenuously and successfully aimed
at, and in which the general mortality is lowest; and it may
be believed to be in great part owing to this cause that Cholera
has shown so little power to exist as a general and severe
epidemic in London, except during a somewhat elevated
temperature. On the other hand, the prevalence of Cholera,
with some though diminished degree of intensity, during the
winter in Moscow and St. Petersburgh, accords with the
higher rate of general mortality in those cities, and may
with much likelihood be ascribed in great measure to their
defective sanitary conditions; for though there are special
circumstances in St. Petersburgh, if not in both those cities,
which doubtless tend to increase the ravages of an epidemic
such as Cholera amongst the inhabitants during the winter,
namely, the high temperature maintained in the dwellings of

the poor as well as of the rich by close stoves, and the impediments to ventilation offered by the double windows and doors so generally used to exclude cold, these would hardly account for the disease continuing to exist through the winter in an epidemic form.

The other exceptions to the general rule, as to the relation existing between epidemics of Cholera and the external temperature, must now be more particularly noticed, with the view of determining how far they can be ascribed to variations in the state of the air produced by known conditions of insalubrity. The exceptional facts alluded to are, the decline of the epidemic in several instances while the temperature was still high and even still rising, the fluctuations in the intensity of the epidemic not connected with corresponding variations of the temperature, and generally the absence of accordance in the rate of their rise and decline between the epidemics of Cholera and the indications of the thermometer. Instances of all these facts have already been given.

In the endeavour to explain these facts the first idea that suggests itself is, that the arrest or retarded rise of the epidemic may have been due to a strong wind setting in and sweeping away the impure atmosphere. And some support to this notion is found in the case of the last epidemic in London, where, just as the rise of the epidemic seemed to be accelerated from time to time by a still atmosphere, so it was retarded on more than one occasion on the wind acquiring greater force (see the Table at page 26, and the Diagram, Plate 2, in Mr. Farr's Report). Very imperfect information is available respecting the force of the wind in London during the epidemic of 1832, or at Paris during the visitations in that city. But it is quite clear that in neither case was an adequate cause of the sudden decline of the epidemic during a high temperature to be found in the strength of the wind. During the sudden and rapid subsidence of the epidemic in Paris between June 10th and 25th in 1849 (Diagram No. 3), the wind is not once stated in the Meteorological Table given in M. Blondel's Report to have been "strong;" and in the instances in which a strong wind is mentioned as having prevailed, only a check in the rise of the epidemic, no remarkable diminution of it, followed*.　The temporary subsidence of the epidemic in London in 1832 after the first week of April (Diagram No. 4), is not better explained by the notices of the state of the wind in the Meteorological Tables, published by the Royal Society.　On the 6th, 7th, and 8th of April there was a "light wind;" but no wind is noticed on any other day of the month before the 19th; while during the early part of March, at the time when the epidemic was increasing, there was "wind" noticed on four successive days, and on one of these days "light brisk wind," and on another "brisk wind."

An inquiry into the quantity of rain that fell, and the changes of the barometer at the periods referred to, has led to no more satisfactory result,

The conclusion seems inevitable that, in these and other similar instances, the great and more or less continued decrease in the force of the epidemic has been due to some other agency than the ordinary meteorological conditions: and at present the nature of this agency is unknown.　It may act by directly destroying or removing the cause of the disease itself.　But inasmuch as the local conditions of unhealthiness have power to determine the spots where Cholera shall be most destructive of life, and since the tendency of all these conditions is to render the atmosphere impure,—while the variations of the intensity of the epidemic in any place are, moreover, as a general rule, dependent on influences which must produce corresponding variations in the degree of impurity of the air, it is not unreasonable to imagine that the unknown agency in question produces its effects by destroying the atmospheric impurities; and the extraordinary prevalence of the disease in some instances, in the cold season, may be supposed to arise, in part, from this agent not being present in its normal amount. Ozone, which

* See Table III., in the Appendix.

has been shown by Professer Schönbein to exist in the atmosphere in varying quantities, has the power of destroying the impurities resulting from the decomposition of organic matter, and has so far the requisite attributes of this unknown agent. But the agent which checks in so mysterious a way the destructive work of Cholera, can scarcely have so general an action on all impurities of an organic origin as ozone seems to have ; for, if that were the case, all diseases which are fostered by an impure air ought to be more or less repressed by it at the same time with Cholera*.

The results of the foregoing examination of the circumstances, apparently determining variations in the intensity of a Cholera epidemic in a place where it already exists, are, then :—

1. That a high temperature has a decided tendency to increase, and a low temperature to diminish, the prevalence of the disease; although no particular degree of its prevalence is connected with a given height of the thermometer, and the rate of increase and decrease of the epidemic is not strictly regulated by the rapidity with which the temperature rises or falls.

2. That a stagnant state of the air has, in several instances, appeared to exert the same influence as atmospheric heat, while rapid horizontal movement of the air seems, like cold, to cause a temporary subsidence of the epidemic, or, at least, to check its increase.

3. That the influence of temperature is subject to marked exceptions ; the disease occasionally prevailing with much severity in the cold season, and, on other occasions, subsiding rapidly while the heat is still great and even increasing.

4. That as the conditions which determine the spots in which Cholera causes the chief mortality, all tend to produce

* The subject of ozone is one of great interest, since it shows how important an influence the electrical state of the atmosphere may indirectly exert on animal and vegetable life. At present, however, there is no satisfactory evidence that the electricity of the atmosphere bears any relation to Cholera epidemics.

an impure state of the air, and as a high external temperature and absence of wind tend to increase the impurity of the air of such spots, it is probable that the varying degrees of impurity of the air are, at least, one cause of the varying intensity of the epidemic in any given place.

5. That, on the other hand, no known influence effecting alterations in the degree of purity or impurity of the air will explain the exceptional cases above referred to, especially the occasional rapid subsidence of the epidemic while the external temperature is high; and it is, therefore, necessary to admit the agency of an unknown cause, capable of producing even more remarkable variations in the intensity of the epidemic than those caused by fluctuations of temperature.

How do these results affect the principal theories with regard to the cause and mode of diffusion of Cholera?

The theory of a general state of the atmosphere or atmospheric influence, acting in spots fitted for its manifestation by "localizing conditions," may certainly be reconciled with them. For this general influence would be manifested more intensely in proportion as the "localizing conditions" (the conditions of insalubrity) were increased by a high temperature and a stagnant state of air. And the unknown cause, which, in modifying the severity of the epidemic, occasionally overrules the influence of temperature, might be simply the varying intensity of the atmospheric morbific influence itself. Other features, however, of a Cholera epidemic make it difficult, as we have seen, to admit that the cause of the disease is such a general condition of the atmosphere.

The theory that Cholera is propagated and diffused by means of human intercourse, receives no support from the facts relating to variations in the intensity of Cholera epidemics, and the circumstances determining those variations. These facts tend, on the contrary, to establish the close resemblance borne by Asiatic Cholera to the common summer Cholera and Diarrhœa of this country and Remittent Fever, which there are such good grounds for believing to be purely of malarious origin, and not to be in any way communicable; while they present a striking mark of distinction between Cholera and the best-known contagious diseases of this country, Small-pox, Measles, Scarlatina, and Hooping Cough. The Table at page 8, showing the mortality from English Cholera and Diarrhœa in the several quarters of the year, and the Table of Cholera epidemics, at pages 30–31, may be compared with the annexed Table, which gives the mortality from the contagious diseases just referred to, and from Continued Fevers, in the several quarters of thirteen years. It will be seen that, instead of becoming more intense in the hot season of every year and declining in every winter, epidemics of the latter diseases (excepting Hooping Cough *) most frequently extend through cycles of two or three years, and have their most fatal period more frequently in the colder than in the hotter season of the year. How different must be the laws of increase and decrease of these contagious diseases from those regulating the rise and decline of a Cholera epidemic, is clearly shown, too, in the annexed Diagrams of the mortality from Small-pox, Measles, and Scarlatina in London in 1849; where, on the other hand, an epidemic of Diarrhœa and Dysentery is seen to resemble very closely one of Cholera, in the time and mode of its rise and decline.

Cholera, then, differs from the contagious diseases of this country in being far more under the influence of temperature and other conditions of the atmosphere. And if its cause be really a contagious virus, reproduced and multiplied in the bodies of the sick and emanating from them, certain conditions of the air must be necessary for its continual existence out of the body, or must greatly affect its power of propagating the disease from one person to others, or (a still more improbable supposition) must render persons proof against this disease, and this disease only. The

---

* The fatality of Hooping Cough is so much increased by the cold season, that no conclusion as to the time of its chief *prevalence* can be drawn from the number of deaths in each quarter.

1840-52.

Years.	Small-Pox, in the quarter ending				Measles, in the quarter ending				Scarlatina, in the quarter ending				Hooping Cough, in the quarter ending				Continued Fever, in the quarter ending			
	March.	June.	Sept.	Dec.	March.	June.	Sept.	Dec.	March.	June.	Sept.	Dec.	March.	June.	Sept.	Dec.	March.	June.	Sept.	Dec.
1840	106	171	254	709	202	283	311	356	530	518	524	419	298	296	198	287	342	390	305	310
1841	608	256	139	76	160	148	260	409	170	133	193	181	656	537	463	653	324	353	297	291
1842	74	59	196	108	311	388	313	346	123	196	392	522	731	408	180	309	255	266	309	359
1843	145	105	75	114	272	374	352	456	299	325	548	718	509	625	336	468	508	690	446	400
1844	259	425	556	571	334	208	255	385	586	601	1020	872	487	361	167	277	482	455	424	885
1845	481	246	70	106	381	322	688	927	421	201	194	269	411	463	385	557	363	308	273	358
1846	77	87	51	42	401	168	78	105	221	177	208	329	767	545	355	868	410	364	403	619
1847	82	181	320	372	99	277	521	881	196	174	316	747	544	392	238	426	442	566	895	1279
1848	388	381	435	413	465	306	154	218	615	816	1560	486	374	449	340	472	922	882	882	883
1849	328	118	78	99	173	368	274	383	776	497	386	273	905	739	428	273	699	512	710	558
1850	95	103	109	191	303	282	178	264	199	234	316	429	442	406	300	424	404	426	414	619
1851	275	209	248	339	363	495	260	204	206	169	291	603	781	734	360	286	521	428	627	770
1852	889	472	231	74	151	199	129	121	366	543	668	953	539	466	244	316	527	483	530	634
The 13 years.	3390	2808	2683	3218	3615	3713	3773	5010	4658	4604	6616	6798	7443	6421	3908	5115	6148	5965	6565	7525

probability, however, founded on analogy, is very much against the increase and spreading of Cholera being due to contagion; and in addition to the facts already mentioned, on which this inference from analogy is based, the case of Continued Fever may be adduced in support of it.

It will be observed in the Diagram No. 5, that an increase in the number of deaths from Continued Fever occurred in the third quarter of the year, but especially in the month of August and September, 1849. Now inasmuch as two fatal diseases, Typhus and Typhoid Fever, are included under the head of Continued Fever (termed Typhus in the Registration Returns), it appears probable that this increase of deaths at the end of summer was due to the Typhoid Fever, which seems to be produced chiefly, if not entirely, by endemic miasms*, and not to the highly contagious Typhus. And this conjecture is entirely confirmed by information kindly furnished by Dr. Sankey, with reference to the statistics of the London Fever Hospital. Of the cases of the two diseases admitted into that institution during the last three years, the cases of Typhus have been more numerous in the first and second quarters of the year than in the third and fourth; while the cases of Typhoid Fever have been fewest in the first quarter, have increased in the second, and still more in the third or summer quarter, and have again diminished in the fourth quarter. Moreover, in the three years taken separately, Typhus furnished the largest number in three different quarters; whereas Typhoid Fever in every year furnished by far the largest number of cases in the third quarter. So that these two fevers, in the fluctuations of their

* At Millbank Prison, where deaths from Continued Fever occur every year, no case of Typhus, certainly no fatal case of that disease, has appeared within the last 13 years. The fever has in every case had the characters of the enteritic Typhoid Fever. The contagious Typhus has not gained an entrance, probably in consequence of the prisoners coming to Millbank not direct from their own homes, but after passing some weeks in county and borough gaols, in which, for the most part, cleanliness and good ventilation are now maintained, and the prisoners very generally kept apart in separate cells.

amount of prevalence, seem to follow respectively the rules of contagious and non-contagious epidemics; and the decidedly contagious fever bears in this respect no resemblance to Cholera.

An additional reason for believing that the diffusion of Cholera through a town is independent of contagion, is furnished by the extraordinary rapidity of its increase in some cases. To take one example of this from many that might be referred to; the epidemic of 1832 in Paris commenced on the 26th of March, and increased so rapidly, that in 18 days (on the 14th of April) it had reached its climax, had already extended to all the quarters of Paris, and had been fatal to 7000 people. It is scarcely possible to believe that this was the effect of contagion, of the re-production and increase of the morbific poison solely within the bodies of the sick, and its subsequent communication from the sick to other persons previously healthy.

But, though the theory of true contagion cannot with any degree of probability be made to explain the facts which have been reviewed in relation to the rise and decline of a Cholera epidemic, it must not hastily be assumed, that the disease is in no cases and under no circumstances communicable. Plague and yellow fever, like Cholera, take their rise in hot climates, are in a similar manner under the influence of temperature, and are undoubtedly, in the main, dependent on endemic miasms; yet there are reasons for believing that both plague and yellow fever are in some way propagated by human intercourse.

The view of the cause of Cholera which seems most consistent with the variations of intensity of a Cholera epidemic, and with what is known of the circumstances determining those variations, and which at the same time accords with the other characteristics of Cholera previously considered, is the " miasm" theory,—that, namely, of a material substance distributed through the air and undergoing increase in the air or on surfaces exposed to the air. For as this Cholera miasm is supposed to find the *pabulum* for its increase in the im-

... ...
... ... of temperature
would ... the increas
... ... Since ...
... the process ...
reproduced and ...
theory afforded ...
in hot seasons, as w
... between the
fluctuations of ...
the unknown caus
the course of C
distinct agent. I
strewing either
the air, which i
present in le ...
crease both ...
Cholera matte
the influence
an objection
otherwise to
membered, :
tions in the
known met
ferred to a
a " health
cording as
over, no
account ...
Cholera.

V. A fifth
is, that *after*
In England,
reappeared part
again in the sum
epidemic in this co..

...blic institution, and then after a short in-
...as many persons suffer... in the
...in the former one. At ... of this
...se of Sunderland, where a short attack,
...ths of October, 1848, and January, 1849,
...er more than a month's ...
...x of far greater severity; this again being
...months' interval, by a third interval of a
... character. It is not likely that in the
...ease ceased in the two earlier ...
... persons still susceptible of the disease,
...strange concurrence of circumstances, ...
...the contagious influence.

...place, the supposition that Cholera, if pro-
...after a time cease throughout the country, or at
...throughout a large city, from the absence of any
...susceptible of the poisonous influence, is con-
...experience respecting the best known contagions,
...seem at no time to become entirely extinct
...ion, and still less throughout England.

...considerations, then, with other facts relating to the
...of the epidemic, which will be noticed in the
...though they by no means prove that Cholera
...communicated from one person to another, make
...improbable that the cessation of the epidemic
...the country, or even in a town or village, is the
...of subjects for the contagious influence.

...disappearance of **Cholera** from the country,
...would be most readily explained by the theory
...is produced and maintained by a peculiar
...ieric influence, which, at
..., leaves the country free
this view, the slighter re...
...ld involve the neces...
h visitation of the
But inasmuch
and in

and the duration of the disease in different towns and villages, and it has been argued, that " if the Cholera cases were not connected one with another, there would be no reason why the few cases which happen in a village should not be scattered over as long a period as the thousands which occur in a great metropolis." * The fact referred to is indisputable,—and the same general rule obtained to a certain extent in the epidemic of 1849. For in 41 registration sub-districts, of which the population was under 10,000, the average duration of the epidemic was 81 days; in 44 sub-districts, which contained from 10,000 to 20,000 inhabitants, the disease continued to prevail on the average 108 days; and in 35 sub-districts or districts comprising large towns, the population of each of which exceeded 20,000, the disease lasted 117 days. The contrast with these larger places would be more strongly seen in single villages or small towns, several of which are often included in one sub-district.

These facts, however, are intelligible, without reference to contagion,—to the reproduction of the Cholera poison in the human body, and its communication from one affected person to others. It will presently be shown, that Cholera during its prevalence in a town does not affect all parts simultaneously, but rather attacks them in succession; the localities thus attacked being, for the most part, spots in which certain conditions abound. Now, in a large town, such localities are of course more numerous than in a small town, and hence it would be expected that, in whatever way the successive attacks of the different localities were produced, a longer time would generally elapse before the disease had run its course through the more populous and more extensive place.

Moreover there are reasons for believing that the cessation of the disease in a town is *not* owing to all persons susceptible of it having already been exposed to its cause and affected by it. In the first place, the disease may cease in a

* On the Mode of Propagation of Cholera, by John Snow, M.D., London, 1851, p. 2.

town, or a large public institution, and then after a short interval be renewed,—as many persons suffering from it in this renewed outbreak as in the former one.   An example of this is met with in the case of Sunderland, where a slight attack, between the months of October, 1848, and January, 1849, was succeeded, after more than a month's complete interval, by a second attack of far greater severity; this again being followed, after two months' interval, by a third outbreak of a still more serious character.   It is not likely that, in this instance, the disease ceased in the two earlier outbreaks, because all the persons still susceptible of the disease, through some strange concurrence of circumstances, failed to be exposed to the contagious influence.

In the second place, the supposition that Cholera, if contagious, must after a time cease throughout the country, or at any rate throughout a large city, from the absence of any more persons susceptible of the poisonous influence, is contrary to past experience respecting the best known contagions diseases, which seem at no time to become entirely extinct, even in London, and still less throughout England.

These considerations, then, with other facts relating to the cessation of the epidemic, which will be noticed under the next head, though they by no means prove that Cholera cannot be communicated from one person to another, make it at least improbable that the cessation of the epidemic throughout the country, or even in a town or village, is due to the failure of subjects for the contagious influence.

The entire disappearance of Cholera from the country, regarded alone, would be most readily explained by the theory that the epidemic is produced and maintained by a peculiar state of the atmosphere, or atmospheric influence, which, at length, passes away, and, of course, leaves the country free from the disease.   According to this view, the slighter renewed outbreaks in 1833 and 1834 would involve the necessity of supposing that there was a fresh visitation of the atmospheric influence in each of those years.   But inasmuch as the epidemic prevailed in Spain both in 1833 and in

1834, and was present in Sweden also in the latter year, these renewed outbreaks of the disease oppose no great difficulty to the reception of the theory.

If, on the other hand, the view be adopted that Cholera depends on a material poison conveyed by the atmosphere, but only partially distributed through it, this poisonous matter increasing wherever there are the conditions of damp and foul air, the cessation of the epidemic must, it would seem, be ascribed to some other cause, which either frees the entire atmosphere from matters essential to the existence and increase of the Cholera poison, or destroys the poison itself. At all events, this is the kind of agency which, if the theory of a material Cholera poison be adopted, would seem best adapted to bring about the ultimate cessation of the epidemic; and the influence of a similar agency has already been inferred as the most probable cause of those partial and temporary fluctuations in its intensity, which cannot be ascribed to known meteorological phenomena. The cause of the cessation of Cholera in each particular spot, house, or group of houses, will come under consideration at a future page.

VI. The characters of Cholera thus far discussed have been—1, the distribution of the epidemic in respect of extent and intensity; 2, the distinguishing features of the spots in which it has especially manifested itself; 3, its duration; 4, the varying degrees of its intensity at different periods of its persistence in a given place; and, 5, the fact that in each place, and even throughout the whole country, it ultimately ceased. The next character of the disease which must be inquired into is, *the manner of its dissemination as regards time; that is to say, the degree in which its appearance, its period of greatest intensity, and its cessation were severally simultaneous in different places.*

The epidemic made its appearance in England at the end of September, or the very beginning of October, 1848; fatal cases of Cholera having certainly occurred at this time in the

Metropolis, Hull, and Sunderland. The question, how soon the country generally was visited by it, must be determined, if possible, by means of the Registration Returns. The common summer Cholera in most years rapidly diminishes in prevalence after the month of September. Wherever, therefore, the number of deaths registered as due to Cholera decidedly increased in the month of October, there is *primâ facie* evidence, that the epidemic had already affected that place. And in the instances where the number of deaths assigned to Cholera remained stationary, it may with little doubt be admitted, that the epidemic disease was present, if the deaths occurred in groups of two or more in limited spots, and were those of adults, as well as of infants. On the other hand, wherever the number of deaths registered in October, was much less than the number in the preceding month, there is strong ground for believing that the epidemic had not then appeared. (See Table V. in the Appendix.)

Now when the 44 counties and equivalent Registration Divisions of England and Wales (North Wales, South Wales, and the three Ridings of Yorkshire,) are examined from this point of view, it is found that four counties, Durham, the East Riding of Yorkshire, Cheshire, and Middlesex (exclusive of the metropolis), certainly suffered in October; ten others, namely, Buckinghamshire, Lincolnshire, Northumberland, Kent, Cornwall, Hertfordshire, Warwickshire, Cambridgeshire, Suffolk, and the West Riding in November; five others, Essex, Norfolk, Lancashire, Cumberland, and North Wales, in December; and two, Gloucestershire and Shropshire, in January.

On the other hand, it would appear, from the data referred to, that ten counties, Sussex, Oxfordshire, Dorsetshire, Huntingdonshire, Rutlandshire, Northamptonshire, Herefordshire, the North Riding, Westmoreland, and Monmouthshire, escaped throughout the entire seven months from October, 1848, to April, 1849, inclusive.

With regard to thirteen others, Surrey, Berkshire, Hampshire, Devonshire, Wiltshire, Somersetshire, South Wales, Staffordshire, Bedfordshire, Worcestershire, Derbyshire, Nottingbamshire, and Leicestershire, it would remain doubtful whether 'they were visited by the epidemic during this period.

The twenty-one counties distinctly attacked by Cholera in the course of the four months, October, 1848, to January, 1849, inclusive, lie, with few exceptions, on the eastern coast, or at least in the eastern half of the country; while of the ten apparently not attacked before May, 1849, only one is situated on the eastern coast, the rest being southern, western, and midland counties. These facts, therefore, suggest the notion not only that the epidemic affected a few counties first, and gradually extended to others, but also that it did not, during the winter of 1848 and 1849, reach the south-western part of England; the sole apparent exception to this rule being the case of Cornwall, and the deaths registered there as due to Cholera having been but ten during the whole period.

There are other facts, however, which throw some doubt on this view of the matter. It may be shown, that even in the counties which presented no marked increase in the deaths from Cholera after September, 1848, and in which the deaths occurred singly in different towns or districts, or were almost entirely those of infants, the total mortality registered as due to Cholera during the last three months of the year 1848, and the first three months of 1849, was considerably above the normal amount. The data from which this conclusion may be drawn are, the number of deaths from the disease registered during the different quarters of the year 1848 and the first quarter of 1849, in the different counties, and the proportion borne in other years by the deaths during the first and the last quarter respectively to the annual deaths from Cholera, in London. It will be seen in the Table given at page 8, that the deaths from sporadic Cholera occurring in London in the last three months of the year have, according to the average of a series of years, amounted to only 10 per cent. of the annual mortality from the disease, and the deaths occurring in the first three months of the year to less than 4 per cent.; and that in no year in which the mortality was at all considerable, was the proportion in the last three months above 16 per cent., or in the first three months of the year above 8 per cent.   Now in the year 1848, 61 deaths from Cholera were registered in the ten counties named at p. 53, as those in which no decided outbreaks of the epidemic disease were noticed; and 17, or nearly 28 per cent., of these deaths occurred in the last three months of the year.   In the 13 counties, again, in which the appearance of epidemic Cholera during the winter of 1848–49 seemed on other grounds doubtful, 206 deaths from Cholera were registered during the year 1848, and 91 of them, or 44 per cent., in the last three months; while in the 21 counties in which the effects of the epidemic during the winter of 1848–49 were most decided, the proportion of deaths in the last quarter of the year 1848 was less than 52 per cent. of the mortality of the whole year, namely, 519 out of 1005 deaths[*].   These facts, then, afford grounds for the suspicion that the influence of the epidemic was exerted, though with different degrees of intensity, in nearly all parts of the country, in the course of the last three months of the year 1848.

In the first three months of the year 1849, the deaths from Cholera became less numerous, except in a few counties.   But yet the mortality was generally much above the average ratio, or even the highest ratio of other years in London.   In the 10 counties least severely visited, the deaths in the first three months of the year 1849 were equal to 18 per cent., instead of 4 per cent., of the total number of deaths in the previous year.   In the 13 other counties where there were still no decided outbreaks, the proportion was 30 per cent.   In those most severely visited, it was 74 per cent. (See the Table at page 56.)

There is a third series of facts also tending to the conclusion that epidemic Cholera extended throughout the country in the course of the winter of 1848-49.   It is certain that during the whole period of the epidemic many deaths, especially of children, due to the same cause, though often

* Table showing the number of Deaths registered as due to Cholera in the different Counties of England and in the Metropolis, during the

not presenting all the ordinary features of Cholera, were registered as deaths from diarrhœa. And it is most probable that a very considerable part of the great excess of deaths registered as caused by diarrhœa during the year 1849, was due to this circumstance.

It is true that, for nearly three years previous to the inva-

whole year 1848, in the last three months of that year, and in the first three months of the year 1849.

Counties.	Deaths from Cholera.			Counties.	Deaths from Cholera.		
	In the whole year 1848.	In the last three months of 1848.	In the first three months of 1849.		In the whole year 1848.	In the last three months of 1848.	In the first three months of 1849.
London (comprising parts of Kent, Middlesex, and Surrey)	662	478	512	13 counties in which the outbreaks were of doubtful character......	206	91	54
				Surrey (extra-Metropolitan).	5	3	5
				Hampshire.............	31	14	11
21 counties in which decided outbreaks occurred during the winter of 1848-49	1005	519	764	Berkshire	12	8	6
				Bedfordshire	12	7	1
				Wiltshire	6	4	3
				Devonshire............	33	12	7
Kent (extra-Metropolitan).	46	24	11	Somersetshire.........	7	4	1
				Staffordshire	28	10	1
Middlesex (do.)	43	26	11	Worcestershire	12	5	1
Hertfordshire.........	21	15	37	Leicestershire.........	20	3	2
Buckinghamshire ...	60	48	6	Nottinghamshire ...	11	7	5
Cambridgeshire	45	36	8	Derbyshire............	11	4	3
Essex..................	20	11	14	South Wales	18	10	8
Suffolk	19	10	6				
Norfolk	26	13	48	10 counties in which only isolated deaths from Cholera occurred during the winter, 1848-1849 ...	61	17	11
Cornwall	21	7	2				
Gloucestershire	14	5	6				
Shropshire	7	...	7				
Warwickshire....... ..	38	12	7	Sussex	14	3	1
Lincolnshire	42	25	4	Oxfordshire	4	3	...
Cheshire..............	39	15	2	Northamptonshire ...	17	3	3
Lancashire	188	52	55	Huntingdonshire ...	5	2	1
West Riding	139	54	69	Dorsetshire............	1	1	1
East Riding	55	36	18	Herefordshire.........	2	...	...
Durham	66	48	266	Rutlandshire	1	1	...
Northumberland......	76	65	131	North Riding..........	13	4	4
Cumberland	21	9	44	Westmoreland	...	...	...
North Wales	19	8	2	Monmouthshire	4	...	1

sion of Cholera, the deaths from diarrhœa had been much more numerous than they had been previously. Other diseases of the epidemic class likewise had begun to be productive of increased mortality in London about the year 1846, and had continued very fatal till the year 1850, when, like diarrhœa, they again, in nearly every instance, declined in prevalence or in fatality[*]. So that some condition favourable to the ncrease of such diseases would seem to have arisen in the year 1846, and to have ceased or abated at the end of 1849. Still it will be observed in the subjoined Table that the increase in the deaths ascribed to diarrhœa in the year 1849, was incomparably greater than the increase of deaths from the other epidemic diseases; and that, excepting dysentery, the diminution in the following year was also much more considerable.

These facts, therefore, on the whole, lend support to the view that a large part of the mortality ascribed to diarrhœa in the year 1849, was due to a new cause, namely, the cause

[*] The data for the subjoined Table are derived from the summaries of the London Returns of Mortality for the several years.

Years.	Yearly deaths in London from					
	Diarrhœa.	Dysentery.	Cholera.	Remittent Fever.	Continued Fever.	Erysipelas.
1844	705	125	65	33	1696	320
1845	841	99	43	32	1301	308
1846	1152	156	228	71	1796	347
1847	1976	307	117	96	3184	525
1848	1913	334	652	96	3569	579
1849	8453	370	14,125	80	2479	459
1850	1884	182	127	87	1923	374

The next Table shows, as far as the data serve, that the recent increase in the mortality from Diarrhœa was not confined to London.

Mortality from Diarrhœa in several years in		
Years.	London.	All England.
1838	393	2,482
1839	376	2,562
1840	452	3,469
1841	465	3,240
1842	704	5,241
1847	1,976	11,595
1848	1,913	11,067
1849	8,463	18,887

which produced Cholera; and if this were the case, it follows that a great excess in the number of registered deaths
from diarrhœa in any part of the country may be taken as
evidence that the cause of Cholera was there in operation.
Now the number of deaths registered as due to diarrhœa in
different counties of England and Wales during the last
three months of 1848 is not known; but these data are
available with respect to the different months of the year
1849. It is possible, therefore, to compare the actual number of deaths from diarrhœa in each county during the first
three months of 1849, with the number that would have
occurred in the same period, if the mortality from diarrhœa
during the whole year had been the same as in the year 1848,
and had been distributed over the different quarters of the
year in the same proportions in the counties as in London *.

* This Table, with the exception of the last four lines, is extracted
from the Eleventh Report of the Registrar-General, p. xxxii.

Deaths in London from Diarrhœa in each of the four quarters of the years 1840–48.					
Years.	Quarters ending				Totals in the several years.
	March.	June.	September.	December.	
1840	57	62	279	62	460
1841	68	65	228	112	473
1842	81	63	489	87	720
1843	69	50	455	268	842
1844	79	83	414	129	705
1845	109	84	449	199	841
1846	119	153	1549	331	2152
1847	178	202	1196	400	1976
1848	244	239	1048	375	1906
Total	1004	1001	6107	1963	10,075
Annual average	111	111	678	218	1119
Proportion per cent. in each quarter, cal- culated from the an- nual average.........	9·9	9·9	60·6	19·5	100·
Proportion per cent. in each quarter of the year 1848	12·8	12·6	55·0	19·6	100·

It will be seen * that the mortality from diarrhœa during the first three months of 1849, was excessive in almost every

* The subjoined Table is constructed from data derived from the Eleventh Report of the Registrar-General, and from Mr. Farr's Report on Cholera.

Deaths in London and in the different Counties of England from Diarrhœa, during the year 1848, and during the first three months of the year 1849, with the Estimated Number of Deaths from the same disease during the first quarter of the year 1848 in the different Counties.

| Counties. | Deaths from Diarrhœa. | | | Counties. | Deaths from Diarrhœa. | | |
	During the year 1848.	Estimated No. during first 3 months	During the first 3 months of 1849.		During the year 1848.	Estimated No. during first 3 months.	During the first 3 months of 1849.
London (comprising parts of Kent, Middlesex, and Surrey).	1906	244 (the actual No.)	396	13 counties in which the outbreaks were of doubtful character ...	2027	253	505
				Surrey (extra-Metropolitan).	77	9	18
33 counties in which decided outbreaks of Cholera occurred during the winter of 1848-49 ...	5718	837	1164	Hampshire	204	26	42
				Berkshire	73	9	35
				Bedfordshire	81	10	12
Kent (extra-Metropolitan).	255	32	48	Wiltshire	84	10	33
Middlesex (do.)	104	18	22	Devonshire	173	22	33
Hertfordshire	57	7	21	Somersetshire	149	19	60
Buckinghamshire	62	7	18	Staffordshire	566	72	128
Cambridgeshire	110	14	24	Worcestershire	128	16	27
Essex	189	17	26	Leicestershire	130	16	19
Suffolk	151	19	37	Nottinghamshire	128	15	25
Norfolk	189	24	42	Derbyshire	84	10	19
Cornwall	74	9	17	South Wales	155	19	64
Gloucestershire	250	32	52				
Shropshire	82	10	26	10 counties in which only isolated deaths occurred during the winter of 1848-49 ...	519	60	151
Warwickshire	626	80	69				
Lincolnshire	175	22	44	Sussex	138	17	45
Cheshire	313	40	42	Oxfordshire	77	9	21
Lancashire	2409	303	394	Northamptonshire	74	9	21
West Riding	848	106	152	Huntingdonshire	26	3	3
East Riding	232	29	17	Dorsetshire	35	4	8
Durham	227	29	44	Herefordshire	20	2	5
Northumberland	132	16	29	Rutlandshire	7	...	2
Cumberland	104	13	18	North Riding	52	6	11
North Wales	69	8	22	Westmoreland	10	1	8
				Monmouthshire	77	9	27

county in England, and most so in those 23 counties in which the effects of Cholera were least apparent; the number of deaths in them being, in the majority of instances, nearly or quite double the normal amount.

The statistics of the mortality ascribed to diarrhœa tend, therefore, to strengthen the belief that epidemic Cholera had existed generally over England and Wales during the first four months of 1849, and that its effects merely differed in degree in different parts, but were not really absent over any considerable portion of the country.

That Cholera in the first months of its visitation was spread very generally over the country may, then, be admitted, at least, as highly probable. But the fact still remains, that at this period its effects were much more decided in some parts of England than in others; and another fact, too important to be overlooked, is, that those tracts of the country in which its early appearance was most unequivocal, and the particular localities in which it was most fatal, had, as a general rule, certain distinguishing characters.

The counties which have already been named as those distinctly visited by the epidemic between October, 1848, and January, 1849, lie for the most part on the coast, border large rivers, or have a generally low level, with a damp soil and atmosphere; and where such are not their natural features, they are in most instances remarkable for density of population, especially for the preponderance of the town population over the rural population, and for activity of traffic, either maritime or inland. On the other hand, the counties in which the appearance of the disease was more or less doubtful, had, as a rule, characters of an opposite kind. This is shown in the subjoined Table *.

There are, however, marked exceptions to this rule. Hertfordshire and Buckinghamshire, though decidedly visited— the latter as early as November, the former in December— have not the characters just mentioned; while, amongst the counties in which only very slight outbreaks or isolated

* See Table * on next page.

deaths occurred, several, as Monmouthshire, South Wales, and Staffordshire, were by the density and character of their population apparently as well fitted as any others in England to experience an early and severe visitation.

In regard to the particular towns and villages, the same general rule prevailed. The influence of the characters above indicated on the period of the attack of Cholera seems indeed to have been in them more clearly manifested.

During the winter of 1848–49 the disease had four principal seats, represented in Map I., one of which has London for its centre, while the second comprehends Norfolk, Suffolk, and Cambridgeshire; the third has Hull and.Liverpool at its extremities; and the fourth extends around Sunderland and Newcastle. In all these "Cholera fields" the epidemic appeared in October; but in each of them the outbreaks, in the individual districts, towns, or villages, were

* The names of the Counties included in the three different classes described in this Table have already been given at page 53.

Classes of Counties.	Counties in which decided mortality from Cholera occurred between October, 1848, and January, 1849.	Counties in which mortality from Cholera appeared doubtful between October, 1848, and April, 1849.	Counties in which the occurrence of deaths from Cholera in the same period appeared still more doubtful.
Number of Counties in each class	21	18	10
Counties situated on the Coast, or bordering a navigable river, or having a generally low level.	17	4	4
Counties in which the population exceeded 300 to a square mile	8	5	...
Counties in which the town population formed more than 44 per cent. of whole population	11	4	1
Counties in which traffic is very active, at least in parts	11	7	1

apparently far from simultaneous. In the subjoined Table*
are given the names of all the places in these principal " Cholera fields," and in other parts of the country where two or
more fatal cases of Cholera were registered within a month,

* The facts on which this Table is based were extracted from the
manuscript returns of Deaths from Cholera belonging to the office of
the Registrar-General.

Towns and other smaller places in which Cholera was more or less fatal during the seven months, October, 1848, to April, 1849, inclusive.						
District, or Cholera Field.	1848. October.	November.	December.	1849. January.	February.	March.
London Cholera Field.	London Brentford Chiswick Hillingdon Ingatestone Chatham Edmonton	Isleworth Sunbury Gravesend Chesham Missenden	Waltham Abbey Stratford Chatham Hertford Hemel-Hempstead Reading	Edmonton Margate Eastry		
Norfolk and Cambridgeshire Cholera Field.	Newmarket Lowestoft Rudham	Gorlestone Upwell	Cambridge Mileham Peterboro'	Swaffham Prior Rudham		Chatteris
Hull and Liverpool Cholera Field.	Hull Gainsbro' York Bradford Halifax Dewsbury Doncaster Knottingley Liverpool Stockport Poulton-cum-Seacombe Macclesfield	Grimsby Selby Huddersfield Manchester Prestbury Clarebro'	Liverpool Horncastle Pontefract Barnsley	Goole Howden York Wakefield Bradford Sheffield		Goole
Durham and Northumberland.	Sunderland Westoe Middlesbro' N. Shields	Blyth Bedlington	S. Shields Gateshead Newcastle Norham Berwick	Durham N. Shields	S. Shields Hexham	Sunderland
Wales, Gloucestershire, and Midland Counties.	Cardiff Llandaff Pennygladfa Caernarvon Bristol Kingswinford	Shipton-on-Stour	Holyhead Stroud Radford Offchurch	Market-Drayton	Neath	
Devon, Hampshire, and Cornwall.	Plymouth Gosport St. Just	Churchtown	Exeter	Sheet Tithing		
Cumberland ..			Carlisle Longtown			

between the 1st of October, 1848, and the 30th of April, 1849; the names being arranged according to the months in which the first death occurred, and repeated where the places experienced a second outbreak within the above period. And it will be observed that in thirty-five places, the first registered deaths from Cholera occurred in October; that in seventeen they occurred in November; in twenty-four in December; in eleven in January; in only two in February; in two in March; and in none in April. It will further be perceived that the manufacturing towns and seaports not only form a large proportion of the whole number of these places, but especially predominate amongst those earliest attacked. Thus, of the thirty-five attacked in October, thirteen are seaports, and seven cities or large towns, chiefly manufacturing towns; while, of the sixteen first attacked in December, only four are seaports, and two large manufacturing towns.

In connection with this result it must not be overlooked that beyond the limits of the chief "Cholera fields" there are several places in which two or more deaths from Cholera occurred during the month of October, 1848; and that the larger number of these (as is shown in Map I. and in the Table at page 62) were great seaports or other places on or near the coast of the south-western part of England, namely, Gosport, Plymouth, St. Just in Cornwall, Bristol, Cardiff, Llandaff, and Caernarvon.

The outbreaks in these several places were very slight, and their nature was equivocal; but, taken together, and compared with the more decided outbreaks in the "Cholera fields" in regard to the site and other characters of the places in which they arose, they undoubtedly lend some additional corroboration to the view that the epidemic on reaching England in the autumn of 1848 very soon extended itself over the south-western as well as other parts of the country.

A fact opposed to this view is the apparently total escape

of the principal towns and mining districts in South Wales, and in the counties of Monmouthshire and Staffordshire, during the winter of 1848–49. No deaths from Cholera were registered during this period in Merthyr, Aberystwith, Bilston, and Wolverhampton, though, from the density and character of their population and from other local conditions, they would appear to have been as well fitted as towns in the eastern part of England, or as some of the mining districts of Durham, to experience the early ravages of the epidemic, and in the following summer did suffer from it most severely. But too much weight must not be ascribed to this fact; for, in the first place, many deaths from diarrhœa were registered in these places during the first four months of the year 1849; and, in the second place, there were remarkable instances of places, within the chief "Cholera fields," escaping entirely during the whole seven months previous to May, 1849. This, for example, was the case with Leeds in the Hull and Liverpool "Cholera field," and of Alnwick in that of Durham and Northumberland.

Results very similar to the foregoing are obtained when the inquiry is directed to the manner of revival of the epidemic throughout England in the summer of 1849, after its almost complete extinction in the months of March and April.

At the commencement of May the epidemic was already distinctly prevalent in London and in the counties of Lancashire, the West Riding, and Durham. In nine other counties the disease distinctly appeared in the course of May; in eleven counties it became prevalent in June; in ten in July, and in two in August. There remain nine counties in which there were no deaths or in which the mortality was below 5 in 10,000 inhabitants.

The subjoined Table * gives the names of the counties, and

* This Table is abstracted from Table VI. in the Appendix, which gives the mortality from Cholera alone. The rise of the epidemic is

shows the months in which they severally began to experience a decided increase in the mortality from the epidemic.

The counties attacked early in the summer of 1849 differed from those attacked late, in the same respects as the counties in which the epidemic appeared distinctly in the autumn and winter of 1848–49, differed from those in which it did not then declare itself by well-marked outbreaks. Most of the counties earliest attacked in a severe degree were situated on the coast or traversed by large rivers, and densely populated, including large towns, and remarkable for activity of trade*. In other words, they had the cha-

assumed to have commenced when two or more deaths were recorded in the month, and when the number of deaths increased in the succeeding months. Herefordshire and Westmoreland are not named, Cholera not having been fatal in those counties.

Some difference would be made in the times assigned for the commencement or revival of the epidemic in the different counties if the deaths from diarrhœa were included. (See Table VII. in the Appendix.) But no essential difference would thereby be produced in the main results stated in the text.

	Counties in which the Epidemic of the Summer of 1849 commenced in the several months.			
	May.	June.	July.	August.
Counties in which the mortality from Cholera during the year 1849 was 40 or upwards in 10,000 inhabitants.	Durham Lancashire Monmouthshire South Wales	Staffordshire	Northumberland East Riding	
Counties in which the mortality during the year was 30 to 10,000, but under 40 in 10,000 inhabitants.	Middlesex Kent Hampshire Gloucestershire	West Riding	Cumberland Hertfordshire	
Counties in which the mortality during the year was 10 to 30, but under 30 in 10,000 inhabitants.	Cheshire Lincolnshire Somersetshire Devonshire	North Wales Worcestershire Warwickshire Berkshire Wiltshire Dorsetshire Essex Surrey Sussex	Shropshire Nottinghamshire Norfolk Cambridgeshire Buckinghamshire Oxfordshire	Bedfordshire Northamptonshire
Counties in which the mortality from Cholera during the year 1849 was below 5 in 10,000 inhabitants.	Derbyshire	North Riding Suffolk Cornwall	Leicestershire	Rutlandshire Huntingdonshire

* This is an abstract of Table VI., in the Appendix. Only those

F

racters which distinguish those parts of a country which are known to be more liable than other parts to suffer severely during an epidemic of Cholera; and, in fact, as the Table at page 65 shows, the counties which had begun distinctly to suffer in May did experience a higher rate of mortality than the other counties.

There are, however, marked exceptions to the rule just now indicated. The East Riding of Yorkshire and Northumberland, which, from their position on the coast and the activity of their maritime trade, at least in parts of their extent, might have been expected to suffer early, and which ultimately stood first and third amongst the different counties in the scale of mortality, did not apparently experience the ravages of Cholera in a severe form until July. In Northumberland no death from Cholera, and only seven deaths from diarrhœa were registered in June; and in the East Riding of Yorkshire only two deaths from Cholera and nine deaths from diarrhœa during the same month. Similar exceptional cases have already been noticed, and others will soon be met with. The causes on which they probably depend will come under consideration at a future page.

counties are enumerated in which the mortality amounted to at least 5 in 10,000 inhabitants.

	Number of Counties in which Cholera became prevalent in the month of			
	May.	June.	July.	August.
Total number of Counties in which Cholera was epidemic	12	11	11	2
Counties situated on the Coast, bordering a navigable river, or having a low level	9	5	5	...
Counties in which the population exceeds 300 to a square mile..................................	7	3	1	...
Counties in which the town population form more than 40 per cent. of the whole population	8	4	3	...
Counties in which traffic is very active............	11	3	3	...

By a glance at Map II. it will be perceived that during the summer of 1849 there were seven different tracts of the country which chiefly suffered from the epidemic—seven " Cholera fields ;" and by observing the initial letters of the months from May to December attached to the names of the places in which the mortality from the epidemic was above the rate of 5 in 10,000 inhabitants, it will be seen that the different towns and smaller places in each " Cholera field" were not attacked by any means simultaneously. In the South Devon and Cornwall "Cholera field," for example (Table VIII. in the Appendix), 2 places, Newton Ferrers and Noss Mayo, both in the Yealmpton registration sub-district, were attacked in May, 5 were attacked in June, 11 in July, 16 in August, and 11 in September. In others of the " Cholera fields" there was less diversity in the times of the attacks, or, to speak more correctly, a larger proportion of them occurred within the space of two months. Thus in the Shropshire, Staffordshire, and Worcestershire " Cholera field" (Table IX. in the Appendix) no place suffered from the epidemic in May, 2 began to suffer in June, 10 in July, 22 in August, and 12 in September. And in the London "Cholera field," comprising 7 counties, 5 places, including the metropolis, were attacked or began to suffer severely in May, 16 were attacked in June, 51 in July, 54 in August, 17 in September, and 8 in October. But in these instances the absence of simultaneousness in the renewed influence of the epidemic in different places is still obvious. And the fact remains essentially the same when the deaths recorded as due to diarrhœa are also taken into the account; the commencement of the epidemic in the summer of 1849 in the different places being dated from the first deaths whether of diarrhœa or of cholera. In this case the result merely is that a greater number of places appear to have been attacked in May, June, and July ; fewer in August and September.

The question then arises whether the order in which

places in the same "Cholera field" were attacked can be referred to any differences in their characters similar to those which seem in a great measure to have determined the periods at which different counties were visited by the epidemic.

The Map II. and the Table XI. in the Appendix both illustrate two principal facts bearing on this question. First, throughout the country, seaports and places in the course of large rivers form a large proportion amongst the localities affected by the epidemic during the two earliest summer months, May and June ; and, on the contrary, a very small proportion amongst those in which the disease began to appear in the later months, August and September; places lying inland and on a higher level being for the most part attacked at the later period. Secondly, in each "Cholera field" where a large seaport existed the epidemic very generally affected this first, and then seemed to advance gradually up the river at or near the mouth of which the seaport was situated, or from the coast towards the interior, attacking different towns successively in its course, and reaching, last of all, those on the highest level.

In illustration of the former fact it will be sufficient to mention that the 118 places in which Cholera was fatal in May and June, include 42 seaports and towns on large rivers; while amongst about 140 places attacked in August and the following months only 16 were towns of the same description, and these generally smaller, less densely populated, and in other respects less unfavourably circumstanced than those which first fell under the influence of the epidemic.

The following passage, quoted from Mr. Farr's Report, describes the order in which some of the principal places in the several "Cholera fields" were attacked ; and his statement may, as far as regards the months of attack, be verified by means of the Map and Table above referred to.

" The epidemic," Mr. Farr says, " made little progress until the spring of 1849, when it gradually spread from the coast and river mouths to the interior of the country. Noticing only the great eruption, it appeared at Liverpool, on the Mersey, March 10th; Manchester, in the interior, June 25th; and Wigan, July 9th. As it went from Cardiff to Merthyr Tydvil, so ascending the Usk, it broke out at Newport, on May 29th; Abergavenny, on June 3rd; Crickhowell, on July 21st. On the Lower Avon it was at Clifton on May 24th; Bristol, June 1st; Bedminster, July 8th. Gloucester, on the Severn, was attacked on May 4th; Shrewsbury, higher up the river, on July 25th. The great Wolverhampton cholera field, in the interior of the country, was attacked late; Wolverhampton, on July 17th; Stourbridge, August 10th; Walsall, August 25th; West Bromwich, August 31st. On the south coast the chief epidemic broke out at Plymouth, on June 5th; Stoke Damerel, July 4th; Tavistock, higher up the country, July 24th. Southampton was attacked on June 30th; the low Portsea Island, July 2nd; Alverstoke, July 6th; Salisbury, July 10th. The epidemic in the London field began to be fatal in London itself about May 25th; in Brighton, June 13th; Gravesend, June 29th; Brentford, June 29th; Rochford, July 5th; Thanet, including Ramsgate and Margate, July 14th. Up the river Lea, Hertford was attacked August 21st; Hitchin, farther north, August 27th. The first cases on the Humber, and its tributaries, occurred at Hull in 1848; but the outbreak of the great epidemic occurred first at Leeds, on June 14th; Hull, July 7th; Sculcoates, July 23rd; Gainsborough, August 4th; Howden, August 2nd; Selby, August 13th; Goole, August 6th; Thorne, August 19th. On the river Tees the epidemic began at Stockton, July 7th; at Teesdale, higher up the country, on August 17th.

" The epidemic appeared, it will be recollected, at the port of Sunderland, on the Wear, October 4th, 1848. The epidemic of 1849 broke out at Durham, higher up the river, on May 12th; at Sunderland there was one outbreak on March 4th, and a second on June 28th. The seaport was first invaded; and in the *great outbreak,* the inland town, on the Wear, was neither the first nor the greatest sufferer. The low ports of the Tyne were the first attacked on that river; the epidemic appeared at South Shields on June 2nd; Tynemouth, July 1st; higher up the river, at Newcastle-upon-Tyne, on July 30th; Gateshead, August 11th."

The general results then are, that in the spring and summer of 1849, different towns began to be affected in succession, and not simultaneously; and that the order in which they felt the effects of the epidemic was, as a general rule, connected with certain characters of site, density of population, and trade. Those towns were usually affected first which lie on or near the sea-coast or on navigable rivers, and consequently on a low level, which have at the same time a dense and poor population, and which, as a consequence of this, have a large accumulation of ill-constructed, and ill-ventilated dwellings surrounded by all kinds of impurities. These, it need scarcely be said, are likewise the characters distinguishing most of the localities in which Cholera during its prevalence produces the greatest mortality.   There seems, however, to be this difference between the circumstances attending a high degree of mortality, and those associated especially with an early period of attack, that an early appearance of Cholera, at all events in a severe degree, has been induced more certainly by the conditions peculiarly characterising sea-ports, than by mere density of population, and the sanitary evils ordinarily associated with large accumulations of men in inland places; while the latter circumstances have, in the end, appeared at least equally effectual in determining the severity of the epidemic's ravages.   This, at least, is the inference suggested by the fact, that several towns in Staffordshire and South Wales, although they ultimately experienced a much greater proportional mortality than the majority of the seaports, were not attacked by the epidemic until the months of August or September.

There are, however, some decided exceptions to the general rule which cannot be referred to this head: for example, the late rise of the epidemic in Northumberland* and the East Riding† in the summer of 1849, and consequently in the seaports of Newcastle, Wallsend, North Shields, Blyth, and many places on the banks of the Humber, as well as in the large inland towns of Morpeth, Alnwick, and York; the appearance of the disease in the city of Durham and its neighbourhood, two or three months before it showed itself at Gateshead; and its outbreak at South Brent, Plympton, and Egg Buckland, earlier than at Torquay and Brixham, in Devonshire, the latter places, though on the coast, not being visited until September‡.

These instances, and numerous others of the like nature, as well as the exceptions to the order in which the different counties suffered, both in the last three months of 1848, and in the summer of 1849, prove that the obvious local conditions which are generally present in tracts of country and towns early attacked by the epidemic, either do not in all cases and at all times include the essential element which determines the manifestation of the disease in a given place, or are liable to have their influence counteracted by some other agency.

The facts and the conclusion to which they lead are found to be very much the same when the enquiry is directed to the mode of appearance of Cholera in different parts of towns. It does not appear simultaneously in all the parts ultimately affected, but begins in one spot, or in a small number of spots, and increases by attacking a larger number of localities. In large cities, it is true, it may appear in nearly all quarters or divisions within a few days, but still in each quarter it affects one spot first, and others in succession;

---

* There were four isolated deaths in Northumberland in May, none in June (Table X. in the Appendix).

† The only cases previous to July in the East Riding were two cases in May, and two cases in June, at Hull.

‡ It is necessary to state, that, in the places where the appearance of Cholera was thus remarkably delayed, there were no deaths from diarrhœa, or only a very few, registered in the previous months.

and the localities which it first visits have usually those characters which are known to distinguish generally the seats of its most severe ravages.   In seaports and towns situated on large rivers, it commonly first appears close to the harbour or river, and, in the case of seaports, often amongst the shipping.   This fact is too well known to need any extended exemplification.   It is sufficient to refer to the appearance of the disease in London in 1848, at Rotherhithe; and in 1832, nearly at the same time, at Rotherhithe and at Limehouse, and on board two ships in the river; and to the first cases at Sunderland, which occurred in similar situations both in 1831 and in 1848.   In towns not situated on the coast or on large rivers, in villages, and in the several quarters of towns, Cholera usually appears first in some low spot where there are damp and filth around the houses, with poverty, dirt, often crowding of the inhabitants, and almost always defective ventilation, within; or in some public establishment such as a prison, a lunatic asylum, or a workhouse, in which a large number of persons are congregated together.

One of the questions proposed in the letter issued by the Cholera Committee on the 13th October, 1849, related to the characters of the particular locality in which the first case in a town or village occurred, as regarded elevation, drainage, supply of water, density of population, ventilation, and cleanliness.   Abstracts of the answers to this question are given in Table XII. in the Appendix; and it will be seen that few amongst them mention exceptions to the rule, that Cholera, in visiting a town or a village, shows itself first in spots having the characters above described. It would, however, be an error to suppose that the spots in which the epidemic first manifests itself, are always the worst, in a sanitary point of view, that could be found in the town. For although the spots first visited usually present the characters of unwholesomeness in a marked degree, it frequently happens that other localities which, at least for a time, escape, have the obvious features of insalubrity more decidedly marked.

Here again, therefore, it appears that these obvious conditions of insalubrity do not necessarily include all that is essential for determining the spots in which an epidemic of Cholera shall produce its first effects.

Another division of the subject must now be investigated; namely, the relation that existed between the outbreaks of Cholera in different places in regard to the *periods of their greatest intensity.*

During the winter of 1848–49, the epidemic in England reached its highest point in January; and in a majority of the counties where the mortality from the disease rose to a certain height and then fell, January was likewise the month of greatest intensity. In two, Buckinghamshire and Cambridgeshire, the greatest mortality occurred in December; in Hertfordshire, Norfolk, the West Riding, Northumberland, and Cumberland, it took place in January; in Durham, in March (see Table V. in the Appendix). This fact, that the early period of the epidemic had a faintly-marked climax in January, is interesting, since January was the month in which Cholera was so fatal in several of the towns in the south of Scotland; and some ground is thereby afforded for the belief, that even in the winter the intensity of the epidemic was in some measure regulated by a general influence.

But it was in its second period, that the epidemic had its decided climax, and the Diagram, Plate III. in Mr. Farr's Report, demonstrates very clearly, that this climax occurred in the eleven great divisions of England nearly at the same time, but was not exactly simultaneous in all. Table VI. in the Appendix gives the same information with regard to the different counties, and shows that of the 35 counties which were at all severely affected by the epidemic (suffering a mortality from Cholera during the year 1849, of 5 deaths or more per 10,000 inhabitants) 22 had the greatest number of deaths in September, 11 in August, 1 in July, and 1 in October. In London, the month in which the greatest number of deaths occurred was August, but the mortality in London really reached its highest point at the very commencement of September, though it afterwards declined rapidly.

The period of greatest intensity of the epidemic even in the individual towns and smaller places within each of the chief " Cholera fields" was likewise, in the large majority of instances, August or September, as the annexed Table shows.

	Number of Towns which suffered the most severe effects of Cholera in the months of							
	May.	June.	July.	August.	Sept.	Oct.	Nov.	Total No. of places.
Northumberland and Durham		1		1	17	3	1	23
Yorkshire, Lancashire, and Cheshire		1	2	11	32	10	?	56
Staffordshire, Shropshire, and Worcestershire..............			?	4	14	3		21
South Wales, Gloucestershire, Somersetshire, North Devon, and North Wilts....	1	2	4	15	11	1	3	37
South Devon and Cornwall			1	9	14	3		27
Dorsetshire, Hampshire, South Wilts, and Sussex.			6	3	3			12
London Cholera Field			2	18	27	3		50
All these " Cholera Fields."..............	1	4	15	61	118	23	4	226

But the exceptions to the rule were here more numerous.

In the Northumberland and Durham " Cholera field" the epidemic was far more fatal in the city and registration district of Durham in June, than in any subsequent month, while, on the other hand, at Bedlington in Northumberland, it was fatal to 25 persons in November, although it had caused only a single death there previously.

In the great "Cholera field" of the manufacturing counties, Yorkshire, Lancashire, and Cheshire, two exceptional cases are especially to be noticed; one, that of Nantwich, where 108 deaths occurred in July, and only 18 in August, and 21 in September; and the other, that of the Stanley subdistrict, where, in the West Riding Lunatic Asylum, 100 deaths occurred in October, there being only 16 deaths in the sub-district in the two previous months taken together.

In the "Cholera field" occupying either side of the Bristol Channel and the Severn, Gloucester and Cardiff suffered their greatest mortality in June, Keynsham in May and June; and, on the other hand, Bridgewater in October, and Taunton in November.

Lastly, in the Hampshire "Cholera field" it is remarkable, that although the Cholera epidemic in no place reached its climax before July, yet in that month it attained it in 6 out of the 12 places which suffered any considerable mortality; amongst these 6 being, the large seaports of Portsmouth, Gosport, and Southampton.

These facts show that the general tendency of the epidemic to reach its climax in August or September, and perhaps the influences producing that tendency, were in the instances of many towns or registration districts counteracted or interfered with by special causes.

When different parts of the same town are compared one with another, in respect of the time at which they suffered most severely from the epidemic, it is found that, in the case of the largest towns or cities, there was the same general approach to simultaneousness as appeared in a comparison of different counties, and of different towns, one with another. But this statement applies for the most part, only to considerable districts of these towns. In proportion as the subdivisions of the town examined and compared are smaller, the character in question becomes less apparent and at length is lost altogether.

The weeks of the chief mortality of the 36 districts of London during the height of the epidemic in 1849, are shown in the subjoined Table * to have all occurred within a period of five weeks, and to have coincided in 21 instances, with the most fatal week of the epidemic in the whole metropolis; in 6, to have fallen only a week earlier; and in 6 others, a week later.

In the smaller subdivisions of the metropolis,—the different sub-districts,—the weeks of grea test mortality from Cholera were in much smaller proportion simultaneous. They were spread over nearly three months; and scarcely more than a third of them occurred in the week of the general climax of the epidemic in London †.

Lastly, when the progress of the epidemic in each sub-district is examined, it appears to have produced the general result of an augmented mortality at a particular time rather

* The data for this Table were published by the Registrar-General in the last Weekly Returns for the year 1849.

Table showing the Districts of London which suffered the greatest Mortality from Cholera in the several weeks ending				
August 18th.	August 25th.	September 1st.	September 8th.	September 15th.
Hampstead	Holborn	Westminster	Chelsea	Kensington
Strand		West London	St. James's, West-	St. George's Han-
		London, City	minster	over Square
		Shoreditch	Marylebone	St. Martin's-in-
		Bethnal Green	Pancras	the-Fields
		Stepney	Hackney	Islington
			St. Giles	Clerkenwell
			East London	St. Luke
			St. George's-in-	
			the-East	
			Whitechapel	
			Poplar	
			St. Saviour	
			St. Olive	
			Bermondsey	
			St. George's,	
			Southwark	
			Newington	
			Lambeth	
			Camberwell	
			Rotherhithe	
			Greenwich	
			Wandsworth	
			Lewisham	

† See Note * on next page.

by affecting then a larger number of individual spots, than by producing an increased mortality in all the localities previously visited by it, and to have exerted its fatal influence in the several seats of its chief action in succession,—not simultaneously.   Thus, in the sub-district of St. John's, Westminster, the localities in which the epidemic was most destructive to human life, were the Millbank Prison, Regent Street (Westminster), Douglas Street, and Duck Lane. Now in Duck Lane, 9 deaths occurred between the 5th of July, and the 4th of August, besides 7 fatal cases admitted within that period from the same locality into the Westminster Hospital, and no other deaths occurred subsequently before the 19th of October; while in Douglas Street (with Emery's Cottages), no fatal case occurred before the 25th of August, and then 16 deaths occurred, the last on the 1st of September.   In Regent Street the greater number of deaths occurred at the same period.   But, in Millbank Prison, which is contiguous to both these streets, there was a lull in the epidemic at that time; yet immediately afterwards, namely, on the 4th

* This Table is derived, like the one given at the last page, from the Registrar-General's Return for the last week of the year 1849.

	Number of Sub-Districts in which the weeks of greatest Mortality coincided with the several weeks ending										
	July 14.	July 21.	July 28.	Aug. 4.	Aug. 11.	Aug. 18.	Aug. 25.	Sept. 1.	Sept. 8.	Sept. 15.	Sept. 22.
30 Western Sub-Districts	1	...	...	1	...	...	2	3	7	5	...
30 Northern Sub-Districts	...	...	...	...	1	2	3	2	7	5	...
26 Central Sub-Districts	...	...	...	...	...	2	5	6	7	3	1
27 Eastern Sub-Districts	...	1	...	...	...	4	3	11	6	1	1
42 Southern Sub-Districts	...	3	1	2	2	1	1	4	20	7	...
135 Sub-Districts	1	1	1	3	3	8	13	26	47	21	1

of September, the most fatal outbreak ensued, 8 prisoners dying within five days.

Now what is here described as having taken place in one sub-district of the metropolis, seems to have been a common character of the progress of the epidemic in smaller towns. In Lancaster four parts of the town, namely, the Quay with Lune Street, Henry Street, Brewery Yard, and the suburb Skirton, especially suffered, affording two-thirds of the mortality of the town. Lune Street on the Quay, was affected chiefly between the 26th of July, and the 15th of August. In Brewery Yard the most fatal period was from the 10th to the 17th of September; in Henry Street it was from the 29th of September to the 11th of October; while in Skirton the epidemic did not begin till the 18th of October, and then prevailed severely until the 14th of November.

In Canterbury Cholera prevailed from the 17th of July to the end of the month, in the neighbourhood of the river; and when it had nearly ceased there, namely, from the 2nd of October to the 10th, it raged with great violence in Burgate Lane in St. George's parish, which is distant from the river.

In Hertford the epidemic was fatal in the town during August and the beginning of September, without affecting the prisoners in the Gaol, where there had been considerable mortality in the previous winter. But in October, when it had ceased in the town, it reappeared in the Gaol, and was in a short time fatal to 9 of the inmates.

In the town of Wakefield the epidemic was at its height in September; but it caused then only one death at the House of Correction, where 16 had occurred in January. It did not appear in the neighbouring County Lunatic Asylum till the last day of September, and it raged there violently during October, when it was becoming extinct in the town *.

* The facts respecting St. John's Westminster, Lancaster, Canterbury, Hertford, and Wakefield, have been chiefly derived from communications received from Mr. Pearse, Mr. Harrison, Dr. Locheé, and Mr. James Reid, Dr. Davies, and Dr. Wright. Facts of a precisely similar character have

however this fact may be explained, it offers another example of the most severe effects of the epidemic being manifested in different localities within a limited sphere at different times.

These facts relating to the manner in which different parts of towns or of large public establishments fell successively under the influence of the epidemic have the same import as some of those before stated relative to counties and entire towns, inasmuch as they infer the existence of an agency which is capable of determining the appearance of the disease in different localities at various times, and which is at least in a great measure independent of the influence bringing about the general climax. It is not certain, however, that the agency producing the phenomena is the same in the two cases; and it will be necessary to examine both series of facts again at a subsequent page, to ascertain their bearing on theories of the cause and mode of diffusion of the disease.

The question how far the *cessation* of the epidemic throughout England, or throughout parts of the country, was simultaneous, or occurred at divers times in different localities, remains to be examined.

The facts may be stated briefly. In London the epidemic became extinct in November; 8 of the 35 counties* which

* Names of the Counties in which Cholera ceased in the several months.		
October.	November.	December.
Surrey	Hampshire	Hertfordshire
Sussex	Middlesex	Wiltshire
Kent	Northamptonshire	Devonshire
Berkshire	Bedfordshire	Somersetshire
Buckinghamshire	Cambridgeshire	Gloucestershire
Oxfordshire	Dorsetshire	Staffordshire
Essex	Cornwall	Worcestershire
Shropshire	Norfolk	Nottinghamshire
	Warwickshire	Cheshire
	Lincolnshire	Lancashire
	East Riding	West Riding
	Northumberland	Durham
	Cumberland	South Wales
	Monmouthshire	

suffered a mortality of 5 deaths or upwards in 10,000 inhabitants, were freed from it in October; 14 in November, and 13 in December. In the course of these three months the epidemic disappeared from all parts of England. And the reason why it left some counties sooner than others is in a measure elucidated by obvious differences between those it first quitted and those in which it remained longest.

The former are nearly all counties of small extent and small population. But a more important fact is, that the counties in which the disease remained to the end of the year, include most of those which have a very dense population, a large town population, and a very active traffic, and which are traversed by large rivers; that they have, in fact, the same characteristics which distinguish the parts of the country most severely affected by the epidemic. Accordingly it is found when the different counties in which the epidemic was decidedly prevalent, are compared and regarded from this point of view, that while those first freed from the epidemic suffered in all but one instance the lowest, those which experienced its ravages to the latest period, in a large proportion of cases, suffered the highest rate of mortality. The mere relation of the counties to the sea-coast seems to have influenced the time of cessation of the epidemic less than it did its time of commencement.

There was, as might be expected, more diversity in the time of cessation of the epidemic in towns than in counties. In about half of the whole number of towns distinctly attacked, the last deaths occurred in October, and in a very large proportion of instances, namely, 309 out of 371, the last deaths occurred in the course of the months September, October, and November. But in 34 instances the disease continued to be fatal in December; while in 21 it ceased to be so in June; and in 4, in July. Even in the same "Cholera field" and in the same county, some towns were freed from the epidemic several months earlier than others.

The conditions determining the late persistence of the epidemic in certain towns, or sub-districts of the country

o

were apparently in part the same as those that occasioned the
early appearance or development of the disease in particular
localities. For, as a general rule, the towns in which the
disease tarried latest had all the obvious characters of site,
density of population, and sanitary condition which distinguished the towns earliest and most severely visited; and in a
large number of instances, the places that suffered longest
were those which had been earliest attacked. There are,
however, many exceptions to this rule—or, at all events, many
facts relating to the time of cessation of the epidemic in different places, which cannot be thus entirely explained.

The most remarkable instances of the late persistence of
the epidemic are the following:—

In the Northumberland and Durham " Cholera field" 16
deaths from Cholera and 2 from diarrhœa occurred amongst
miners at Longbenton in December; although no death at
that place had been ascribed to either disease during the
two previous months, and although the epidemic had very
nearly ceased in the whole " Cholera field," the number of
deaths from Cholera and diarrhœa together, during December,
being in Northumberland 4, and in Durham 29.

In the Staffordshire and Worcestershire " Cholera field,"
the mortality from the epidemic continued in December in
Dudley and Stourbridge, and in a less degree in two or
three neighbouring towns, while in the northern part of Staffordshire, and in Shropshire, it had almost entirely ceased as
early as November.

In the South-Wales, Gloucestershire, and Somersetshire
" Cholera field," the epidemic was still severe at Taunton
and Bridgewater, and in the neighbourhood of Bath, in
November, when it had subsided in the " Cholera field"
generally, and even in the mining districts of South-Wales;
and it was fatal still later in Midsummer Norton, and in
Poulton, near Bath—in the latter place 13 deaths occurring
in December, when it had virtually ceased throughout the
" Cholera field."

In the London " Cholera field" the epidemic generally

subsided in October; even in London only 22 deaths were recorded as due to Cholera in November and December; and the only place in which any remarkable mortality occurred in November was Baldock, with Weston and Norton in Hertfordshire, where the first death took place in October, and where, after 30 deaths in that month, 13 occurred in November.

The instances of the opposite kind—of the early cessation of the epidemic in particular localities, while it still prevailed in the country generally, and even in the same " Cholera field " or county—are numerous among the smaller towns, but few among the larger and more densely populated towns.

In several towns in Shropshire, namely, Shrewsbury, Condover, Madely, and Bridgenorth, the epidemic ceased in September; but the deaths caused by it after that month in any part of the county were few, and it was rapidly subsiding in other neighbouring counties. The same remark does not apply to the instance of Keynsham in Somersetshire, Wootton-under-Edge in Gloucestershire, and Devizes in North Wiltshire ; in the first of which places the disease ceased to cause deaths in July, and in the latter two in September, though in neighbouring places it still continued to be fatal two months later. In several places in South-Wales, too, the epidemic, after causing many deaths, ceased in August or September. In Dorsetshire the epidemic produced no deaths in Poole after July. In many places in Essex there were no deaths after September. The mortality ceased at Boston, in Lincolnshire, in August; and at Wisbeach, in Cambridgeshire, in September ; although in most places in both these counties it continued a month later.

On the whole these cases are less remarkable than those of the long persistence of the disease. But both series of instances present decided exceptions to the rule that the early cessation or late persistence of the epidemic in different places was determined by the degrees in which they seve-

rally presented the known local conditions of unhealthiness.

With regard to the mode of cessation of the epidemic
within individual towns, little need be said. In the different
districts or quarters of large cities the disease has ceased in
most cases nearly simultaneously. On the other hand, the
instances already adduced to show how different parts of the
smaller towns, and different parts of the several districts of
large cities suffer rather in succession than simultaneously,
may serve to illustrate also the absence of simultaneousness
in the disappearance of the disease from the different localities within such limited spheres. But it may further be
noticed, that at the close of the epidemic in London, as well
as at its commencement, the disease very commonly manifested itself by attacking two, three, or more persons in succession in the same house in various parts of the metropolis,
rather than by single attacks in a greater number of distinct
houses; and that these groups of cases frequently occurred
in houses which had not previously been visited by the epidemic, and, though usually situated in low and ill-drained
spots, were often in site and in internal sanitary condition
not apparently worse, frequently better circumstanced, than
many others that escaped.

The foregoing facts have been detailed with the view of
illustrating the manner in which Cholera rises in a country,
reaches its climax, and afterwards subsides and disappears.
They have shown :—

1. That the epidemic of 1848–49 in England was very
widely diffused over the country, though with very different
degrees of severity in different parts, within three months
after its first appearance at the end of September; that the
renewed rise, or, more strictly speaking. the increase, of the
epidemic at the beginning of the summer of 1849 took place
in different counties in June, in July, and in August, its climax in a large majority of the counties in September and in
nearly all the remainder in August, and its ultimate cessa-

tion in almost all cases in one or other of the three months September, October, and November; that there was considerable diversity in the times of the commencement and of the cessation of the epidemic, and some diversity even in the times of its climax, in the different towns of each division of the country taken separately ; and that, although it began, reached its climax, and ceased at nearly the same time in the several chief divisions, registration districts, and even sub-districts of the metropolis, it affected the different streets, groups of houses, or public establishments within each sub-district and the different parts of the smaller provincial towns by no means simultaneously, but rather in succession, and often manifested the same migratory character in its mode of affecting different parts of a large public institution.

2. That the earliness of its rise in different counties, and the lateness of the period to which it lingered in them, seemed, as a general rule, to be determined by their levels, their nearness to the sea-coast, and their relation to the mouths of large rivers or inlets of the sea, and in a less degree by the density of their population, and especially by the comparative number of their town population; and that the order in which different towns were attacked, and the degree of persistence of the disease in them during the decline of the epidemic, were obviously in a great measure dependent on the same circumstances, the time of attack of towns, as of counties, being, however, apparently influenced by lowness of site and nearness to the coast or to the mouths of rivers, more decidedly than by the density and character of the population.

3. That in numerous exceptional instances the times of the commencement and of the cessation of the epidemic in counties, towns, and parts of towns were imperfectly, if at all, accounted for by any circumstances of site, or population, or sanitary conditions; and that the absence of simultaneousness, and, indeed, the absence of any rule as to the order of succession in the outbreaks in the different parts of

small towns or of the several sub-districts of the metropolis, also found no satisfactory explanation in such circumstances.

It will be necessary to inquire into the degrees of consistency that may be traced between these results and the several schemes proposed to explain the diffusion of Cholera; but before this is done, some examination of the relation borne by the facts last set forth, and the results previously elicited, may with advantage be instituted. It will show the close agreement subsisting between the main features of a Cholera epidemic, and will lead to inferences which may aid in deciding on the comparative probability of the different theories.

In an epidemic of Cholera, the localities especially and most severely visited by the disease, have certain distinguishing characters, which are for the most part wanting in those other parts of the country or of an individual town which escaped the ravages of the epidemic or suffered only in a slight degree. The characters referred to are, in the case of tracts of country, a low level, proximity to the coast, the presence of large rivers, and a dense population, in great part collected in towns: and in the case of towns they are of similar nature—namely, a low site on the coast, or near the mouths of rivers, where the soil is alluvial and damp; a dense population often engaged in maritime traffic, and living in ill-constructed and ill-ventilated houses; want of sewerage; often a deficient supply of water, and accumulation of filth of various kinds. Now all these circumstances are such as tend to render the atmosphere of the localities where they exist more or less damp and impure. On the other hand, the tracts of country spared by Cholera have a high level, and, lying far inland where the rivers take their rise, have a comparatively dry climate, and have usually also a thin population; and the towns which escaped more or less completely the ravages of Cholera, being situated in these tracts of country, share in their characters, and are likewise free from the great sanitary defects of those towns where Cholera found its most numerous victims. In these tracts of country and these towns, it is clear, the atmosphere must be comparatively pure.   The parts of large towns in which the mortality was great and those in which it was trifling in amount, likewise differed in the same way, in level, in the degree of cleanliness and ventilation of the dwellings, and in other conditions affecting the purity or impurity of the atmosphere.   The inference suggested by these facts alone was, that the cause of Cholera finds the conditions for its increase or for its action in impure and damp air, and either cannot exist, or can exert its morbific power but feebly, when the air is pure.

Facts which came under examination in relation to another feature of a Cholera epidemic, its variations of intensity, led to the same conclusion.   All the known influences to which the rise of a Cholera epidemic to a great degree of intensity could be ascribed, were found to be such as tend to increase the impurity of the atmosphere; namely, in most cases a rise of the temperature of the atmosphere and want of wind with or without great moisture of the air; and, where the influence of a high temperature was wanting, local circumstances productive of great impurity of the air either within or without the dwellings.   From these facts, taken in conjunction with the relation known to subsist between the degree of mortality produced by Cholera, and the degree in which the sources of impure air existed in different localities, it seemed reasonable to conclude that the rise of an epidemic of Cholera to a climax during the summer season was due to the increased impurity of the air, occasioned by the meteorological conditions above referred to, and its subsequent decline to the diminished impurity of the air under opposite meteorological conditions; and the further inference was drawn, that great variations in the intensity of an epidemic, not explicable in this manner or by temporary local causes of impure air, were due to some unknown agency or agencies in the atmosphere, either affecting the degree of its purity or acting more directly on the cause of the disease.

Now the general rules which have been found to prevail

respecting the times at which different parts of England began to suffer distinctly from Cholera, experienced its effects in the greatest intensity, and were freed from the visitation, are in entire accordance with these foregoing conclusions.

If the influences which occasioned the rise of the epidemic in the summer of 1849, acted by increasing the impurity of the air in certain localities, it would seem to have been a necessary result that they should produce both those effects soonest in those tracts of country where the sources of impure air most abounded, and last in those where the same conditions were in the greatest degree deficient. If the decline of the epidemic was occasioned by influences tending to remove or diminish the impure state of the air, it was likewise a necessary consequence that this change in the atmosphere and repression of the epidemic ensued, *cæteris paribus*, soonest in places where there were fewest sources of foulness, and latest where these were rife. Since, moreover, the influence of the meteorological conditions bringing about the climax of the epidemic would be at its height, as a general rule, in all parts of the country about the same time, the greatest development of the atmospheric impurity and the greatest mortality from Cholera could not fail to be everywhere nearly simultaneous. The main facts, then, which have been detailed relating to the order in which different places were attacked during the summer of 1849, and ceased to suffer during the following autumn and winter, are in complete accordance with, and therefore in a measure corroborate, the conclusions previously arrived at with regard to the influence of the atmosphere. The three series of facts, then, alike lead to the general conclusions that an essential condition for the action of the cause of Cholera is an impure and damp atmosphere, and that the degree in which this condition exists, *cæteris paribus*, regulates both the time and the intensity of the epidemic's effects.

Even those exceptional cases in which severe local outbreaks of Cholera occurred at times when the epidemic manifested as yet no great power, or was rapidly declining, afford further confirmation of the view that a damp and impure state of air is a chief condition for the development of the disease. Very many of these local exceptional outbreaks, as has been before pointed out, occurred in public establishments, lunatic asylums, workhouses, and prisons, and these establishments have usually within them conditions for the production of an impure state of air which compensate for the want of external warmth in the very early or late periods of the year. Indeed, as the ventilation of these buildings is usually less effectually provided for in cold than in warm weather, it is, on the principle assumed, quite intelligible, why they occasionally have suffered so severely in the winter.

In the same way the severity of the outbreaks in several towns and villages during the winter of 1848–49, and the earlier months of the summer of 1849, namely, in Sunderland, Rodruth, Chesham, Poulton, Bedlington, Norton and Baldock, Keynsham and Poole, may be ascribed in great part to local conditions of unhealthiness, which in most instances were sufficiently flagrant to explain the great mortality. It is true that, neither in these cases nor in those of the public establishments before referred to (the Taunton Workhouse, the Wakefield Lunatic Asylum, the Hertford Prison, and the Pauper School at Tooting), do the mere local conditions, regarded as sources of foul air, account for the sudden occurrence of some of the outbreaks after the epidemic had subsided elsewhere, and for the continued absence of the disease from others of them after the first early outbreak had ceased, although the epidemic was increasing in other places. But this is a difficulty which does not materially affect the matter now under consideration, namely, the position that impure air is an essential local condition for the severe manifestation of Cholera; in other words, the principal condition by virtue of which individual localities, and the persons inhabiting them, are susceptible of the influence of the epidemic.

Certain other facts relating to the times at which different localities began and ceased to suffer from Cholera, suggest

a further inference as to the part played by an impure
atmosphere in regard to this epidemic disease; namely,
that not merely the state of the air in the particular localities affected, but also the condition of the more general
atmosphere, influences the times of attack of different places.
It has been mentioned as in some respects apparently an
anomalous fact, that during the summer of 1849, districts
and towns situated in the interior of the country, and on a
higher level than the coast districts, though, by density of
population and deficiency of sanitary provisions, fitted to
suffer severely, and in the end visited most severely, were
attacked late. Now the influences producing the general
increase of the disease at the period referred to would act on
the sources of impure air in each of these places, as soon as
elsewhere ; why, then, did not the disease appear in them at
an early period? It seems most in accordance with other
facts to believe that it was because the general atmosphere
of these higher districts was purer than that of the lower
districts nearer the coast, and, by virtue of its greater purity,
interfered with or obstructed the action of the epidemic.
And if this be the correct explanation of the fact, it of course
follows that the impure air of the lower districts in some way
facilitates the action of the epidemic on the localities within
its range.

   The statistics of the rise of Cholera in the different districts of London in the summer of 1849, afford facts of a
strictly analogous kind, which need, or at least admit of, a
similar explanation. The epidemic began first in the districts on the lowest level, and last in those on the highest
level. This was in general accordance with the various sanitary conditions of the different localities, and with the different rates of mortality which they ultimately suffered. But
among the districts which are not on the lowest level, and
which were comparatively late in experiencing the attack of
the epidemic, there were some, as those of St. Giles and
Bethnal Green, which presented the worst local conditions,
and ultimately suffered a very high rate of mortality. Here,

again, supposing the state of the air to be an important condition for the action of the epidemic, the inference seems a just one, that not merely the state of the air in the particular localities (for example, the interior of houses), but the state of the general atmosphere of each district of a large city, regulates, in some measure, the time of outbreak of the disease in that district.

Other exceptional facts in the history of the epidemic, which have as yet been only cursorily alluded to, extend as well as corroborate the same view respecting the influence of the state of the general atmosphere over a more or less extended tract of country, or part of a large city, since they render it probable that the time of the climax as well as of the attack in the particular localities within certain areas may be thus determined. The cases in which both the rise and the climax of the epidemic were extraordinarily late over entire counties, obviously find in this assumption their readiest explanation. In the cases, too, where towns have been adduced as examples of departure from the rule as to the time of the attack, of the climax, or of the disappearance of the epidemic, further examination likewise traces the effects of an influence extending over a large tract of country, and with great probability referable to the state of the atmosphere. Two examples taken from the south coast may be instanced. The disease appeared two months later at Torquay and Brixham, on the coast of Devon, than at several inland places, South Brent, Plympton, and Egg Buckland. But the latter places lie in the western part of the county near Plymouth, where the epidemic commenced early in the summer, while Torquay and Brixham are situated in its eastern part, where no deaths from Cholera occurred before August or September, except a single (imported?) one at Exeter and three single deaths at Chudleigh, St. Thomas, and Dartmouth. Here, then, likewise it seems most probable that Torquay and Brixham, and the other places on the east coast of Devon, were protected during the months of May and June from the inroads of the epidemic by the state of the atmosphere which surrounded them. Again, in the instance of the large ports of Hampshire—Gosport, Portsmouth, and Southampton—in which the epidemic reached its climax so early as July, the dependence of this upon a particular state of the atmosphere is rendered most probable by the fact of Ryde, on the opposite coast of the Isle of Wight, suffering its chief mortality in the same month, and of other places in the island being also visited severely at the same time. This instance, indeed, affords stronger evidence than the former one, for while different views might be entertained as to the manner in which the disease is brought early or late to a tract of country, there seems no plausible mode of accounting for an early climax of the disorder over a particular region except by ascribing it to an early intensity of the same general conditions on which the climax everywhere depends, and that condition has been seen to be almost certainly an increased impurity of the atmosphere.

Instances are met with in the history of the winter period of the epidemic where the disease, although generally in abeyance, manifested itself with comparative severity over considerable tracts of country, as if from the influence of some agency or condition which was present over a corresponding area. Thus, in Norfolk, during the months of January and February, 1849, the deaths from Cholera amounted to 45, and 18 of these deaths from Cholera were registered in the village of Mileham (between the 3rd and 31st of January), and 17 in the two small parishes of East and West Rudham (between the 5th of January and the 13th of February). But the occurrence of the disease in these places at this particular time, seems not to have been entirely due to local conditions; for the remaining 10 deaths from Cholera in Norfolk during these two months were registered in the same north-western part of the county, where, moreover, scarcely a death was caused by the disease during the rest of the year. Again, in Cambridgeshire there were 28 deaths from Cholera during the months of November and December, 1848, and 15 of this number occurred in the single parish of Upwell, but there were contemporaneous, though less fatal, outbreaks in the neighbouring places of Downham, Southery, and Peterborough, with single deaths in other spots. Lastly, in Buckinghamshire, 50 persons died of Cholera during November and December, 1848, and January, 1849, and 44 of them died in the village of Chesham, between the 13th of November and the 18th of January, but in the month of November two other deaths were registered in the adjoining parish of Missenden; and the only outbreaks in towns in the same part of the " Cholera field," namely, St. Albans, Hertford, Hemel Hempstead, and Reading, occurred in December and January. These instances may, too, be contrasted with a group of small outbreaks in Middlesex; namely, at Chiswick, Brentford, Isleworth, Hillingdon near Uxbridge, and Sunbury, in which places several deaths from Cholera occurred between the beginning of October and the 4th of November, no others following during the entire winter.

In these cases, then, as in others that have been adduced, an influence seems certainly to have been exerted over tracts of country of some extent, including many separate localities; and all the best-established facts respecting Cholera being considered, it is most probable that this influence was exerted through the medium of the atmosphere.

The exact nature of the part played by the atmosphere is not obvious in the instances hitherto noticed, but others will now be referred to in which it seems to be apparent that the atmosphere, if it at all participated in the production of the results, most probably served as the means of communicating or transmitting the cause of the disease from one locality to another.

One fact of this kind is the almost complete simultaneousness of the climax of the epidemic of 1849 in the different registration districts of the metropolis south of the Thames, the weeks of greatest mortality being the same in all these districts (see Table, page 76); while the periods of greatest

mortality in the several districts north of the Thames fell
in different weeks of the two months, August and September.

To perceive the bearing of this fact on the point now
under consideration, it is necessary to remember that the
climax of the .epidemic in each district and each division of
London, was due to the increased number of particular localities affected at one time. It must be borne in mind, too,
that the atmosphere of the low districts on the south side
of the Thames was more impure than that of the districts
on the opposite side of the river. If, then, it be admitted
that the greater severity of the epidemic in the southern
districts was due to this state of the atmosphere as well as
to the defective sanitary state of the courts, houses, and other
particular localities, while the less severity in the northern
districts was owing to the comparatively pure state of the air
on the north side of the river, it follows almost as a necessary consequence, that the impure atmosphere of the southern
districts contributed to the simultaneous production of the
climax in all of them by causing the disease to appear in
each of them in many spots at one and the same time;
while it is equally apparent that the different dates of the
climax in the different northern districts must be due to the
air of that part of London not being uniformly in the same
state of impurity even at the time of the general climax, and
consequently, not able to determine very numerous outbreaks
in every district at the same time.

When further with this fact is coupled the successive
mode of attack of the individual localities, houses, groups of
houses, and public establishments within each sub-district,
the further inference suggests itself, that the impure atmosphere of a district determines the occurrence of numerous
outbreaks within its area by rapidly communicating the disease from one locality to another.

Additional support to the same view is afforded by the
contrast which the more severe summer period of the epide-

mic presents to the winter period in respect of the degree of simultaneousness of the outbreaks in different localities. In the winter comparatively few places were attacked, and those at very various times, while many which appeared to possess the necessary local conditions escaped. In the summer period of the epidemic a much larger number of places were attacked,—few, indeed, that presented the conditions of insalubrity escaped, and those attacked began to suffer within a comparatively limited period. This, moreover, is true, not only of the different towns in the several " Cholera fields," but also of the different localities affected in the metropolis. Thus during the height of the epidemic 21 of the 36 districts suffered their chief mortality, owing to the increased number of localities affected, in the same week, and 33 of them within three weeks; whereas during the winter period the different districts or groups of districts had the greatest number of deaths at very different times: the south districts (except that of Wandsworth) between October the 21st and November the 6th, 1848; the east districts between the 10th of November and the 30th of December, and again between the 5th of February and 10th of March; while the great outbreak in the Wandsworth district fell in the intermediate period, namely, between the end of December, 1848, and the 27th of January, 1849. Other modes of explaining the fact might perhaps be found, but the idea that the generally impure state of the air produced by the influences determining the climax causes a larger number of places to be affected at nearly the same time, by conveying the disease, or permitting it to be conveyed, from one locality to another, affords, at all events, a sufficient solution of the problem, and a solution of it which is in accordance with other features of the epidemic.

One illustration of the supposed participation of the atmosphere in the spread of Cholera remains to be noticed.

It has been stated that the order in which different parts of the country began to suffer severely from Cholera in the beginning of the summer of 1849, is explicable on the principle that the general causes which then determined the extension of the epidemic acted by increasing the quantity of the impurities poured into and detained in the atmosphere, and necessarily produced this result, together with the consequent increase of the disease, first in those parts where the sources of foul air were most abundant, last where they were wanting. But this principle does not entirely explain the facts of the case; for when the disease increased in the country at the time referred to, there was not a gradual increase of it in the several localities affected, varying in degree according to their differences of site and sanitary condition, but for the most part a succession of sudden outbreaks in the different localities, which could hardly be accounted for by mere differences of degree in the gradually increasing impurity of the air in the localities themselves. The facts are rather indicative of sudden changes of condition in the spots affected, and would be better explained by the assumption that the air in the several low tracts of country, in proportion as its impurity increased, acquired the power of transmitting the cause of the disease from one locality to another within its range.

At the period referred to, the disease seemed, as the summer advanced, to spread from many centres, but with great irregularity, the probable cause of which will be noticed at a future page. In the winter of 1848, the extension of the epidemic from London, one of its first seats, to the places situated around, took place with a more regular progress, as may be seen in Map I. and in the subjoined table*; the different places being attacked generally in the order of their nearness to the centre, not merely in the order of their nearness to the river, or to the coast. And the probability that the disease was here really communicated from one place to another, is strengthened by the circumstance that many of the smaller places attacked were, neither by the natural character of their site nor by sanitary condition, ap-

---

* The subjoined Table will exemplify the fact stated above. The places are arranged in the order of their attack by Cholera :—

parently such as the epidemic would have been expected to visit thus early.

This remark is applicable likewise to the smaller towns and villages attacked in the summer of the year 1849, in parts of the great Cholera fields most distant from their centres, and to the still smaller spots affected in the immediate vicinity of each town which became a seat of the disease. Of the numerous places attacked in healthy and comparatively elevated parts of Middlesex, Hertfordshire, Buckinghamshire, and Kent, many would most probably have escaped had it not been for their proximity to the already existing foci of the disease, formed by London and other places near the Thames. It can scarcely be doubted that the disease was transmitted to many of them more or less directly from these centres, and all the facts relating to the epidemic hitherto examined tend to the conclusion, that its transmission was in some way or other facilitated, if not effected, by the atmosphere.

A few words may here be said with regard to the state of atmosphere which has been spoken of, in the preceding pages, as in all probability favouring not only the development of the epidemic with intensity over a tract of country, but also its diffusion from one place to another. The condition of air which is known to be most constantly attendant on the severe ravages of the disease, and its rapid spread in towns

In London	.	first death	.	.	September.
Uxbridge	.		.	.	October 5th.
Guildford	.			„	7th or 30th.
Chatham	.				9th.
Edmonton	.				11th.
Brentford	.			„	23rd.
Chelmsford				„	26th.
Sunbury				November 1st.
Chesham				„	11th.
Gravesend	.		.	„	11th.
Stratford	.	„	.	.	December 3rd.
Chatham		second outbreak	.	„	8th.
Reading	.	first death	.	.	„ 10th.
Hertford	.	„	.	.	„ 12th.
Hemel Hempstead	„			„	16th.

H

or public buildings, is undoubtedly one of dampness, and impregnation with animal effluvia, or with the products of the decomposition of organic matter, especially animal matter. The same condition, in a less degree, is acquired by large bodies of air when their movement is sluggish, and when they pass over surfaces where there is much moisture, and much decomposing animal and other organic matter. It is of course especially in the lower parts of the country, where they are densely populated, that the lower strata of the atmosphere acquire these characters. In the more elevated regions, the air more rarely approaches to the stagnant state, and also finds less moisture and less impurity to absorb. If, therefore, this damp and impure air is a necessary medium for the diffusion of Cholera, the difference between the atmosphere of the lower and that of the more elevated districts, explains the difference in the rate of diffusion of the disease in the latter and the former respectively.

Our conception of the share probably taken by the atmosphere in extending the ravages of the epidemic is aided, too, by remembering that the air in the low districts, though it may seem to be nearly motionless, is not really so, or, at all events, is so only for very short periods ; and that portions of the damp and impure air are constantly passing off in the direction of the atmospheric currents on one side, while fresh portions enter on the other, and acquire the same characters. After passing a longer or shorter distance (which will vary according to many variable conditions), a portion of this damp and impure air will become diluted, and lost amidst the purer and drier air of other and more elevated tracts of country. But there are good grounds for believing that, in certain states of the atmosphere, a body of damp and impure air may travel over the surface of the country for many miles, still preserving its original properties. · It is quite possible, therefore, that such air, if capable at all of transmitting the disease or its cause from place to place, may convey it from one town to another some miles distant.

It must not, however, be assumed as certain, that mere

moisture and impregnation with animal and other organic impurities are all that distinguish air which favours or effects the diffusion of Cholera. Reasons have been given at a former page, for the belief that there are qualities of air at present scarcely known but by their effects, which, according as one or other is present, may repress the epidemic when other circumstances are favourable to its continued rise, or promote its increase in a degree out of proportion to any obviously existing conditions capable of producing such a result. Whether these qualities of the air depend respectively, the one on the absence, and the other on the presence in unusual quantity, of ozone, or some matter having a more special relation to the cause of Cholera, is a question yet to be determined. But all the facts relating to the subject render it probable, that the unknown condition of the air which represses Cholera is most frequently associated with comparative dryness and purity of the atmosphere, and the unknown condition that promotes it with the presence of moisture and impurities.

The foregoing inquiry has been directed to the discovery of the relation borne by the atmosphere to the spread of Cholera. The results which have been arrived at will now be found to lend much support to that-theory of the cause of Cholera, which regards it as a morbific matter or poison, reproduced in the air, and diffused, at least in part, by the agency of atmospheric currents.

Such a poison brought by the atmosphere to this country might soon be dispersed over many parts of it, and would meet with a suitable nidus for its reproduction in the lower districts, near the mouths of rivers ; while in parts where the atmosphere, from its dryness and purity, failed to afford the necessary conditions for its increase or maintenance, it would perish.

The *unequal distribution* of the disease over the country in the winter of 1848-49, as seen in Map I., would therefore be quite intelligible. The absence of it in some parts, such as the mining and pottery districts of Staffordshire, Mon-

mouthshire, and South Wales, where the conditions of unhealthiness, without doubt, abounded in the towns and other
inhabited places, would be accounted for; since the supposed
poison, even if it did not perish before it reached those inland
or more elevated districts, would find there an atmosphere
unfit to preserve its active properties, and to communicate it
to the spots in which it could increase and produce its effects
on the inhabitants. The comparative intensity of the epidemic over other parts for short periods in the same season,
would also be intelligible; for the poison, being brought by
a body of moist and impure air, might be distributed over an
area of greater or less extent, infecting particular localities
within its limits, and giving rise to outbreaks of various degrees
of severity, corresponding with the local sanitary conditions.

The lingering of the disease, in the spring of 1849, in
certain spots, for the most part distinguished by the local
conditions productive of a damp and impure air, while
elsewhere throughout the country it had disappeared, is
also in complete accordance with the theory of a poison
which finds the means for its maintenance and increase in
such places, and in such an atmosphere.

The renewed *rise* of the epidemic in the summer might
reasonably be referred to the increase of impurity and
moisture in the air under the influence of rising temperature, and perhaps other meteorological conditions, to the
consequent increase of the poison in the localities where it
already existed, to its distribution with the air from these
different foci to other places more or less distant;—to its
increase in these again, if they afforded the necessary conditions, and to its further diffusion from them to other places,
through the medium of the atmosphere. While the general
atmosphere continued to acquire, more and more, the qualities favourable to the extension and increase of the poison,
and while the number of towns or villages affected would,
as a consequence, continue to increase, the number of
localities affected in each town likewise would, as a general
rule, become greater. Thus the extent of the disease

over the country, and its intensity in each large town, would continue to increase together, and the climax of the epidemic would be reached everywhere nearly at the same time. Lastly, when, with the fall of temperature, the atmosphere had begun to lose the properties favourable to the transmission of the poison, comparatively few fresh places would become infected, and the epidemic would gradually subside and cease.

The *order* in which different parts of the country and different towns were attacked, and ceased to suffer in the year 1849, is also in entire accordance with the same theory. At the beginning of the summer, the poison would find the means for its dissemination as well as for its increase soonest in districts where the sources of damp and impurity most abound; and hence the towns in those parts would necessarily soonest become foci, where the disease would increase, and whence it would afterwards spread to towns in the more elevated and more inland regions. In the autumn and the beginning of the winter, the lowest districts and most crowded towns would likewise continue longest to afford an atmosphere fitted to transmit the poison from spot to spot, and, inasmuch as the epidemic is maintained in each town or sub-district by the successive outbreaks in different localities, it would be expected to survive to the latest period where the conditions for the transference of the poison from one of these localities to another existed longest.

The exceptions to the order of attack, both of tracts of country and of towns, are equally in accordance with the theory. The late attack of some towns abounding in local conditions of unhealthiness, but situated in elevated tracts of country, would be sufficiently explained by the purer atmosphere of those regions rendering it difficult for the poison to reach the damp and foul localities in which it might increase and produce its effects on the inhabitants. And the late appearance of the epidemic in some coast districts scarcely offers greater difficulty; for it is an often-observed fact that the state of the atmosphere varies on different parts of the coast at the same time, and in the same part at different times, so that the morbific matter, while it was spreading rapidly over one such district, might be excluded by the state of the atmosphere from another not far distant one.

The long-delayed appearance of the disease in towns or smaller localities, such as parts of towns, which, from their natural site, sanitary condition, and nearness to a focus of the disease, would have been expected to have received it through the medium of the atmosphere at an earlier period, is in entire agreement with a character which has already been assigned to the supposed Cholera poison, namely, that it has the properties, not of a gaseous substance, but of a matter in the form of solid or liquid particles. Such a poison being distributed only partially through the air, and carried hither and thither by the atmospheric currents, might for a long time fail to reach a spot which was in itself even well fitted to afford it the means of increase.

The fact of the different spots within a registration subdistrict of the metropolis, or in a small town, being, like the different towns of a country, as a rule, attacked in succession, obviously finds a ready explanation in this theory of the cause of Cholera.

Again, the *climax* of the epidemic was more nearly simultaneous in the different localities visited by it, at the season, and in the area, most remarkable for impurity of the atmosphere, and this fact which was exemplified by the case of the registration districts of London (see pages 93-94), seemed itself to suggest the inference, that impure air was the medium through which the disease or its cause was communicated from one spot to another. But it is rendered much more intelligible by the theory of a morbific matter diffused by currents of air. For in an atmosphere uniformly or very generally impure, the poison would find in all parts of a given area an equal medium for its transmission from spot to spot, and consequently the number of spots infected would, under the influence of meteorological or other conditions aggravating the local and general atmospheric impurity, increase everywhere equally, and reach the climax in all at or about the same time.   But in air generally not so impure, the transmission of the poison from spot to spot would be more dependent on, or more interfered with, by accidental circumstances, and would affect the greater number of spots in some parts of a given area at one time, and in other parts at another time.

Lastly, the fact that around or in the neighbourhood of the more considerable foci of the epidemic, slighter outbreaks occurred in places which from natural site or sanitary condition had apparently no special fitness, as it were, inviting the attack, is consonant with the idea of a morbific poison, which, while it undergoes increase in certain foci, is capable of being scattered around them by means of atmospheric currents.

The two other principal theories are consistent with several of the facts relative to the dissemination of the epidemic, but neither of them affords an explanation of all the facts without the aid of assumptions which are opposed to other well-established features of the epidemic, or are in themselves far-fetched and improbable.

With regard to the theory that the cause of Cholera is a general state of the atmosphere, an " atmospheric influence," or " epidemic constitution " of the air, it has before been shown that this theory cannot be maintained in the sense that this general state belongs to the moving mass of the atmosphere, since while the air is constantly moving, and indeed changed by the currents setting in from different quarters in succession, the epidemic is for a long time persistent.   Some modification of the theory must, therefore, be adopted.. One before suggested was, that a mass of atmosphere in a peculiar state, passing over England, determined the production of a more fixed cause of the disease, at different points of the surface of the country.   But as this fixed cause would then necessarily have the properties which have been assigned to the Cholera poison, by the theory already examined, and, after its first production, would be disseminated in the same way, there would be no real difference between this modified theory and the one referred to, except as regards the conveyance of the disease from one country to another, in which alone the supposed atmospheric influence or state would be concerned. This hypothesis need not be further considered here: it will, however, be noticed again hereafter.

Another modification of the theory of an "atmospheric influence" is, that which supposes it to be a power operating in the atmosphere, though not moving with it (just as light or electricity acts in or through the atmosphere), and producing its effect on the human body only in localities where the atmosphere is foul, or on persons rendered susceptible by long dwelling in an impure air. This theory would include the vaguely-propounded notions of a particular " electrical state," and a " telluric influence."

An argument in favour of such a theory as this, might doubtless be based on the great extent to which the epidemic apparently soon reached, on its first appearance in this country in 1848. But, independently of the doubts that still exist as to the extent attained by the epidemic in the month of October, and the certainty, as far as statistical facts can afford it, that large tracts of the country were not visited till the end of November or even December, it is to be observed, on the one hand, that the extent of the epidemic at its outbreak, though accepted with the least limitation, is sufficiently explained by the theory of a Cholera matter partially diffused through the air; and, on the other hand, that if the disease was really thus general on its first appearance in England in 1848, this was an exception to the rule which has more commonly prevailed, as to its mode of attacking a country. Thus in the epidemic of 1831–32, the disease had been very fatal for two or three months in Sunderland and near Edinburgh before it appeared in London, and still longer before it showed itself in other parts of the country; and even in the late epidemic, it tarried in parts of Ireland, as late as the month of March, 1850; although it disappeared two or three months previously from the rest of that island, as well as from England*. The partial prevalence of the disease at the beginning and the end of an epidemic, exemplified in these instances, is its more usual character: so that, in fact, the mode of commencement of a Cholera epidemic must be regarded as less easily reconcileable with the notion of an imponderable influence of the kind supposed than with that of a material agent, the sphere of action of which might be expected to be more partial and at first more limited in extent.

The general fact of the successive outbreak, and disappearance, and nearly simultaneous climax of the epidemic in different places during the year 1849 is consistent enough with the idea of a general imponderable influence producing its effects by the aid of certain local conditions. But all the facts constituting exceptions to the rule of a simultaneous climax, and of an order of attack and cessation connected with the presence of certain known conditions, or on the degree of their presence, while they obviously favour the theory of a Cholera poison partially distributed in and by the air, are so many difficulties in the way of the adoption of the theory of a general atmospheric influence of whatever kind. The sudden outbreak of the disease with great severity and without sufficient local cause in certain small spots at periods when the epidemic was generally nearly extinct, namely, both at the beginning and towards the end of the year 1849; its long absence during the summer of the year 1849 from towns in the worst sanitary condition, and its sudden and violent outbreak in them in the autumn; the successive (almost migratory) mode of its attack of different houses and groups of houses in the sub-districts of London and in small towns, or of different parts of public buildings, and the outbreaks in places situated around the foci of the disease, not explained by the local characters of those places,—all these facts in the history of the epidemic need for their explanation other assumptions than are included in the simple theory of an atmospheric influence. It must be assumed that this influence, though requiring for its action on the human body the presence of a local impurity of atmosphere, yet does not produce its effects everywhere at the same time in different degrees proportional to the amount of the atmospheric impurity in the several localities; but that of the many localities apparently equal in sanitary conditions, only a few at first acquire an unknown cause of susceptibility of the influence, and that certain localities without apparent alteration of condition, or with only an alteration in degree, undergo on a sudden a complete change in some unknown respect, rendering them at once highly susceptible of the influence which previously they had wholly resisted. It must be assumed that this change affects either the air of a limited locality or the inhabitants of it; and in either of these forms the assumption is opposed to probability. It is not probable, that when for months a whole town had been insusceptible of the influence, the susceptibility suddenly acquired by one spot should induce very soon the same susceptibility of other spots in various parts of the same town,—yet, for the explanation of the facts, this must be admitted; or that, after all the inhabitants of a town or of an establishment had resisted the atmospheric influence for a long period, many individuals in several parts of the town or of the public establishment should on a sudden begin to suffer from it, one after another. Moreover, the causes of these sudden changes of condition in localities or in their inhabitants would be as mysterious in their nature and effects, as the hypothetical atmospheric influence itself.

The theory that Cholera is diffused by means of human intercourse affords a ready explanation of some of the more remarkable facts relating to the epidemic which have been detailed in the present section of this report; namely, its early appearance in sea-ports, and in counties and towns where traffic is active, its appearance in different towns in the same county or "Cholera field" not simultaneously but successively, the late attack of some places which for site and sanitary condition seemed obnoxious to an early invasion, the successive mode of attack of different localities in a small town, or in a sub-district of London, and the appearance of the disease in small places around great foci of the epidemic ; it explains, indeed, all those facts which point rather to a morbific poison partially distributed than to an agent or influence existing throughout the atmosphere.

On the other hand, diffusion by human intercourse seems to be by no means the most appropriate explanation of some other facts of great importance. But in relation to these adverse facts, a distinction must be made between the two principal modes in which human intercourse may be the means of propagating Cholera.

The idea usually associated with the diffusion of a disease by human agency, is that the disease is the effect of a virus which is reproduced in the bodies of the sick, and which, emanating from their bodies, infects other persons; and consequently, that a person receiving the contagion in one place, and travelling to another, may convey the infection thither in his own body.

The very close connection between Cholera and local conditions which are productive of a damp and foul state of air, the great influence exerted over the epidemic in a country or town by varying meteorological or other conditions of the atmosphere, the want of analogy with the best known contagious disorders in respect of its varying prevalence at different seasons, and the remarkably rapid spread of the disease through a large city, destroying many thousands of lives in a few days, are grounds already adduced for regarding the "contagion" theory of Cholera with something more than doubt. In the preceding examination of the various facts relating to the time of commencement, climax, and cessation of the epidemic in different places, further reasons have been met with for regarding this theory as less probable than others. For it has been seen, that not only the air of the particular localities, but also the more general atmosphere of an entire city or tract of country, exerts a powerful influence over the diffusion of Cholera. In the case of diseases universally admitted to be contagious, the general atmosphere, without doubt, at one time, by its rapid movement, dissipates the virus emanating from the bodies of the sick, and at another time, from its almost stagnant state, permits the virus to accumulate and become concentrated. But the influence of the atmosphere over the supposed virus of Cholera must be far greater than this, otherwise the appearance of the disease would not have been so strictly regulated as to time by the character of the districts in which the towns were situated, and would not so long have failed to reach the populous and busy towns of the mining and pottery districts of Worcestershire and Staffordshire; nor would the climax of the epidemic have been so nearly simultaneous in all parts of the country. It is, indeed, so much opposed to probability, that any disease, the diffusion of which is thus under the control of different states of the atmosphere, should be essentially and in the strict sense of the term contagious, that this theory must be regarded as inadmissible, unless the communication of the disease from the bodies of the sick to the healthy should hereafter seem to be proved by numerous facts explicable on no other assumption.

There is, however, a second mode in which human intercourse might be the means of communicating and diffusing Cholera: a poison undergoing its increase out of the body might be carried from place to place in the vehicles of men, in their baggage, or even in their clothes. This is, in fact, the fifth theory mentioned at page 5. It is consistent with the history of the dissemination of the epidemic through the country, not only in all those particulars which were mentioned above as favourable to the idea of its diffusion by human intercourse, but also in respect of the power exercised by the sanitary condition of different localities, and especially by the state of the air in them on the extension as well as on the local severity of the epidemic; since, according to this theory, the poisonous matter, though carried to many places by human intercourse, could only increase and produce the disease in those spots where the air is foul. But when this theory is applied to the explanation of some other facts, difficulties are encountered which seem necessarily to limit the share taken by human intercourse in the general result. The simultaneous or almost simultaneous appearance of the disease in several parts of a large city, and its occasional extension through a town or city with extraordinary rapidity, need the admission that the poison may undergo its increase or reproduction not merely in the air of limited spots, but in the general atmosphere of a city, or, at all events, that wherever its increase takes place, it may be disseminated by means of the atmosphere, and independently of human intercourse.   It would *à priori* be most probable, that a poisonous matter which increases in foul air would be at least as capable of dissemination through a limited area by means of atmospheric currents as by the vehicles of luggage or clothes of men.   And the following facts frequently referred to before afford grounds for doubting whether the conveyance of the disease from town to town is always or even generally effected by human intercourse. During the winter of 1848-49, towns of large population, such as Leeds, where local conditions of unhealthiness abound, and where the traffic with places already affected with Cholera was very active, nevertheless escaped infection. And in the subsequent summer the appearance of the disease in the crowded towns and mining districts of Worcestershire and Staffordshire, was long delayed, while it had very rapidly spread through other districts of the country. These facts can scarcely be ascribed to accident; to explain them on the assumption that a material poison transmitted from one place to another is the cause of the disease, it seems necessary to suppose that the poison was destroyed or rendered inert by the general atmosphere of the towns themselves, or rather of the parts of the country in which the towns are situated before it could reach the spots in which it would have found the fit medium for its increase; and it is clearly more likely that the poison would be thus arrested or destroyed on its way, if it were carried by the air than if it were conveyed in the vehicles or about the persons of men moving from place to place.

On the other hand, it must be borne in mind, that the theory of a poisonous matter increasing in impure air, and distributed by atmospheric currents by no means excludes the idea of human intercourse being an additional means by which it is disseminated. The same reasons, in fact, which led to the inference, that the cause of the disease is a matter, not gaseous and diffusible, but solid or liquid, and capable of attaching itself to surfaces, also make it probable that this poison may be and is conveyed from place to place by human beings or in the course of human traffic. Whether there is conclusive evidence of this really occurring is a matter for subsequent inquiry. It need here merely be remarked, that the general and statistical facts of the history of the epidemic in England neither require nor refute the assumption that human intercourse had a large share in the diffusion of the disease.

Two characters of epidemic Cholera remain to be considered in their bearing on the theories of its cause and mode of propagation. One is the manner of its commencement, progress, and cessation in each particular spot visited by it. The other is the manner in which it passes across a continent, or across a sea from one country to another.

VII. The main features of the local outbreaks of Cholera in regard to their progress and duration may be conveniently studied in the history of the visitations experienced by lunatic asylums in England during the epidemic of 1848-49. Returns made to the Commissioners in Lunacy show that deaths from Cholera occurred in 16 asylums. In one of them there were only 2 deaths, which happened at distant dates. But in the remainder there were series of several cases, with a proportional number of deaths. And as 3 asylums experienced visitations of the epidemic both in the winter of 1848-49, and in the subsequent summer, there were in these establishments 18 distinct outbreaks, the features of which may be examined *.

The first thing to be observed in regard to them is, that in lunatic asylums, as in the sub-districts of the metropolis, and as in smaller towns, the disease did not appear in all parts simultaneously; but that, on the contrary, the first cases in the different wards occurred after successive intervals. Sometimes, as at Wakefield, the disease was confined to one ward for two or three weeks, and then extended, within a few days, to nearly every part of the establishment. In other cases, it sooner began to spread from the ward first affected, but afterwards extended neither so quickly nor so widely as in the instance of Wakefield. In a third class of cases, again, it commenced in two or three wards on the same day, though its subsequent extension to other wards took place, in accordance with the general rule, after successive intervals. In almost every asylum some parts escaped altogether; and this fact, which has already been noticed as an instance of the partial operation of the epidemic, was the more remarkable when an entire section of the establishment, devoted to all the patients of one sex, remained, during the entire outbreak, free from the disease; while the section occupied by the patients of the other sex was more or less severely visited; as happened in the instances of the Grove Hall Asylum, Bethnal House, and the St. Marylebone Infirmary.

The cessation of the outbreak was usually as gradual as its commencement, the disease lingering some days, or even weeks, longer in a few wards than in the majority of those affected. In some instances, indeed, the effects of the epidemic had ceased to be felt in one part of the institution before they had begun in other parts.

It was owing to this successive attack of the different wards that, in the more severe outbreaks, the numbers of the cases occurring in successive weeks showed distinct periods

* See Tables XIII. and XIV. in the Appendix, which have been constructed from the data furnished by the Commissioners in Lunacy.

of rise, climax, and decline. For here, as in the wider sphere
of a sub-district of the metropolis or a provincial town, the
greater number of cases and the greater mortality at the
time of the climax depended not so much on an increase
of the disease in each part as on the increased number of
parts then affected, while the subsequent decline was owing
to the disease having again become restricted to fewer parts.

The duration of the outbreaks in these institutions varied
very considerably ; but while the most protracted one—the
summer outbreak in Peckham House—lasted 72 days, few
exceeded 45 days or six weeks. In 3, however, as was
before mentioned, the disease appeared twice, namely, in the
winter of 1848-49, and in the subsequent summer.

When the progress of the epidemic in the separate wards
of lunatic asylums is examined, the cases are found to have
occurred, for the most part, in succession, but with very irregular intervals. Sometimes single cases followed each other
at intervals of from three to seven or more days. In the instances where the outbreak was more severe, or the number
of patients in a ward greater, the cases occurred day by
day ; and occasionally two or three happened on the same
day. But even where the cases were most numerous, no
distinct evidence can be perceived of the epidemic having,
as a general rule, increased for a time, and subsequently declined, in power in the individual wards. It did, however,
sometimes seem to linger in them after its chief force was
spent ; for it not infrequently happened that in wards where
several cases had occurred during a week or more in quick
succession, there was afterwards an interval of ten days or a
fortnight, and then, unexpectedly, the appearance of one or
two cases of the disease. The duration of the epidemic in
one ward seldom exceeded three weeks, and, in the majority
of instances, did not extend to more than ten days or a fortnight.

The course of the disease here described, as it occurred
in lunatic asylums, is exactly that which obtained in prisons
and workhouses, and groups of the houses of the poor. It

is, therefore, unnecessary to enter upon any further examination of the particular facts. Respecting one of the characters described, however, some information was elicited by the second circular letter issued by the Cholera Committee, which may be here briefly stated. To the following question —" In the instances where several cases have occurred in the same house, have they been simultaneous or successive ?"— 41 answers were received ; and in 28 it was stated that the cases were successive, or generally so ; in 6, that the cases were simultaneous, or nearly so ; while in 7 the question was left undecided. It is obvious, therefore, that the rule in this matter is the same in individual houses as it is in the individual wards of a lunatic asylum.

The relative probability of the different theories of Cholera must now be again tested by their respective capabilities of explaining the facts which have been detailed.

The commencement of the disease, usually, in one limited part of a public establishment, or in one of a group of houses, and its extension to others in succession, is not easily reconcilable with the theory of a general and persistent atmospheric state or influence. To adapt this theory to the facts, one of two hypotheses must be adopted : either it must be assumed that a peculiar condition of localities is necessary for enabling the general epidemic influence to produce its effects, and that when one part of a public establishment or a group of houses, previously free from this condition, has on a sudden acquired it, other parts are very liable to participate in it in more or less quick succession; or else it must be supposed that a peculiar state of susceptibility is necessary in the persons who are to be affected by the hypothetical epidemic influence, and that when one or more among the inmates of a public establishment or group of houses, who have all hitherto resisted that influence, chance, from whatever cause, to acquire the necessary state of susceptibility, those in different parts of the building or in contiguous houses are apt successively to fall into the same state.

A much more probable explanation of the commencement

of the epidemic in one part of an asylum, or other public establishment, and of its subsequent extension through other parts, is obviously afforded by either of the other theories, which suppose the cause of the disease to be a material poison, transferable from spot to spot, and from person to person, by human intercourse, or by currents of air.

Again, if the theory of the production of Cholera by a general atmospheric influence were adopted, the continuance of the disease in each ward of a lunatic asylum for a certain time, its cessation in some wards sooner than in others, and its final disappearance from almost all before the epidemic in the neighbourhood had come to an end, could be explained only on the supposition of the temporary existence, in each ward in turn, of that supposed condition, either of the locality or of the patients, which was necessary to excite the general atmospheric cause to action. The difficulties in the way of this hypothesis are obvious.

On the other hand, the explanation of these last facts by those two theories which appear to be the more plausible, implies the assumption, either that the material poison, after existing for a time in each ward, was removed or destroyed, or spontaneously perished, or else that, among the persons living there, only a certain number were susceptible of its morbific influence. And here the preference at first sight seems due to the th ory of " contagion," which supposes that Cholera is propagated by means of a poison emanating from the bodies of the sick, and that it continues to exist in each locality as long as there are persons within the reach of the contagious virus who are susceptible of the disease, and consequently capable of reproducing the poison. For this theory would explain not only the continuance of Cholera for many days or weeks in each ward of an asylum or prison, or in each of a group of houses, and its ultimate cessation there, but likewise the various duration of the outbreaks in different asylums; since, as a general rule, the duration of outbreaks of the disease was certainly proportioned, though not strictly so, to the number of patients resident. In other particulars, however, the facts do not so clearly favour this theory. Some qualification of it, or the admission of a large participation of external conditions, such as different states of the atmosphere, in the production of the results, seems necessary, for example, to explain the extremely different rate of succession of the cases of Cholera in a house or ward of a public establishment in different instances, (the intervals being sometimes only a few hours, at other times many days,) and likewise the very different proportions of persons affected before the disease ceases in a house or ward.

These difficulties are, it is true, in themselves far from insuperable. But they add somewhat to the improbability which on other grounds has already been attributed to the theory of contagion. Moreover, it must be noticed that one fact adduced in support of that theory is otherwise explicable. The duration of each outbreak bore as close a proportion to the number of wards successively affected as to the number of patients, and the different wards being attacked in succession, the duration of the disease in the whole establishment would, *cæteris paribus*, be regulated by the extent of the buildings, even though the disease were not strictly contagious, and though the poison were communicated from one part of the establishment to another rather than from one person to another.

If, on the other hand, the theory of contagion be rejected, and the cause of Cholera be regarded as a poison not reproduced within the bodies of the sick, but existing and increasing independently of human bodies, the comparatively protracted duration of the epidemic in one ward of a lunatic asylum, while it was spreading to other parts of the establishment, seems to require some such assumption as that the poisonous matter attached itself to the surface of the walls, or furniture of the ward, or to the clothes of the patients, and remained there for a time, its quantity increasing more or less, and that while one portion of it was imbibed in some way or other by patients in the ward,

I 2

another portion was conveyed to other parts of the establishment. According to this view, too, the ultimate cessation of the disease in each ward must be ascribed either to the destruction of the poison by a spontaneous process such as might be supposed to take place in the most simple vegetable organism after it had thrown off germs, or to its destruction or removal either by an altered state of atmosphere or by the ventilating, cleansing, or other sanitary processes adopted. The hypothesis of the susceptibility of only a limited number of persons would not here suffice to explain the entire cessation of the disease, inasmuch as it would leave the cause of the disease still existing and ready to affect any persons newly exposed to its influence.

If, then, the doctrine of contagion be rejected, it is undoubtedly difficult to find a mode of explaining the cessation of the epidemic in each limited spot which would not be simply conjectural.

There is another question, too, which the general history of the progress of the epidemic in public establishments, or groups of houses, seems inadequate to determine, namely, the question whether the transmission of the disease from one ward to another, or from one house to another, was due to, or independent of, human intercourse. But the fact of this progressive extension of the disease is itself of great importance, from its giving increased probability to the belief that the cause of the disease is a material poison. And the fact of the cessation of the disease in each locality after a limited duration, though unexplained, throws light on the more general fact of the cessation of the whole epidemic in a large city or a country. It has been shown that, from some general cause, which there is reason to believe is an altered state of the atmosphere, the epidemic, after reaching a certain degree of intensity, declines and ultimately becomes extinct. It has been shown, too, that while the epidemic is rapidly declining, it often lingers in the interior of some public institutions and ill-ventilated dirty houses of the poor. It has further been shown, that the atmosphere appears to have a great influence over the transmission of Cholera from one spot to another, certain states of the air favouring or effecting its transmission, and others arresting or checking it; and, lastly, the fact has been noticed that, in each spot visited by it, the disease always ceases after a limited period. If these premises be all well founded, the conclusion is inevitable, that the extinction of the epidemic is the conjoint result of this limited duration of the disease in each spot visited by it, and of the supervention of a condition of the atmosphere which no longer favors its communication to new spots. If this explanation of the extinction of the epidemic be the true one, it follows that the share taken by human intercourse in its diffusion is a partial and subordinate one, or that it is dependent on other conditions. It does not, however, follow that human intercourse is quite inoperative, for the decline of the epidemic is always more or less gradual, and when it is obviously repressed by some general influence, outbreaks still occur for a time in new spots, and these outbreaks, so far as can be judged from the present tendency of this inquiry, may with great probability be referred to the introduction of the morbific cause of Cholera by human agency.

VIII. The main features presented by an epidemic of Cholera in a single country have in the preceding pages been deduced from the facts collected during the prevalence of the disease in England in the years 1848–49. The history of the disease during a longer space of time, and in relation to a wider extent of the world's surface, must now be glanced at with the view chiefly of determining what is *the manner of its progress across a continent, or across a sea* from one country to another.

The first fact to be noticed in the more general history of epidemic Cholera, is its progressive march. This is obvious in the dates of its first outbreaks in the different countries lying between the Delta of the Ganges, where it originated,

and this country. Having spread over the valley of the
Lower Ganges in 1817, it passed in the summer of 1818 across
the northern part of the peninsula, and reached Bombay in
August or September of that year. It was not till July,
1821, that it appeared at Muscat at the mouth of the Persian
Gulf, but in September of the same year it was at Bagdad.
It extended through many parts of Persia and the eastern
provinces of Turkey in 1822. In 1823 it passed the Caspian
Sea, and in the month of September showed itself at Astracan. It made no further progress, however, in Europe until
the year 1830. In that year, having appeared again at
Astracan in June or July, it extended rapidly through the
eastern part of Europe, reaching Moscow in September. In
the following year it extended to Riga and Dantzic in May,
then to St. Petersburg in June, to Berlin in August, and to
Sunderland in this country in November. So, again in the
later invasion of Europe, starting from Astracan, where it
appeared in June, 1847, it was felt at Moscow in September
of the same year, at Berlin in June, 1848, at Hamburgh in
August, in London at the end of September, and at Belfast
in Ireland in December.

When the progress of the epidemic is thus traced from
India to England, its general direction appears to be from
the south-east towards the north-west, and hence the notion
has been entertained of its progress depending on an influence passing across this hemisphere in the direction named.
But the history of the epidemic affords abundant evidence
of the incorrectness of this supposition. The disease has
travelled from its original source towards all points of the
compass: southward to Ceylon, towards the south-west as
far as the Mauritius, to the islands of the Indian Archipelago
in the south-east, and to the north of China and Tartary in
the north-eastern direction. In many parts, too, of its course
through Asia and Europe, it has manifested its power of
advancing in any direction, and within the circuit of one
country in several directions at the same time. Thus, in
India, the epidemic in 1817 and 1818 seemed to radiate towards all points of the compass from its source in the Delta

of the Ganges; in the year 1846, its course in Persia, Turkey, and Arabia was most singular and capricious*, and in this country in 1849 its extension took place simultaneously from several centres and in various directions.

It is next to be observed that the epidemic, though not compelled to move in any definite direction, has shown a decided tendency to follow certain tracks, or tracks having certain conditions, namely, the ramifying and tortuous lines of large rivers, and the low or flat districts in their neighbourhood, the lines of the sea-coast, and, less decidedly or less frequently, also, the great roads or lines of communication over land; while it has appeared to be arrested or checked in its course by mountains, and sometimes by seas, although at other times a sea or ocean has seemed to afford facilities for its extension.

In its westward progress it spread in 1817 and 1818, especially along the valley of the Ganges†; and in 1821 and

---

* It is described in the following words in the report of the Board of Health from dispatches received from foreign ministers and consuls: " By the month of July it reached Teheran. . . . From Teheran it proceeded by a north-west course to Tabreez. . . . From Tabreez it turned off in a south-east direction towards Ispahan, which it reached in September. . . . Then proceeding westward, it reached Bagdad at the latter end of the month. . . . From Bagdad, instead of pursuing its westward course, it again turned directly back in a south-east direction, taking the road through Cashan to Sheerez. . . . In October it entered Asiatic Turkey, breaking out at Mossul, and reaching as far westward as Diarbekr. At the same time penetrating into Syria, it spread to Damascus, in a few days reached Aleppo, and in the following month (December) it extended its ravages over the whole of the Upper Tigris, and the Lower Euphrates; thence advancing into Arabia, it reached Mecca early in January, 1847." A similar account, but with some slight differences in the dates, is given by M. Verollot, physician to the French Embassy at the Sublime Porte, in the Echo de l'Orient, and is quoted by Dr. Dickson, in the New York Journal of Medicine, January, 1849.

† Its progress is thus described by Mr. Jameson:—" From the rise of the disorder on the banks of the Ganges and Burrumpooter to its arrival at the mouths of the Nerbudda and Taptee, it" (the marked disposition of the disease to follow the course of rivers) " excited the surprise of the medical

1822, along the shores of the Persian Gulf and the rivers Tigris and Euphrates. The intervention of the sea had apparently delayed the progress of the epidemic from India to Arabia, and Persia; and now the mountainous regions of Circassia and Georgia, and of Asia Minor, seemed to retard its transmission to Europe. Having found its way, however, to the shores of the Caspian Sea, it soon extended to the European port Astracan at its northern extremity. In its subsequent march through Europe, it spread chiefly along the tracks of the Volga*, the Don, the Dneiper, and the

observer. Thus, from Sonergong, in the Dacca district, where the epidemic broke out in July, 1817, it crept along the banks of the Megna to Naraingunj and Dacca, attaching itself chiefly to the ferries and market-places in its vicinity. In like manner it afterwards step by step advanced up the Burrumpooter, affecting during its transit the villages situated on both its margins. From the mouth of the Hooghly to its termination in the Ganges, near Moorshedabad, the same peculiarity was observable. The shipping at the new anchorage, at Diamond Harbour, and along the whole channel as high as Hooghly, was particularly affected, and almost every village adjacent to its banks buried many of its inhabitants. In the Bhaugulpore district the propensity was so strong, that the virus scarcely ever spread into the interior, whilst it almost depopulated the low lands near the Ganges. Again, in the autumn of 1817, Moozufferpore, and the villages along the Gunduk River, in Tirhoot, and the station of Chupra, on a branch of the Ganges in Sarun, were alone visited; while at a subsequent period the disease was thence communicated along the Gogra to numerous cities in the north-east quarter of our territories. From Allahabad upwards, along the channel of the twin branches there forming a junction, until the virus was lost under the hills. it wavered so little from the line of those rivers, that hardly a town or village lying remote from their course was brought within its influence. Without going further over our old ground, let us briefly state that the same rule held yet more unexceptionably in Raj-pootana, through the province of Bundlekund, and all along the Ner-budda to the numerous branches of the Chumbul."—Report on the Epidemic Cholera Morbus, &c., by James Jameson, Assistant Surgeon, &c. Calcutta, 1820, pp. 102, et seq.

* Thus, on the Volga it appeared at
        Astracan, on the 20th of July, 1830.
        Donbooka, on the 7th of August, 1830.
        Samara, on the 13th of September, 1830.
        Novogorod, on the 27th of August, 1830.

lower Danube, advancing gradually from the towns at or near their mouths to those at higher points in their course, or on their tributaries; and in the north of Europe it followed the lines of the Vistula*, Oder, and Elbe, from towns on the higher parts of those rivers to the ports at their mouths, thus reaching the northern shore of the European continent.

In Europe the influence of mountains in checking the progress of the epidemic was again manifested in the escape of the south-western part of Germany, Switzerland, Italy, and Spain, for a long period after the parts of the continent traversed by the rivers above-named, as well as France and England, had suffered severely. And on the continent of America the preference of the epidemic for the course of large rivers was exemplified in the ravages committed by it along the river St. Lawrence, and the lakes beyond it, in the years 1832 and 1834, and along the Mississippi and its tributaries in the year 1840 †.

> Kostroma, on the 3rd of September, 1830.
> Yaroslaff, on the 6th of September, 1830.
> Ribinsk, on the 11th of September, 1830.

See Dr. Hawkins's History of Epidemic Cholera, p. 187; Moreau de Jonnès' Rapport sur le Cholera Morbus, p. 290; Dr. Christie's Treatise on the Epidemic Cholera, p. 23; and the maps in those works.

  * On the Vistula it attacked
> Lublin, at the end of March.
> Warsaw, on the 10th of April.
> Dantzic, on the 29th of May.

  † The epidemic of 1832 and that of 1834, alike ascended progressively the St. Lawrence River, and the lakes beyond, from Quebec.

	Date of appearance of Cholera.	
	1832.	1834.
Quebec	8th June	7th July
Three Rivers between Montreal and Quebec	escaped	9th July
Montreal, 180 miles above Quebec . .	10th June	11th July
Kingston, 190 miles above Montreal .	16th June	26th July
Toronto, 184 miles beyond Kingston .	28th June	30th July
Fort George, 40 miles from Toronto . .	14th July	13th August
Detroit and Amerstberg at the extremity of Lake Erie	6th July	End of August

(See

Of the asserted march of Cholera along great roads or lines of communication overland, there is much difficulty in citing satisfactory instances.   There are, in fact, no clearly-established cases of the disease affecting many places successively along a single line of road of great extent, without appearing in other places on either side ; while, from the way in which roads communicate one with another in most countries, it must, except under special circumstances, be most difficult to indicate the particular roads which the disease had followed.   Moreover, in the cases where there has been the nearest approach to a succession of outbreaks along a line of road, the track of the epidemic has generally coincided likewise, either with the course of a river, or with a line of sea-coast.

It is certain, however, that the disease can cross a large extent of country where there are no great rivers.   Thus, in the spring of 1831, it crossed Arabia from Muscat to Mecca; and in India it seems to have made its way from the banks of the Ganges to Bombay independently of the course of the rivers, attacking large places in the interior of the

(See Col. Tulloch's Report on the Sickness among Troops in British America, p. 32.)

In the United States of America, the epidemic of 1849 advanced from New Orleans to the different towns situated on the Mississippi, and its tributaries, successively, as far as Chicago, on the Michigan Lake.   Thus it appeared first at—

New Orleans	on the 11th of December.	
Memphis, on the Mississippi . . .	„	22nd of December.
Nashville, on the Cumberland River		20th of January.
St. Louis, on the Mississippi		5th of January.
Louisville, on the Ohio .	„	1st of May.
Cincinnati, on the Ohio .	„	27th of December.
Chicago, on the Lake Michigan, communicating by canal with St. Louis	„	29th of April.
Buffalo, on tributary of Ohio River .	„	30th of May.
Quincy, Illinois, on the Upper Mississippi	„	20th of March.
Galena, Illinois, ditto, ditto .	„	Middle of April.

(See Dr. Wynne's Report to the General Board of Health, and Dr. Evans, on the Spread of Cholera, Chicago, 1849.)

country between the two points named, such as Nagpoor and Jalnah, earlier than it appeared at the mouths of the only rivers by which it could have ascended to these places from the east coast of the peninsula.

The next point to be noticed in the general history of Cholera is, that in invading a new continent or new island, it almost invariably makes its appearance first in sea-ports, and not indifferently in any town on the coast, but usually at ports having considerable maritime traffic. Thus, in its course from India in the north-western direction, the following ports were the places in the respective countries at which it first appeared—Muscat, in Arabia; Bassora, in Turkey; Astracan, in Europe; Leith, Sunderland, Hull, and London, in England; Dublin and Belfast, in Ireland; Quebec, New York, and New Orleans, in America.

A further fact of importance is, the varying rate of its progress in different situations and at different times. The influence of mountains in arresting the course of the epidemic, and of flat districts, and the course of rivers, in favouring its extension, has already been mentioned. It remains to be noticed, that in different countries not presenting so great a difference in the character of the surface, the rate of extension has been very different. When first extending its ravages through India, its progress was comparatively slow: thus it occupied more than nine months (from March to the end of December) in passing from Ganjam, on the east coast of India, to Pallamcotta near Cape Comorin, a distance in a straight line of about 875 miles, travelling, therefore, at an average rate of about 21 miles a week; whereas, in Europe, in the year 1847, it advanced from Astracan to Moscow, a distance of about 700 miles, in less than two months, consequently at the rate of 87 or 88 miles in a week. In crossing the ocean, again, its rate of travelling has, in several instances, been very rapid. From Ceylon, which it reached in January, 1849, it passed to the Mauritius in November of the same year, traversing a distance of 2500 miles in ten months,—the rate of transit, allowing the longest period, being 62 miles in a week. And in ten weeks after it had reached the eastern parts of England and the north-eastern departments of France, it appeared in the United States of America at New York and New Orleans, having travelled to New York at the rate of 350 miles, and to New Orleans at the rate of 450 miles in a week.

The rate of progression of the epidemic in the same country, and at the same season of the year, seems to have been tolerably uniform in its different invasions. But in each country its rate of progress has been very different at different seasons. At a very early period of its history, it was observed to be one of its best-marked characters, that its extension, which had been comparatively rapid during the summer, was checked during each winter. And in its way to invade Europe, in the year 1847, the disease, having spread rapidly through Persia and Turkey during the summer and autumn of the year 1846, was in the following winter arrested at the Russian frontier. During the summer of 1847, it again advanced with great rapidity, reaching Moscow in September, when it again paused during the winter of 1847–48. Its active extension was renewed in May, 1848, but in September or October, when it had reached England, its march was a third time retarded.

Lastly, in regard to the influence of season, there must be noticed the striking exception presented in the progress of Cholera over the sea. During the winter months from October to March, when the disease had extended so little on land, especially in countries within the temperate zone, it has travelled with great rapidity across the Atlantic. For it was at this season, namely, between October and December, that Cholera crossed the Atlantic Ocean in 1848, appearing at New York and New Orleans in about ten weeks after its invasion of the eastern coast of England, and of a few towns in the north-eastern part of France.

In the foregoing outline of the general facts relating to the extension of the epidemic over many parts of the globe, all mention of particular facts has, as far as possible, been omitted; but enough has been already stated to show that several of the more general laws of its diffusion, namely, the preference of the disease for places in low districts, in the tracks of large rivers, or on the sea-coasts, the arrest or retardation of its course by mountainous districts, and the influence of season on the rate of its extension, are in complete accordance with some of the main features presented by the epidemic in this country. The features referred to formed a strong ground for the belief that the state of the atmosphere has a paramount influence over the extension as well as the degree of local intensity of the disease; and these facts in the general history of the epidemic being essentially the same in their nature, of course strengthen the grounds for that belief, and in a corresponding degree affect the probability to be assigned to different theories.

The bearing of these facts on the view to be adopted with regard to the nature of the cause of Cholera, and the mode of its diffusion, must be considered first in relation to the theory of an atmospheric state or influence producing the disease in the spots where certain conditions exist. Three modifications of this theory have been noticed, and not one of them recommends itself as the probable explanation of the manner in which Cholera has travelled over the surface of the globe. The position that the actual cause of the disease is attached to the moving mass of air, is quite untenable in the face of such facts as the gradual and comparatively slow progress of the epidemic, its slower progress or complete arrest in winter, and its pursuit of certain tracks, over many hundred miles of country, leaving the regions on either side unaffected.

It might, indeed, be supposed that the moving atmosphere merely serves to communicate the disease from one country to another by acquiring a peculiar state in the country where the disease already exists, and producing, in the country to which it communicates it, a more fixed morbific matter in those spots in which the " localizing conditions" are present. But this hypothesis, even if it explained the facts equally well, would have no advantage over the more simple view that a portion of that fixed morbific matter was conveyed from one country to another, and it would therefore be an unnecessarily complex scheme. The hypotheses of a peculiar " electric state" and of a " telluric influence" are almost too vague to be refuted; for it is scarcely possible to say what properties such causes might not possess. It is, however, certainly very difficult to conceive that such an agency as either of these hypotheses supposes, could be the cause both of the slow and step-by-step progress by which the epidemic advances across a continent, and of the great leaps it makes in traversing an ocean ; of its uniform appearance at the sea-ports of a new continent or island, of its arrest for a time in them, before it extends further, and of the capricious character of its course in several instances, as, for example, in its extension through Persia, Turkey, and Arabia in the year 1846, described in the passages already quoted from the Report of the General Board of Health*.

All these facts, and other general features of the progress of the epidemic not here alluded to, are obviously much more consistent with the theory of a material poison conveyed from place to place, increased or reproduced in those places in which it finds the necessary or favourable conditions, and thence transmitted to other places ; its transmission as well as its increase being promoted by damp and impure air, and by warmth, and being impeded by a dry and pure air, and by cold. In relation to this theory of the cause of Cholera, the facts referred to evidently have the same general import as the main body of evidence collected in this country.

But the statistical evidence which has been examined relative to the diffusion of Cholera in England tended to the conclusion that the transmission of the morbific matter was not merely favoured by a particular quality of the air, but was also effected, at least in greater part, by currents of air, though it seemed to leave as an undecided question whether the same result was not in part brought about by human intercourse. Now, in relation to the share taken by currents of air and by human intercourse respectively in the diffusion of

* See note at page 118.

Cholera, some facts in the general history of the epidemic are apparently of great importance, and at all events deserve to be particularly considered. These facts are—1, the rapid progress of the epidemic across the Atlantic Ocean in 1848, and its passage from Hamburgh and Riga to England in 1831, before it had visited countries nearer than England to those ports; 2, the continuance of the disease in ships which had sailed from infected ports for many days or weeks; 3, its appearing in every new continent or island first at the principal sea-ports; 4, its extension down the east coast of the peninsula of India in a south-western and southern direction, and across the north-west part of it during the summer of 1818, in the teeth of the prevalent wind, the south-west monsoon; 5, its continued prevalence amongst troops during long marches over land; 6, the varied rate of its march in different countries, yet its restriction in all within the limits of the rate of human intercourse; and 7, the occasional sudden arrest of its progress, as at Bombay in 1818, and at Astracan in 1823.

From all these facts, except the last, which has a contrary tendency, inferences favourable to the theory of diffusion by human intercourse have been drawn by different writers. They must be examined separately, in order to estimate their individual and collective importance.

The more rapid transit of Cholera across the ocean than overland during the winter season might, of course, be in part explained by the difference of temperature between the ocean, especially the Atlantic Ocean, and the continent of northern Europe, at that season. The importance of the fact, therefore, consists rather in the disease having crossed the Atlantic much more rapidly than it travels overland even in the summer season. Dating its transit across the Atlantic, from its appearance on the east coast of England, and the north-east of France, it was completed in about ten weeks, and as in this time it traversed 3500 miles to reach New York, and 4500 to reach New Orleans, it advanced at the average rate in the one case of 450, in the other of 350 miles a week. During the summer of 1847 it moved at the rate of 87 or 88 miles a week in advancing from Astracan to Moscow, and in the summer of 1848 at the rate of about 100 miles a week in extending to Hamburgh from Moscow, where, after having subsided in the winter, it became active again in May. The rate of transit of the disease across the Atlantic was thus fourfold greater than the rate at which it has moved over the continent of Europe. And the only explanation of this fact that has any positive argument in its favour seems undoubtedly to be that which refers it to conveyance by ships from England to America. The intercourse between different countries by sea is less frequent than it is by land. Yet, supposing that the disease could be conveyed by ships, that mode of transference would, it is obvious, be less interrupted, and in long voyages more rapid than any ordinarily available on land; since journeys of many thousand miles overland are very rarely, if ever, made without interruption.

The fact, that in ships leaving ports where Cholera prevailed, the disease has been developed, and has continued to prevail for many days, sometimes for several weeks, after they put to sea, supports the same view. Many cases of this kind have been recorded: some, observed in ships leaving infected ports in the Baltic, are related in Dr. Berg's " Report on Cholera in Sweden in 1850," and some remarkable instances derived from official sources have been published by Dr. Bryson. The case of the ship *Apollo* must especially be noticed, since it seems to afford incontrovertible evidence of the fact that the very cause of the disease may be conveyed by a ship some thousands of miles, infecting one person after another in the ship during several weeks. The *Apollo*, leaving Spithead on the 4th of June, 1849, arrived in the Cove of Cork on the 7th. On the 11th of the same month, 513 men, 43 women, and 40 children, all of them belonging to the 59th Regiment, were embarked for a passage to Hong Kong, and on the 17th she sailed for her destination. Cases of Cholera had occurred, if not in the regiment, at least in the barracks from which it came, a short time previous to its leaving them, and the disease was also prevalent in the neighbourhood. On the morning of the 18th, the day after the ship left the Cove of Cork, a case occurred, and in a few hours terminated fatally. On the 26th, one of the women was attacked, but recovered. On the 29th, a third case appeared, and was fatal. The fourth case occurred on the 2nd of July, after the ship had passed Madeira, and anchored off Teneriffe. The fifth, sixth, seventh, eighth, and ninth cases, occurring on the 6th, 7th, 8th, 9th, and 10th, all recovered. Two fatal cases occurred on the 16th and 18th. On the 19th there was an aggravation of the disease; and now, thirty-two days after the vessel left Cork, it began to spread to the ship's company, and cases, several of which were fatal, occurred amongst them until the 23rd of July. Amongst the troops cases occurred at intervals until the 11th of August, two days before they landed at Albroo-bay, on the coast of South America, and fifty-five days after they left Cork. The disease, which had caused 16 deaths, then ceased.

Now, in this and other similar instances the persistence of Cholera on board ship, is exactly parallel to its continued prevalence in inhabited buildings on land, at the time of the decline and near extinction of the epidemic in the surrounding country. In neither case can it be supposed that the persons who suffered last had received the germs of the disease into their systems at the same time as those first attacked; for it is certain that the Cholera does not lie dormant in the body for so long a period as several weeks; the usual term of its incubation not exceeding a very few days.*

* It is scarcely possible to define exactly the limits of the period which elapses between the reception of the infection of Cholera and the development of the disease. For the time at which the cause of the disease really exerted its action on the system can rarely be known. The most satisfactory data for deducing the probable period of incubation are, perhaps, those cases in which persons have been exposed to the atmosphere of an infected place for a single day, or part of a day, and have been afterwards been attacked with symptoms of the disease. Among the accounts of the mode of origin of the Cholera in different places, communicated to the Cholera Committee (see Tables XV. and XVI.) twelve

In the case of a ship, therefore, which, like the *Apollo*, had left the seat of the epidemic many thousand miles behind, it must be assumed that the cause of the disease had been carried in the ship. If this assumption is well grounded, it follows that ships are, at all events, adequate means of transporting the epidemic from one continent to another. And although it is, of course, not a necessary result that the disease should always be communicated by infected ships to the inhabitants of the ports they enter, a particular state of the atmosphere being requisite for the reception of the infection, it yet cannot be doubted, that if a favourable atmosphere be present in any port at which such a ship arrives, the

instances of this kind are mentioned with more or less accurate details. And in all of these the interval between the exposure to infection and the attack was under six days, while in half of them it was under three days (see Nos. 2, 4, 9, 11, 19, 22, 26, 37, 50, and 58, in Table XV., and No. 18 in Table XVI). A second series of data are the cases where persons going from a healthy district are attacked with Cholera soon after reaching an infected locality. There are only two distinct instances of this kind in the Tables (No. 5 in Table XV., and No. 19 in Table XVII.) in both of which the attack ensued during the first 24 or 36 hours. A third series, which will be admitted as evidence, however, only by those who believe in the communication of the disease by human intercourse, consists of the cases where the interval between the arrival of an infected person in a locality or house previously free from the disease, and the first case ensuing there, is fixed. There are sixteen such cases in Table XV., (Nos. 6, 8, 10, 18, 22, 23, (bis) 24, 26, 27, (bis) 29, 30, 33, 36, and 46), and in eleven of them the interval did not exceed three days ; in two it was five days, while in the remaining three it was seven, eight, and thirteen days. It may be objected to these data, that cases, in which the intervals were short, have, perhaps, been more frequently recorded than those in which the interval was longer. But, on the other hand, the first symptoms in many of the cases given have probably been overlooked, and consequently the interval between the exposure and the attack represented as longer than it really was. It is, moreover, very probable, that in several instances the poison was not received into the system until several days after the first exposure to the risk of infection. Although, therefore, these data are of course too scanty and imperfect to justify the deduction of a law respecting the period of incubation of Cholera, they are sufficient grounds for the belief that the period usually does not exceed two or three days. This inference is corroborated by other facts. It is communication of the disease hitherto confined to its crew and passengers will extend to the population on shore.

The fact, at all events, that Cholera, and, apparently, its cause, can be conveyed by ships for long distances, strengthens much the probability that the epidemic crossed the Atlantic in the winter of 1848, by the aid of human traffic.

A third class of facts, favouring the belief that this is at least one of the ways in which Cholera is conveyed across the sea to a new continent or island, is the constancy with which, in reaching an island or continent, it makes its appearance first in seaports, and not indifferently in any town on the coast, but at those ports which have most intercourse with a country where the disease already exists. It is unnecessary to refer to the instances presented by the progress of Cholera in Eastern countries, since ample evidence is afforded by the history of the two great epidemics in the British Isles and North America. It will, indeed, be a more satisfactory and safer method of inquiry, to examine all the facts relating to the origin of the disease in these countries, than to refer merely to instances selected from a wider field.

With regard to England, then, the facts are well known. It appeared in 1831, first at Sunderland, and in 1848, almost simultaneously at Sunderland, Hull, and London, and, in Scotland, at Edinburgh, all towns having frequent commer-

mentioned in various original reports on Cholera in India, that troops landing at infected parts of the coast have been attacked within three days by the prevalent epidemic, and that troops marching into quarters, or encamping on ground just before occupied by infected troops, have been attacked the same night or the next day. The immediate diminution in the number of cases of the disease that follows a change in the state of the atmosphere of a town, or that often ensues upon a ship leaving an infected port, also leads to the same conclusion. The fact, too, that outbreaks in towns and public institutions often come to an end in less than a month or six weeks, and outbreaks in parts of towns and public institutions in a still shorter time, though the number of persons attacked is very considerable, obviously limits very much the maximum duration of the period of incubation.

cial intercourse with the ports of the north of Europe, where
Cholera was raging.   In Ireland it showed itself in 1832,
first at Dublin, and in 1848, at Belfast, the ports at which
the traffic with England and Scotland is most active.   And
in North America it appeared in 1832, first at Quebec in
Canada; and in 1848, almost simultaneously at New York
and New Orleans.   Quebec was, in 1832, the great port for
ships conveying emigrants from Great Britain and Ireland to
North America, and it is needless to say that New York and
New Orleans are the two great centres of traffic between the
United States and Europe, the one for the southern, the
other for the northern states.

Cholera, then, in these countries, has in both the epidemics appeared in the ports having the most active traffic
with the countries which were already seats of the disease;
and it is especially remarkable that several of the ports first
visited by it, London, Quebec, and New Orleans, are situated
many miles up rivers, or at a great distance from the line of
coast which would be first exposed to progressive atmospheric
influence, or to a miasm conveyed by the wind.   In 1848, to
reach London, it passed Sheerness and Chatham near the
mouth of the Thames, Gravesend half way up the river, and
many towns on the coast nearer than London is to the north
of Europe, whence the epidemic travelled towards England.
In 1832, to reach Quebec, on the St. Lawrence, it passed all
the ports of New Brunswick and Nova Scotia; and in 1848,
when it invaded the southern states of North America, it
passed over the extensive coasts of Florida, Georgia, North
and South Carolina, and Virginia, and showed itself unexpectedly at New Orleans, the great port of the southern
states in the Gulf of Mexico.

It should be added, that when the epidemic thus crossed
the German and the Atlantic Oceans, it had as yet extended
to few of the countries which lay in its way between the
north-eastern part of Europe on the one hand, and England
and America on the other: it had not shown itself in Hol-
land or Belgium when it appeared in England; nor in

Ireland, the greater part of France, and Spain, before its ravages began in America. But it had reached the great ports of Russia and Northern Germany, and this seemed to be all that was needed to enable it to pass at once to English seaports, and thence to American seaports, as it were, in the lines of maritime traffic.

All these facts, then, relative to the transit of Cholera from one continent to another, and to or from an island, concur in affording strong presumptive evidence of its connection in some way with intercourse by shipping. The value of any corroborative evidence of a more direct nature that can be adduced, must be inquired into hereafter.

Those general facts must now be examined which seem most strongly to support the view of the conveyance of Cholera, by human means, across continents or large tracts of country. The lines of human intercourse, formed by rivers, have undoubtedly, in many instances, been followed very closely by the epidemic; but this fact, though of course consistent with the theory in question, cannot be urged as a strong argument in its favour. It might be explained by other theories, since those conditions which the whole history of Cholera shows to be most favourable to its development and extension exist in the course of rivers in a high degree.*

* Mr. Jameson remarks:—"It is to be recollected that in India, as in all other countries, the inhabitants flock to the neighbourhood of rivers for the purposes of commerce; and that the greatest number of towns and cities will thus be found near navigable streams; whilst the banks of every rivulet, affording the prospect of gaining a livelihood by fishing, will be crowded with villages. It is perfectly plain, that the population being more thickly gathered in such situations, must always suffer more, on occasion of any general mortality, than more thinly inhabited portions of the country. This cause alone would appear sufficient to explain away the apparent anomaly now under consideration. But there is yet another reason of equal force. The vicinage of rivers, from the action of the sun upon the great body of water contained in their beds during the day, and from the influence of the water on the circumambient air during the night, must always be peculiarly subject to those vicissitudes of temperature, which are known so powerfully to influence the state of the epidemic. Hence great evaporation by day, and falling of fogs, and heavy dews by night; and hence

But the extension of the disease along the roads over land is not so well explicable in this manner.

Here, too, the presence of large towns undoubtedly might enable the disease to manifest itself earlier, or, at least, more distinctly at an early period, than it would do in the tracts of country where the population is more scattered.

But the physical conditions of a low level and damp atmosphere are not always, and perhaps not generally, present. The course of the disease along the main roads of a country is, therefore, a fact which demands careful examination. Well-marked instances of it are undoubtedly rare, but one has already been referred to, namely, the passage of the disease along the great road leading from Nagpoor to Jalnah, and thence to Aurungabad and Bombay. And it is with reference to this example of the transit of Cholera in the line of roads that one of the arguments in favour of its dependence on human intercourse has principally been urged.

The general direction of the roads leading from Nagpoor to Bombay is from the north-east to the south-west; and Cholera extended along that line between the months of May and August, 1818. At the same period, namely, between the 15th of May, and the 8th of October, the disease travelled along the east coast of the peninsula from Chicacole and Vizagatapam to Madras, in nearly the same general direction. Now, the south-west monsoon prevails from the middle or the end of May till October. In both these instances, therefore, the disease seems to have travelled "in the teeth of the monsoon." The direction of the wind during the prevalence of the monsoon is modified, from time to time, in the interior of the peninsula, and also on the east coast, by the influence of high lands and by thunder-storms, generally attended by a constant interchange of hot and cold currents: all strong exciting causes of the disorder. To all which, if we add their low, muddy, sedgy banks, and the other numerous sources of miasma usually found in their confines, we shall be at no loss to account for the great sickliness of those residing on their banks, without searching for any more hidden causes of the fact."—Report on the Epidemic Cholera Morbus of Bengal, pp. 105–106.

north-west winds, but it does not appear to be reversed so completely or so frequently, even in limited spaces, as to countenance the belief that the progressive passage of the disease from the south-east towards the south-west, over several hundred miles during the summer season in India could be due to the agency of currents of air passing in that direction.

If, then, the extension of the disease in these instances was not effected by atmospheric currents, to what agency was it due? The numerous well-established facts, tending so strongly to show that the cause of Cholera is a morbific poison, the increase of which is dependent on certain conditions of the atmosphere, leave two hypotheses as the only alternatives; one that the poison was carried by men, or through their influence, and the other that it diffused itself, in the manner of the admixture of gases, through the atmosphere more rapidly than the air itself moved. The latter hypothesis is of course opposed to all those facts already examined, which afforded apparently such firm grounds for the belief that the poison was not diffusible in its nature. On the other hand, the hypothesis of the conveyance of the poison by human means is not inconsistent with the history of the epidemic in England, and as applied in these instances to explain the march of the disease in opposition to the atmospheric currents, certainly finds support in facts which must now be noticed.

Of these facts the most important is, that Cholera has frequently attached itself to bodies of troops on their march in India, and has remained with them during many days in their passage over long tracts of country, the inhabitants of which were not suffering from the epidemic. The duration of the epidemic in marching regiments is stated by Dr. Lorimer,[*] who has collected the largest number of instances, to be, in the majority of cases (in 88 out of 121), less than 30 days. It has often, however, been longer, and in the more severe outbreaks, the epidemic reached its

[*] Quoted by Mr. Scot, in his Report on the Epidemic Cholera in Madras, Edinburgh and London, 1849, p. 17.

climax in the regiment about the eighteenth day,. Many points relating to these attacks of marching troops in India are matter of dispute. But the fact that the disease remained with them for many days, when it did not prevail in the country around, seems not to be gainsaid; and here again the inference is irresistible, that the cause of the disease travelled with the troops, and affected different men in succession.

It seems equally certain that Cholera has attended cara-vans of Mahommedan pilgrims in their journeys to and from Mecca. But accurate details of the circumstances in which these bodies of people were attacked and continued to suffer are wanting.

Another argument in support of the view that Cholera is conveyed by men, and that this is the principal means by which its ravages are extended over continents, is based on the different rate of its progress in different countries. The fact already referred to, that in its passage through Europe it travelled at a much more rapid rate than it did in its first extension through India, has been thought to be connected with the greater activity, and more abundant and rapid means of intercourse in Europe than in Eastern countries. The fact, indeed, appears the more remarkable, when it is considered how favourable the climate of India is to the spread and persistence of the disease; it having never been entirely absent since its first epidemic appearance there in 1817. And additional support to this argument is indeed lent by the observation, that when the advance of the epidemic is most rapid, it does not exceed the ordinary rate at which men travel.

But a different explanation may be given of these facts on the assumption that both atmospheric currents and human traffic ordinarily serve to transmit the disease from one place to another.

The slower rate of progress in India, in the instances adduced, might be ascribed to its advance then depending entirely on human intercourse, the monsoon being opposed to the course the disease took; while in Europe, the wind being very variable, if it sometimes opposed, it would at other times promote the extension of the disease in the direction which human traffic and other causes were giving it. And the limitation to the rate of progress, even in Europe, might be explained on the principle that the poison, when carried by the atmosphere, perishes before it can reach very distant places, that, consequently, the stages of its progress, so far as this is effected by the wind, cannot be of great length, and that as time is required for its increase, at each of these stages, to the amount necessary to enable it to reinfect the air which would carry it further, it cannot advance in this way over a line of country very rapidly.

These facts, and the arguments based on them, are not, of themselves, to be accepted as conclusive proofs of the conveyance of Cholera by human means over land; but they certainly constitute stronger presumptive evidence of the diffusion of the disease in this way than was afforded by any of the facts previously examined relative to the history of Cholera in England; and the idea suggests itself that perhaps the climate of India especially facilitates the transmission of the cause of the disease by bodies of men, if not by individuals.

It would, however, be premature to discuss this question here. For all the evidence relating to the probable part played by human intercourse in the dissemination of Cholera in England, has not yet been examined.

One general fact in the history of the spread of Cholera from country to country, as yet scarcely noticed, seems, at first sight, to negative the diffusion of the disease by human traffic. It is the occasional sudden arrest of the progress of the epidemic after it had been progressively advancing. The two most remarkable instances of this occurrence have been cursorily mentioned, namely, the arrest of the epidemic at Bombay, and in the north-west part of India, from 1818 until 1821, when, for the first time, it reached the shores of the Persian Gulf; and its still more remarkable arrest in 1823 at Astracan, beyond which town it did not extend further into Russia until 1830. How can these facts

be reconciled with the idea of transmission by human intercourse? It seems difficult to believe that no opportunity
occurred for the transmission of the poison by human intercourse from Bombay to the towns on the shores of the
Persian Gulf for three successive years. And although the
difficulty is somewhat less in the case of Astracan, since the
disease commenced there in September, and was cut short
in the winter, apparently by a severe frost, and some
attempts, it is said, were made to confine it, by means of a
cordon sanitaire; yet here too, as the disease existed in
other places on the borders of the Caspian Sea, its arrest
seems to be referable, with much less probability, to the
failure of its transmission by men than to an adverse condition of the atmosphere.

A similar obstacle to the application of the theory of the
diffusion of Cholera by human intercourse is met with
again in the preference of the epidemic for certain tracks
in its course through Europe; while it left countries on
either side at least for a long period wholly unvisited,—a
fact which has already been examined and found confirma-
tory of the view that the state of the atmosphere regulates
very much the course of the epidemic.

Neither of these facts can be reconciled with the theory
that human intercourse is the sole or principal means by
which Cholera is spread over the world, unless it be admitted that particular states of the atmosphere exert a
destructive influence upon the cause of the disease, even
when it is thus conveyed. It would, perhaps, be easier to
concede this than it would be to explain the march of the disease in opposition to the monsoon, and all the facts relating
to the passage of the disease across the Atlantic, its persist-
once in ships during long voyages, and its selection of ports
for its first attack in reaching a continent or island, if human
intercourse were altogether excluded from the conditions by
which the epidemic is enabled to pass from country to
country. But these latter facts do not require the belief
that human intercourse is the sole or chief means by which
the diffusion of the epidemic is effected; and if it be one

which only occasionally comes into operation, the difficulty of understanding how it might fail to disseminate the disease in countries in which the atmosphere was at the time unfavourable to the increase, or even to the existence, of the morbific matter is much lessened.

The conclusions, then, from this inquiry into the mode of extension of Cholera over the continents and seas between the Delta of the Ganges and North America are essentially the same with those which were arrived at from the examination of statistical facts relating to its appearance in England. The belief that the cause of the disease is a material poison is strengthened; the great influence of varying states of the atmosphere over the extension, as well as over the virulence of the epidemic, is rendered still more certain; and the probability that the poison is capable of being conveyed, and has been communicated from one place to another, both over land and over the sea, by men, and by means of their intercourse, has been increased by evidence of a much more direct and cogent nature than had previously been met with.

IX. All the generally-admitted features of the epidemic having been considered, those facts or observations must now be examined, which might be expected to afford more direct evidence of the correctness or incorrectness of the view that the dissemination of Cholera is in some way connected with human traffic. Afterwards, any actual observations sanctioning the belief that it or its cause may be conveyed by atmospheric currents, will be briefly noticed.

In examining these particular facts in relation to the part played by human intercourse, it will be safer to limit the inquiry to the experience of the British Isles and America, than to select instances from a wider field. And in relation to these countries it will be convenient to reverse the order of the foregoing inquiry, by noticing first those *facts which bear on the mode of transit of the disease from one country to another, across the ocean*, and subsequently such as tend to elucidate the mode of its dissemination through the interior of an island or continent.

The information available with regard to the introduction of the disease into England, Scotland, and Ireland, is as follows:—The appearance of the disease in Sunderland in 1831 was preceded by the arrival of ships from infected ports of the Baltic; and the persons first attacked in the port resided on the "Quay," and were exposed to intercourse with the shipping.* No communication, however, was satisfactorily traced between these persons and the particular ships referred to, nor were any of the ships known to have persons sick with Cholera on board. In the later visitation of the epidemic in 1848, the occurrence of indigenous cases on shore in Sunderland was immediately preceded by several on board ships in the port, the ships in which the first of these cases occurred having come from Hamburgh, and other infected ports in the north of Europe.† At Hull, the first cases in 1848 likewise occurred in the crew of a vessel which arrived from Hamburgh at the end of September;‡ and the deaths of eighteen persons (only two of whom were mariners) were registered as caused by Cholera in Hull and the adjoining township of Sculcoates, in the month of October, although the disease did not then spread further in this port. The origin of the disease in London in 1848 has been ably and impartially investigated by Dr. Parkes. A seaman, named Harnold, who had arrived on the 18th or 19th of September, in a steamer from Hamburgh, died on the 22nd of decided Cholera. The second engineer of the steamer had died on the voyage, of an attack believed to be Cholera. One of two persons who slept in the same house in Horsleydown,

* See The appearance of Cholera at Sunderland, in 1831, by James Butler Kell. Edinburgh, 1834.

† The particulars of this outbreak of the disease in Sunderland have been communicated to the Cholera Committee by Dr. Brown of Sunderland, and will be found in the Appendix.

‡ See official circular of the General Board of Health, No. 1, Oct. 10, 1848, p. 9.

and, indeed, in the same room, with Harnold, until he was attacked, had decided symptoms of Cholera on the 30th of September, but recovered. On the same day two other cases occurred, one fatal at Lambeth—the other, a very slight attack at Chelsea. During the next week, there were 26 cases, all but 4 fatal; and 18 of them occurred on the river, or close to its banks, between Woolwich and Chelsea, the remainder being scattered over the other parts of the metropolis.*

In the year 1831, the Cholera did not appear in Scotland until some weeks after its outbreak in Sunderland. In 1848, the first cases of it in Edinburgh were nearly contemporaneous with those in Hull, Sunderland, and London; but no very detailed account of their probable origin has been published. Dr. Simpson, however, is reported † to have given the following statement to the Medico-Chirurgical Society of Edinburgh, as " the result of inquiries made by him at Newhaven, near Edinburgh, as to the outbreak of the Cholera. It is well known that the first case of Cholera which appeared in Edinburgh was on Wednesday, the 4th of October, 1848. On the Wednesday before this, three pilots from Newhaven went down to the Isle of May to look out for vessels. One of them was taken on board a vessel from Cronstadt bound to Leith. The other two remained in their boat on the lee-side of the vessel, and were towed to Leith, a distance of four or five-and-twenty miles; both of these men were seized with diarrhœa on their passage. On arriving at Leith, they went on board the ship. One of them died on Sunday of Cholera. The vessel had left Leith, and the existence of Cholera on board the vessel had not

* See An Inquiry into the Bearing of the earliest cases of Cholera which occurred in London during the present Epidemic on the strict theory of Contagion, by E. A. Parkes, M.D., London, 1849, p. 27. A manuscript letter addressed by Dr. Parkes to the General Board of Health, and containing corrections of some statements made in this published pamphlet, was communicated by him to the Cholera Committee.

† Monthly Journal of Medical Science, February, 1849, p. 546.

been ascertained. During the next eight or ten days several cases of Cholera occurred among the relations and immediate neighbours of the pilot that died, and these were the first cases in Scotland."

Of the origin of the disease in Dublin in 1832, no account has been found. In 1848, as it appears from the report of the Health Commissioners for Ireland,* the first case of Cholera in Ireland was that of a man who arrived at Belfast on the 2nd of December, having with his family, a few days previously, left a part of Edinburgh in which Cholera was prevalent. The vessel and the route by which he came are not mentioned; but it is certain that he was for some hours in the Belfast workhouse, before he was removed to the hospital where he died; and that some days later other cases occurred in the workhouse, the disease then extending to the town.

In North America the epidemic in 1832 appeared first at Quebec on the 8th of June,† and the circumstances of its origin are thus related by Colonel Tulloch:—" Cases of it were first noticed at Quebec on the 8th of June, among a party of emigrants who landed there on their way to Montreal, in consequence of the steamboat in which they had embarked being overcrowded. On the following day a person belonging to the same party, but who had proceeded by the vessel to Montreal, was attacked shortly after his arrival there, and within a few days the disease became general in both towns."‡ The emigrants referred to had just come from Europe. It appears, too, that the brig *Carrick*, arrived from Ireland on the 3rd of June at the

* Report of the Commissioners of Health for Ireland on the Epidemics of 1846 to 1850, Dublin, 1852, p. 39.

† The first place attacked in the United States in 1832 was New York, where the first case occurred on the 24th of June. The disease may have reached New York from Quebec, but it is noticed by Dr. Vaché (New York Journal of Medicine, May, 1850) as an interesting circumstance, that late in June, 1832, the ship, *Henry the Fourth*, arrived at quarantine off New York, having had Cholera on board.

‡ Report on the Sickness and Mortality, &c., among Troops in British America, p. 306.

quarantine ground, Gross Island, 39 miles below Quebec, having lost at sea from Cholera 39 passengers out of 133; and that the first two cases at Quebec and Montreal were emigrants landed from the steam-boat *Voyageur*, which plied between the two places, and was employed to convey persons from emigrant vessels anchored in the river.[*]

In 1848 the first places attacked in North America were, as has already been mentioned, New York and New Orleans. The history of the origin of the disease in these two places is a remarkable one. On the 2nd of December, 1848, the ship *New York* arrived at the quarantine ground at Staten Island. She had sailed from Havre on the 9th of November, with 315 French and German steerage passengers, and 31 cabin passengers. All remained well until the sixteenth day after leaving port, when cases of Cholera occurred. When she arrived at Staten. Island, seven of the steerage passengers had died, and twelve sick were landed and put into the hospitals. Immediately, eight cases and five deaths occurred at Staten Island in persons who had never been on board the vessel; but a sharp frost seemed to arrest the spread of the disease at this time. Nearly simultaneously with these occurrences at New York (namely, on the 11th of December, 1848), the ship *Swanton*, with 280 poor emigrants on board, reached New Orleans: 13 passengers had died at sea since the 26th of November, most of them from bowel-complaints—supposed to be dysentery; and on the day after the ship's arrival at New Orleans, a woman labouring under decided Cholera, was landed and taken to the hospital. On the following day, the 13th, a man who had come over in the same ship and had diarrhœa when he arrived, was brought to the hospital in a state of collapse, and died in a few hours. Three other cases of Cholera, all fatal, were admitted from different parts of the city the same day. In these cases no communication with the ship was

[*] Macneven, New York Journal of Medicine, March, 1849, p. 188; Vaché on Cholera, New York Journal of Medicine, May, 1850, p. 302; Evans on Cholera, p. 5.

traced ; and now the disease at once spread rapidly in the
hospital and in the city generally, although it did not
exist at this time in any other part of the United States,
except Staten Island, New York. *

Thus then it appears that in the two great visitations of
1831–32 and 1848–49, Cholera not only appeared first in
those great sea-ports of the British Isles and North America,
which had frequent intercourse by shipping with countries
already suffering from the epidemic, but that, in the large
majority of instances, its outbreak was immediately preceded by the arrival of ships bringing passengers sick with
the disease, or at any rate of ships coming from infected
ports. What conclusion do these facts justify? Is it still
possible that the disease has appeared so constantly in the
principal ports through mere accident, a portion of the morbific matter being conveyed by the wind to each indivi-
dually? or was it that the cause of the disease was widely
diffused through the atmosphere, and that these ports
offered conditions especially favouring its " localization "—
the arrival of infected ships, or ships from infected places
being in either case regarded as a coincidence having no
essential connection with the outbreak of the disease which
followed?

Now the hypothesis, that the morbific matter was
carried to the different ports separately by separate currents of air, cannot for a moment be entertained: it supposes in the currents almost a power of selecting the
places to which the poison should be conveyed, otherwise the
disease would not so constantly have appeared in certain
ports. The second hypothesis does not exclude the idea
of a morbific poison, but would assume that the poisonous matter existed throughout a large body of air, and

---

* Report on the Epidemic Cholera, as it prevailed in the United
States in 1849 and 1850, by James Wynne, M.D., pp. 3 and 77.
On the Spread of Asiatic Cholera, by John Evans, M.D., Chicago,
1849. Dr. Fenner, American Journal of Med. Sciences, vol. 43, April,
1849, p. 541.

was brought into relation with a large extent of country, the infection, however, being received only at those places which had the necessary local conditions. To this assumption little perhaps could be objected, in the case of England, on the ground of the distance which a body of air would have to travel in passing from the north of Germany to the shores of this country; it being comparatively inconsiderable. But in the case of America the very distance is an almost insuperable difficulty in the way of admitting that the disease was thus introduced, especially when it is remembered how small a portion of western Europe was at this time affected, how limited were the sources from which a large mass of air could there derive the infection, and how rarely, if ever, Cholera has overleaped the space of several thousand miles under circumstances, making it probable, that it was conveyed such distances by means of the atmosphere.

Another objection to this mode of explaining the facts is, that it supposes a special susceptibility in the parts where the disease first appears, while in several instances the history of the occurrences seems to show that there was in reality a want of susceptibility at the time when the infected ships arrived. This was remarkably the case at Hull and at New York, where although a few fatal cases immediately followed the arrival of the ships, the disease did not become epidemic. The little progress it made in London, too, during the winter of 1848-49, showed that there was then no special fitness for its reception in the general atmosphere of the metropolis.

A third objection is based on the improbability that the coincidence between the outbreak of the disease and the arrival of infected ships, or of ships from infected ports, in so many instances, could be accidental. This objection, however, has not the same force in all cases. In the instances of London, Hull, and Sunderland, the intercourse with the north of Europe by shipping is so frequent, that no great importance could be attributed to the mere fact of ships having just before arrived from a northern port in

L

which Cholera was prevalent. If, therefore, all the facts
had been such as those of the first outbreak at Sunderland
(as far as those facts are known), they would not have added
much to the probability of the disease being imported. But
the ships having in most instances conveyed to the ports
persons already labouring under the disease, as at Sunderland, Hull, and London in 1848, Belfast in 1848, Quebec in
1832, and New York, and New Orleans in 1848, the state of
the question is altered. For even in the English ports,
during the prevalence of the epidemic in the north of
Europe, the arrival of ships having persons sick with Cholera
on board has not been a very frequent occurrence. The
fact, therefore, that in those ports, in which the epidemics
of Cholera first appeared, the outbreak of the disease in so
large a proportion of the instances followed immediately
upon the entrance of ships thus infected, even did this fact
stand alone, could not, without much hesitation, be regarded
as the result of mere coincidence.

In the case of ships crossing the Atlantic, it is a rare
occurrence for cases of Cholera to be thus imported ; so that
it is said " only two emigrant vessels, the brigs *Carrick* and
Royalist, arrived at Quebec, on board which any passengers
had died of Cholera during the season in which it broke out
in that city. And these two vessels, with the exception of
the brig *Brenda*, at Baltimore, were the only vessels ever
suspected (before 1848) of having conveyed this poison across
the Atlantic." *

It is, therefore, a remarkable fact, that one of these ships
should have arrived at the quarantine station of Quebec in
1832, just five days before the disease appeared in that
city ; and that again in 1848, the outbreak of Cholera at the
quarantine station of New York and at New Orleans, should
have followed immediately the arrival of infected ships.
The hypothesis of accidental coincidence is indeed the less
admissible in the latter cases since the disease appeared

* Byrne quoted by Dr. Macneven in New York Journal of Medicine,
for March, 1849.

some months sooner than it might have been expected according to its usual rate of travelling, or according to the much longer time that elapsed between its appearance in England in 1831, and its outbreak in Canada in 1832.

A further fact, corroborating the belief that the outbreaks of Cholera in the several ports of England, Ireland, and America, were not independent of the arrival of the ships coming from infected countries, or having infected persons on board, is, that in several instances, namely, in London, in Belfast, and in New York, a nearer connection can be traced between the persons brought by the infected vessels, and the residents first attacked.

In London only one person who had direct communication with the seamen from Hamburgh was attacked with the disease. The further spread of the epidemic in London, if it was imported, must be ascribed to the communication of morbific matter to the air about the river from the infected vessel in which he arrived, and perhaps from other vessels at the same time.

In the case of Belfast, the circumstances more obviously point to the importation of infection; since more than one case occurred in the workhouse within a few days after the short stay there of the men who had just arrived from Edinburgh, suffering from the first stage of an attack of Cholera which proved fatal; though there does not appear to have been any direct contact between this infected man and the persons in the workhouse who were next attacked.

At New York the facts are of a more convincing character. " Nothing like Cholera existed at Staten Island (the quarantine station of New York) at the time of the arrival of the ship *New York*. When her passengers were removed to the public stores, they were occupied by about seventy persons, who had just recovered from other diseases. One of these, a man just recovering from a fractured patella, assisted in the removal of the patients. This was on Sunday (December 2nd): on the Wednesday following he was attacked with violent symptoms of Cholera and died the same day. A woman who had been a nurse, without having any communication with these people, but occupying another room in the same building, was attacked and died the same day, with all the symptoms of Cholera.   A man who had been discharged and gone to the city of New York on Monday, and had remained a little over a day in this same inclosure, was returned from the city as a case of Cholera, and died on Wednesday.   On perceiving this communication of the disease to the convalescents, Dr. Whiting immediately sent them away and distributed them through the other hospitals, since which three others have been attacked, two of whom have died, but none other than those at first exposed at the public stores have been affected.   These had all been inmates of the hospital for weeks, were ready to be discharged, and had but a limited exposure for forty-eight hours to the influences of the disease.   Two convalescents from typhus fever were subsequently attacked."   The German emigrants also continued to suffer.   " The whole number of cases including twelve entered from the ship, was on the 19th of December, 63, of which 29 had died."   " The disease has since entirely disappeared from quarantine, and without extending to the city of New York or to its neighbourhood."*

To make the evidence of communication of the disease by human intercourse in this case complete, it is only necessary to add, that the disease had appeared in the ship *New York* while at sea six days before it came to anchor at the quarantine station, and eleven days before the first of the convalescents in the hospital there was attacked.   It surely cannot be questioned, that in this instance, the ship conveyed the infection.   It cannot be believed that the outbreak in the ship at sea, and the subsequent appearance of the disease among persons on shore who were brought into contact or proximity with the sick landed from this ship, and among

---

* From an abstract of a Report of the Sanatory Committee of the Board of Health of New York on the Asiatic Cholera at Staten Island, given in the American Journal of Medical Sciences for April, 1849, page 463.

no others, although a large and very populous city was close at hand, were mere accidental coincidences,—the result of a poison in the air, or an atmospheric influence, affecting the ship at sea, and some days afterwards by chance singling out a few persons at the very quarantine station to which this ship was bending its course, while as yet no other case of the disease had occurred in the whole continent of North America.

Thus far there seems in this case no room for doubt. But circumstances connected with the ship which reached Staten Island, as well as with that which a few days later reached New Orleans, with passengers sick with Cholera on board, may justly bring in question the mode of origin of the disease in the ships themselves. These circumstances must now be examined. The ships had sailed from Havre, where Cholera did not exist. Both had been many days at sea before the disease appeared. In both the disease attacked only the German emigrants, and the emigrants in the ship which sailed for New York are stated to have been living as mechanics in Havre and its environs for some time before their embarkation.[*] This last statement is, however, directly contradicted by another account, according to which the passengers in the ship were emigrants from Hamburgh and other parts of Germany where the disease was prevailing.[†] The latter account is the more probable. For emigrants from Germany certainly do take the packets for American ports at Havre just as they do at Liverpool; and even though the majority of the emigrants who sailed in this ship had been resident at Havre, the probability is greatly in favour of the supposition that some of their relations and friends had come from Germany to join them in their emigration.

---

[*] Dr. Fenner in the American Journal of Medical Sciences, April, 1849, p. 541, and "Abstract of a Report on the Subject of the Cholera at Staten Island, *ibid.*, p. 464.

[†] Dr. Evans On the Spread of Cholera, p. 7. (Reprint from the N. W. Med. and Surg. Journal.)

Supposing it to be admitted that these people or a certain number of them had come from Hamburgh or any infected port of Germany, the difficulty arising from the ship having sailed from a port where Cholera did not prevail is removed; but the other difficulty remains, that the disease did not appear until the ships had been many days at sea. In the ship *New York*, which sailed from Havre for New York on the 9th of November, the first case occurred on the 25th. The *Swanton* sailed on the 2nd or 3rd of November, and no death occurred before the 28th of the month. Now there appear to be only two ways of accounting for these facts. Either it must be supposed that both these ships, while crossing the Atlantic, received the cause of Cholera from the atmosphere which was passing over them, or through which they were passing; or it must be admitted, that they conveyed with them from Europe the morbific agent, which, from some cause or other, was for a time unable to exert its destructive powers.

The disease appeared in the two ships nearly on the same day. This is consistent with the notion of their being struck by some atmospheric influence or infected body of air; and the same view has been thought to find support in the fact that immediately before the disease appeared in the *Swanton*, and on the very day of the occurrence of the first cases in the *New York*, though the two ships were 1000 miles apart, they experienced the same change of the weather from coolness to unusual warmth, a south wind setting in.*

But when it is remembered that Cholera did not at this time prevail in any part of the continent of America, in any island of the Atlantic Ocean, in any part of Western Europe south of England, except two of the north-eastern departments of France, or in Western Africa, it will scarcely be believed that a wind blowing over the Atlantic Ocean from the south could have conveyed to the ships any material or immaterial agent which was the efficient cause of the disease.

* Dr. Wynne's Report on Cholera in the United States, published by the General Board of Health, London, 1852, pp. 77 and 78.

The south wind was, in the case of the *New York*, preceded by a cold north-west wind, by which, likewise, the cause of the disease could not have been brought from any country already infected.

The known facts, then, are altogether opposed to the view that the moving atmosphere was the means of infecting the ships. Any influence operating upon the passengers in the ships from without must have moved independently of the atmosphere. But the belief that an imponderable agent is the cause of Cholera has been already shown to derive little, if any, support from the general features of the epidemic; and arguments against its adoption are afforded by this particular instance. For it is most improbable that such an influence extending across the Atlantic would affect only two ships 1000 miles apart, leaving many others sailing on the same ocean untouched. And yet assumptions still more improbable than this must be adopted by those who believe the outbreaks of the disease in New Orleans and New York to have been independent of the arrival of the infected ships, and all these manifestations of the epidemic to have been alike due to an imponderable influence. They must assume not only that the two ships in question had alone the conditions enabling this influence to produce its effects on the passengers, but that on the whole seaboard of America, and, indeed, on that whole continent, only the two ports to which these ships were on their way were at the time susceptible of it; that after striking the ships it travelled at about the same rate that they did, and thus reached their respective ports just two or three days after them; that it lost its power on the northern part of the continent immediately after producing a slight outbreak of the disease at the particular quarantine station at which the infected passengers from one of the ships were landed; and that in the other instance, as will appear from facts to be related hereafter, it immediately changed its course on reaching New Orleans, since the epidemic having, till then, extended in a south-western direction to reach that city, afterwards

passed directly northwards from the mouth of the Mississippi
towards the sources of that river, and its tributaries.

It seems impossible, then, to believe that in these cases
the disease was due to any agency conveyed by the external
atmosphere, or acting through it. On the other hand, the
view that the cause of the disease was conveyed in the ships
is favoured by several considerations.

In the first place the appearance of Cholera in ships that
have just sailed from infected ports is a frequent occurrence,
while its appearance in ships which have had no communication with, and are not near such ports, is exceedingly rare,
if it ever occurs. Mr. Scot* states, on the ground of his
official knowledge gained in the Madras presidency, that
sixty regiments, conveyed in at least 200 ships to different
quarters, all effected the voyage without Cholera, save in
one instance; and in that one instance the disease had
appeared among the men before embarkation.

Secondly, when the disease has appeared in ships that
have sailed from infected ports, it has not always shown
itself immediately on the ships leaving the ports. In the
instance of the *Havering* convict ship, which sailed from
Deptford on the 21st of June, 1849, Cholera first appeared
among the military guard on board five days afterwards,
namely, on the 26th of June.†   Dr. Berg,‡ in his report on
Cholera in Sweden in 1850, gives instances of the disease
appearing in ships on the 5th, the 6th, the 7th, and the 9th
days after leaving infected ports, and Mr. Lorimer relates §
that "in a ship proceeding from Bombay, where the Cholera
was raging at the time, to Singapore, carrying convicts,
Cholera broke out amongst these people after the ship had
been eighteen days at sea." The very short period during
which the disease usually remains latent in the system after

---

* Report on the Epidemic Cholera, London, 1849, p. xxv.
† Dr. Bryson on Cholera, p. 25.
‡ Cholerafarsoten i Sverge år 1850, pp. 324 and 329.
§ Reports on Asiatic Cholera in Madras, by Samuel Rogers, London,
1848, p. 22.

a person is really exposed to its cause being borne in mind, the only probable explanation of these facts seems to be that the morbific matter may remain dormant in a ship for at least many days, and then, owing to some change of circumstances, be called into activity, and affect the passengers or crew.

These facts and considerations being applied to the outbreaks of Cholera in the two emigrant ships on their way from Havre to the two great ports of the United States in the winter of 1848, it seems most probable that the material cause of the disease, the Cholera poison, was brought by the emigrants from Europe, and as in one of the ships all the persons attacked, with one exception, were Germans, the crew altogether escaping, it may be inferred that it was brought by those German emigrants in their clothes. If this were the case, the development of the disease at the particular time when it showed itself is consistent with one of its established characters. For it occurred just after the change from cool weather to unusual warmth. And the captain of the *New York* states, that immediately before the outbreak in that vessel " the weather had suddenly become colder, and there was a general overhauling of chests for warmer clothing, and this was succeeded by the prevalence of warmth already noticed." This warmth, together with the state of the air which would be present in an emigrant ship, would be conditions obviously most favourable to the increase of the morbific matter when once it was set free.

The subsequent occurrences, when the ships arrived in port, are also consistent with the same view. At Staten Island, the emigrants being landed at the quarantine station, the air of the hospitals, or of the whole " inclosure," seems to have become infected, for persons not known to have been in direct contact with the sick were attacked. The atmosphere beyond the inclosure being, it may be presumed, in a condition unfavourable to the existence or increase of the poisonous matter, the disease did not become epidemic. But

at New Orleans the circumstances were different. Yellow
fever had not quite disappeared, and the weather was, " for
the most part, very warm ; " and here Cholera spread immediately with great rapidity, as if the whole atmosphere had
at once become infected; for, only two days after the ship had
arrived and landed passengers, three or four cases of Cholera
occurred in different parts of the city.   The chief attention
has been directed to the ship *Swanton* as the probable source
of the infection received by the city of New Orleans, because persons sick with the disease were landed from this
vessel.   But it must not be overlooked that two other ships,
carrying emigrants from Hamburgh and Bremen, reached
New Orleans on the 6th and the 8th of December, after
losing several passengers by Cholera, or by a disorder having
similar characters.   These ships may likewise have been
the means of introducing the disease, or, in other words,
have had a share in infecting the air of the city.*

* "The ship *Guttenburg* from Hamburgh, with 250 steerage passengers, after a passage of fifty-five days, arrived at New Orleans on the
6th of December.   Cholera was prevailing at Hamburgh when this ship
left, and six or seven deaths from it occurred on board before she got
out of the Elbe.   As soon as the vessel got out to sea the disease subsided completely."   "As there were no cases of Cholera on board when
she arrived, it attracted no attention, although she came from an infected port ;" but it is said that soon after the epidemic "broke out at
New Orleans, a man died in the hospital," who stated that he had
recently arrived from Germany on board a vessel which had lost several
passengers by Cholera.   Further, " The bark *Callao* from Bremen, having
152 German emigrants on board, after a passage of forty-eight days,
arrived at New Orleans on the 8th December, and anchored on the
opposite side of the river.   The Secretary of the Board of Health was
sent to examine her on the 11th December, and reported that, ' During
the voyage eighteen of the immigrants died, some with purging and
vomiting, others with violent diarrhœa.   The last death occurred on the
30th November.'   Those who arrived were well.   But it is reported in
the log-book that the first that died perished from Cholera.   This is
merely the opinion of those on board, and is not entitled to much
weight."   [Though what this fatal disease could have been, if not Cholera,
it is difficult to say.]—From a letter by Dr. Fenner in the Amer. Journ.
of Med. Sc., April, 1849, p. 542.

The origin of the disease in American ports, and in the infected ships which reached these ports in the month of December, 1848, has been examined minutely and at length, because, when all the facts of these cases are considered in their bearings on the different modes of explaining the transit of the epidemic across an ocean, no room seems left for doubt that here, at least, the cause of the disease was transported by ships from the one continent to the other. If this conclusion be well-founded, it cannot be disputed that in the same way the disease must have been conveyed to ports of this country from the infected ports of Germany, and to Ireland from English ports. It does not necessarily follow that the first introduction of the epidemic into these islands in any one of its visitations, has been due to shipping, for it is possible that the poisonous miasm may have been conveyed by currents of air more quickly than by ships through the distance that separates Ireland from England, or even England from the north of Germany. But the constant appearance of the disease first in the principal ports, and the connection traced between the occurrence of the first cases in these ports and the arrival of ships coming from infected ports, or bringing infected passengers, together with some arguments of a more general nature already advanced, give great probability to the opinion, that at least in most cases the first introduction of the epidemic into England has been due to intercourse with shipping infected in foreign ports.

X. The *means by which Cholera is disseminated through a country after its importation*, must now be investigated by the light of particular facts. It has already been seen, that very many features of the epidemic are equally consistent with the view that the cause of the disease is conveyed from place to place by atmospheric currents, and with the theory of its diffusion by human intercourse. Some instances, too, have been met with in which the progress of the epidemic along rivers and great roads seemed explicable only by the latter theory. But particular facts connecting the introduction of the disease by men, or through their influence, into inland places, have not yet been noticed.

The conditions on land most resembling those favouring the transference of Cholera over seas are afforded by bodies of troops with their baggage, or caravans of traders or pilgrims, journeying from an infected place to others not yet visited by the disease. And the evidence that under these circumstances the disease will sometimes continue with a body of men for several hundred miles is apparently incontrovertible. But whether under these circumstances the infection has been communicated to the inhabitants of the places traversed, or to other bodies of troops not before infected, is still disputed, though the weight of authority is in favour of the occasional communication of the disease in such cases.*

The deficiency of evidence of a conclusive character with regard to this question is of comparatively little importance, since if the affirmative were established, it would only prove the possibility of the occurrence, and would throw little light on the question whether human intercourse is the sole or principal means of disseminating Cholera through a country or town after its first introduction. This question must be decided by evidence of a different kind,—not by selected instances, but by the results of an impartial inquiry into the origin of the disease in a large number of places taken indiscriminately—determining in what proportion of instances the appearance of the disease has followed closely upon direct or indirect intercourse with places or persons already infected; and ascertaining, on the other hand, the proportion of cases in which strict isolation has failed to secure towns, villages, or large institutions from the invasion of the disease.

* Jameson's Report on the Epidemic, Cholera Morbus, p. 143; Dr. Henderson, in Roger's Reports on Asiatic Cholera, p. 143; Scot's Report on the Epidemic Cholera, p. 102, et seq.; Moreau de Jonnès, Rapport sur le Choléra Morbus, pp. 142, 313, et seq.; Orton's Essay on the Epidemic Cholera, p. 321 ; Pruner-Bey, Die Weltseuche Cholera, Erlangen, 1851, pp. 5, 16, and 57.

For the latter portion of the inquiry sufficient data do not exist. But it was with a view to the former object that several of the questions in the second letter issued by the Cholera Committee were framed. A considerable mass of information on the subject was obtained by this means; and additional facts of the same nature have been extracted from official reports of Navy Surgeons, from reports of the Medical Superintendents of Lunatic Asylums, and from the communications made to a Committee of the Provincial Medical and Surgical Association, which Sir W. Burnett, the Commissioners in Lunacy, and Sir C. Hastings respectively placed for a time at the disposal of the Cholera Committee.

The results of an examination of the data thus collected will now be stated, so far as they bear on the simple question of the connection between the outbreak of Cholera in a town and the intercourse with infected persons or places, without reference to any particular theory as to the mode in which such intercourse may be supposed to communicate the disease.

The data comprise accounts of the origin of the epidemic in 119 places, of which sixty-nine are distinct towns or villages, fifteen are parts of towns (parishes or districts), thirty-four are public establishments (prisons, lunatic asylums, and workhouses), and the remaining one is a private house standing isolated in the country. Now, according to the information received by the Committee, the disease appeared subsequently to the arrival of infected persons, or the introduction of other possible vehicles of infection in seventy-three instances out of the whole number, viz. in fifty-five out of the sixty-nine towns or villages, in four out of the ten parts of towns, in thirteen out of the thirty-three public institutions, and in the private country residence. Before, however, any conclusion is drawn from these numbers, the cases respecting which the evidence is least satisfactory must be separated. Thus among the fifty-five cases of towns or villages in which the first patient had come from an infected place, had communicated with persons from an infected place, or had received clothes used by Cholera

patients elsewhere, there are twenty-four cases in which either
the interval between the first imported case and the next
succeeding cases was very long (above fourteen days), or
sufficient details are not given, or, lastly, conflicting evidence
exists as to the facts; and six out of the seventeen cases
of town districts or public institutions being in like manner
supported by insufficient evidence, there remain only forty-
three instances of the apparent introduction of Cholera by
human intercourse which can be referred to with any confidence.   In like manner, among the cases of apparently independent origin of the epidemic, there are several in which
the evidence is unsatisfactory.   But these being deducted,
there are still left thirty-seven instances in which the first
sufferers appear to have been attacked, independently of
infection introduced from without by human means.

The particulars of all the cases are given in abstract (see
Table XV.) in the Appendix, and the histories of some of
them are there added in the very words of the reporters.
The names of those forty-three places are subjoined, in which
the evidence supporting the theory that the conveyance of
the disease is effected through human agency appears least
defective.*

* The numbers affixed to the names of the towns, institutions, &c., indicate their places in Table XV. in the Appendix.

District towns and villages, and public institutions in isolated situations, or in towns not at the time visited by the epidemic.

5. Southend	23. Church Stretton	41. Manchester
9. Lower Whitby	26. Seaham Harbour	42. Boston
10. Long Handborough	27. Gateshead Low	43. Sunderland (Monk-
11. Tichmarsh.	Fell	wearmouth)
13. South Brent	29. South Shields	54. St. Albans
17. Wolverhampton	30. Broomhill (pri-	58. Stockport
18. Barton on the Hum-	vate residence)	62. Stoke Prior
ber	33. Maidstone	65. Dorchester
19. Hedon in Holder-	38. Noss Mayo	66. Northampton
nesse	39. Cairnbulg	70. Newport
22. Pocklington	40. Inveralochy	72. Catterick

15. Swansea Gaol   25. Wakefield Lunatic Asylum
16. Walsall Union Workhouse   56. Wakefield Prison
                69. Margate Pauper School

In many instances, both of towns and of public institutions, the facts cited leave it probable that the cause of the disease was introduced by other means. This must, for example, be admitted when the inhabitants of the place in which the disease newly appears are few, and are in constant intercourse with neighbouring infected places. For under these circumstances, the fact of the first person attacked having recently been exposed to infection might very probably be a mere coincidence, and the fact would lose still more of its importance if it happened in the warm season, which undoubtedly favours the increase and diffusion of the disease, for then the poison, if at all capable of being conveyed by the air, would be likely to have its sphere of action extended independently of the intercourse of men. On the other hand, the probability that the disease did really arise from the introduction of infected persons or things is strengthened when the inhabitants of the place have not frequent intercourse with the town whence the infection is supposed to be brought; when the person said to have brought the infection into the place began to suffer from the symptoms of the disease on his way thither; when communication or near approach was traced between the first patient and those subsequently affected; when the locality, in which the first case appeared, was not particularly insalubrious; and when the season was cool, and therefore not such as would generally promote the increase and diffusion of a disease depending on malaria. Many of the instances both of towns and public institutions offer several of these conditions, and afford as strong evidence as single instances can well give of the introduction of the disease from without by infected persons, clothes, &c.*

Parts of infected towns, and institutions situated in infected towns, in other parts of which the epidemic already prevailed:—

2. South Hackney	24. Stonehouse	45. Bishopwearmouth
4. Sydenham	35. St. George's Parish,	(Sunderland)
14. Swansea	Canterbury	
3. Royal Free Hospital	7. Margate Infirmary	
2. Holborn Workhouse	8. Hertford Gaol	

* It is here necessary to notice an objection which may be urged

With regard to the instances of the apparently independent origin of the disease (Table XVI.), they, taken singly, are necessarily in almost every case inconclusive. For it is scarcely possible ever to prove that infection had not been indirectly conveyed into the place, and to the person first attacked. But this objection does not apply with equal force in all cases. The instances of towns and parts of towns are chiefly obnoxious to it, for the poor inhabitants of towns are much exposed to intercourse with tramps, who are among the most likely vehicles of infection on land. Hence, of seventeen places (towns and parts of towns), of which the names are subjoined*, few can be regarded as of great weight in deciding the question whether Cholera can arise independently of infection conveyed by human intercourse, except the two cases of Shrewsbury and Oxford, where the first cases occurred in public institutions, and those of Notting-Hill and against the validity of the evidence above adduced—an objection based on the difficulty of distinguishing cases of English Cholera from the epidemic or Asiatic disease. It may be supposed that indigenous cases of the epidemic, mistaken for the ordinary summer Cholera, have sometimes occurred previous to the supposed introduction of the disease by human intercourse. And this error has probably been sometimes committed in the hot season of the year. But on the other hand, in some of the instances where the disease has appeared to rise spontaneously at the same season, the first patients may have suffered merely from the sporadic disease, and the really first cases of the epidemic occurring subsequently may have been imported cases, or cases which would countenance the idea of infection by human agency, so that the errors may balance each other. The theory of some writers, that the epidemic is gradually developed, the severe form of the disease being preceded by an unusual prevalence of diarrhœa, is inconsistent with the great mass of evidence on the subject.

* Towns and parts of towns in which the first cases of Cholera appeared to be independent of infection conveyed from other places. (See Table XVI. in the Appendix.)

2. Upper Clapton	13. Dowlais	22. Lancaster
4. Haggerstone District	14. Oxford	23. Part of Leeds.
5. Notting-Hill	15. Southampton	39. Romsey
6. Walham Green	18. Bridgenorth	40. Farnham
8. Brighton	19. Shrewsbury	41. Preston
10. Ilford	21. Holyhead	

Upper Clapton, where the two or more earliest cases occurred simultaneously in different houses.

The outbreak of Cholera in public establishments [*], such as prisons, lunatic asylums, and workhouses, especially the two first, where no known cause of infection had been introduced from without, is a more important fact. For here the intercourse with the surrounding population is limited, and the introduction of infection from without both less likely to occur, and more easily traced if it did happen. Including the lunatic asylums, respecting which information was elicited by the Commissioners of Lunacy, there are nineteen public establishments in which the outbreak of the disease could not be traced to infection brought in by human means. And although in some of these cases possible, or even probable, sources of infection may have been overlooked, yet it can scarcely be credited that this was the case in every instance. If the disease were always introduced by infected persons, clothes, or other similar means, it would surely not have happened that the cause of the outbreak remained undetected in all but one of the sixteen lunatic asylums, and in four out of seven prisons or hulks which suffered from the epidemic.

While, then, the evidence supports the belief, that in many cases the origin of the disease has been attributable to

[*] Public institutions in which the first cases of Cholera appeared to be independent of infection conveyed from other places.

I. Situated in towns already suffering from the disease:—

3. St. Luke's Hospital
25. Bristol Asylum
27. Wrekenton Asylum, near Gateshead
28. Bethnall House
29. Camberwell House
30. Peckham House
31. Grove Hall, Bow

32. St. Marylebone Infirmary
33. Hoxton House
34. Althorpe House, Battersea
35. Cowper House, Old Brompton

37. Hull Borough Asylum
38. London House, Hackney
44. Millbank Prison
45. Woolwich Hulks
46. Dreadnought Hospital.

II. Situated in counties or in towns not previously visited by Cholera:—

14. Oxford County Gaol
19. Shrewsbury County Gaol

19. Shrewsbury House of Industry
36. Vernon House, Glamorganshire.

M

the introduction of infection by human agency, it also seems to show that in many others no such cause could be traced, or probably existed. From a further analysis of the facts, some of the circumstances may be learned, on which this apparent difference of origin probably depends.

The evidence in favour of the introduction of infection by human intercourse is numerically strongest in the case of distinct towns and villages, and of public establishments situated in the open country, or in towns not yet visited by Cholera. In 33 out of 48 detached towns, villages, and public establishments, or 70 per cent., the first indigenous cases of the disease seemed to be immediately consequent on the arrival of infected persons; while among the parts of towns, and the public establishments situated in towns already suffering from Cholera, only 10 out of 32, or about 31 per cent., have appeared to owe the invasion of the disease to such a cause.

A comparison of the distinct towns with the parts of towns of which other parts are already infected, and of public establishments situated in the open country or in towns at the time free from Cholera, with those situated in towns already suffering from the disease, affords results of the same tendency as the foregoing.

The apparent introduction of infection was—

Traced in . . . .   28 towns.
Not traced in 11   „
Traced in . . . . .   . 6 parts of towns.
Not traced in 6   ‥
Traced in . .   5 { public establishments not in infected towns.
Not traced in 4   „
Traced in . .   . . . . 4 { public establishments in infected towns.
Not traced in 16   „

Now, from the different proportions in which the introduction of infection was apparently traced in these different cases, the inference suggests itself that the communication of the disease from one place to another is much less dependent on human agency where the places are contiguous, than where they are distant one from the other. This inference is especially supported by the facts relating to the public establishments situated in infected towns. For, as was before remarked, these establishments being for the most part prisons or lunatic asylums, the intercourse between the persons resident in them, and the population out of doors, is limited, and any means by which infection could have been brought into them, would be, comparatively speaking, easily traced by the medical officers.

On the other hand, the same considerations with regard to public establishments give especial value to those instances, few though they be, in which Cholera without obvious vehicle of infection invaded prisons or lunatic asylums in isolated situations or in towns at the time free from it; instances such as those of the Oxford County Gaol, the County Gaol and the House of Industry at Shrewsbury, and the Vernon House Lunatic Asylum in Glamorganshire. The probability that the disease arose independently of human intercourse is further strengthened in three of these instances by the simultaneous appearance of the disease in the two establishments at Shrewsbury, and by the occurrence of a fatal case of the disease in the city of Oxford at very nearly the same time with the first case in the gaol.

The questions which elicited the information contained in the foregoing pages, had for their object to ascertain in what proportion outbreaks of Cholera could be traced to intercourse with infected places ; but inasmuch as they necessarily directed attention more particularly to the positive facts, and as observers would naturally be more struck by facts of that kind than by those of a negative tendency, it is probable that the proportion of the cases in which the outbreaks appeared to be thus originated, is represented in an exaggerated proportion in the returns received.

This source of fallacy being kept in mind, the evidence

respecting the origin of the Cholera epidemic in towns, parts of towns, and large establishments in England, though not so ample as could be desired, seems, on the whole, to warrant the statement:—1, that in towns, villages, and institutions situated apart from infected places, the disease has in a majority of the cases reported to the committee seemed to owe its origin to the introduction of infection by human intercourse ; 2, that in a moiety of the parts of towns in other parts of which the epidemic was already prevailing, and in a majority of the public institutions situated in infected towns, it appeared to take its rise independently of infection by human agency; and 3, that in a few instances it is satisfactorily shown that the disease was propagated to isolated public establishments independently of the known admission of any probable vehicles of infection*.

With respect to the origin of the disease in the towns of Ireland, it is stated by the Commissioners of Health in their Report, that, having addressed to the several medical officers throughout the country the inquiry " whether the first patients had been long resident, or had lately come from some place where Cholera prevails, or had had communication with persons in that disease, also whether the second case had access to the first one," " thirty-seven replies were received which may be thus classed : eight doubtful, six in support of the view of the first attack in the locality owing its origin to contagion, and twenty-three replies, stating that the attack could not be traced to importation or contagion."

* In the foregoing analysis of the information respecting different localities in Great Britain, only the first outbreak of the disease in each place has been noticed. The renewed outbreaks in places in which it had already existed and died out, would have afforded other instances of the apparent importation of the disease, and of the apparent origin of it independently of human agency; but as the disease might result, in these renewed outbreaks, from the mere revivification of a portion of virus which had for a time remained dormant, owing to the unfavourable state of the external temperature or other causes, another element of doubt would have been introduced, had they been used as evidence for or against any theory of the origin of the disease.

The information published respecting the mode of diffusion of the epidemic in the United States, supports more strongly the belief that human intercourse is a principal means by which it is effected, but at the same time leaves it probable that the poison may be transferred from place to place by some other agency.

In spreading from New Orleans the disease gradually ascended the rivers towards the lakes in the north; at many of the principal towns it reached in its course (Memphis, St. Louis, Cincinnati, Chichago, and Buffalo), the outbreak was immediately preceded by the arrival of boats having persons ill of Cholera on board, and the first indigenous cases occurred in some instances amongst the part of the population living on the river or on its banks, or otherwise exposed.

From New York it found its way up the North River to Albany, and thence pursued its westerly direction along the chief lines of traffic to Buffalo, and up the great chain of lakes. But in the principal places in the northern states visited by Cholera after New York, the communication of the disease by human intercourse has not been traced distinctly, though in the instance of Baltimore it was suspected *.

The information derived from Ireland and America, since it relates to only a few places, would, if it were fully detailed, form a very insufficient ground for the belief that human intercourse is a means by which Cholera is propagated through the interior of a country. Its purport has, therefore, been only so far described as to show its consistency with that view.

The only direct evidence of the conveyance of Cholera from one inland place to another that can be regarded as satisfactory is to be found in the large number of towns,

* The principal facts relating to the extension of the epidemic in the United States will be found in the memoirs, by Dr. Evans, Dr. Wynn, Dr. Macneven, and Dr. Fenner, already referred to. The works published in France and Germany on the subject of the late epidemic, also contain facts, at the first view, contradictory, but really of the same general tendency as those which have been collected in this country.

villages, and public institutions of England, in which the outbreak of the disease has been preceded by the arrival of one or more infected persons from some already existing focus of the epidemic, and in the remarkable nature of the facts in some instances. The value of the evidence afforded by the number of such instances is enhanced by their being proportionally more numerous amongst isolated places than amongst those which would be likely to receive the poison speedily by the agency of the air. With respect to the character of the individual facts, it is unnecessary to repeat here the details which are given in the Appendix. But one series of facts may with advantage be referred to, since it almost fulfils the conditions of an experiment instituted for the purpose of testing the question now under consideration.

It is well known that, on the two last days of December, 1848, an outbreak of Cholera of almost unparalleled severity commenced in the Surrey Hall Asylum, or Drouet's school for pauper children, at Tooting, and that in the first week of January, in consequence of the fearful mortality that was taking place, it was determined to distribute the children among the several parishes to which they belonged. This measure was carried into effect; and the results were most important in relation to the theories of the mode of propagation of Cholera. In four known instances fatal attacks of the epidemic occurred immediately in the workhouses or other asylums into which the infected children were received, and the outbreak of the disease in a fifth institution was traced to communication with one of the dispersed parties of children.

Forty-five of the children being removed on the 6th or 7th of January to the Bellevue House Pauper Asylum at Margate, one of them died there on the 8th of January, and immediately afterwards several inmates of the house, who had not come from Tooting, were attacked, and three died, two on the 11th, and one on the 23rd.

At the Royal Free Hospital, 155 of the children were received from Tooting on the 5th of January; four of them died between the 6th and the 8th of January; five of the attendants were attacked, and two of them died between the 13th and 20th of the month.

At the St. Pancras Workhouse nine of the children died between the 6th and the 20th of January, and, within a few days after their arrival, one other person, who was not, however, resident in the same part of the building, was attacked, and died.

In Park House, at Hackney, where the children belonging to the Islington parish were temporarily placed, four of them died between the 10th of January and the end of the month; and a young woman, brought from the Islington Union House to nurse them, was likewise attacked and died on the 14th of January.

In two other instances in which children were removed from Tooting to asylums on the north side of the Thames, one or two of them died (namely, one in a house in the All Souls' subdistrict of Marylebone, and two in the Kensington Union Workhouse), without any other persons with whom they were brought into contact taking the disease. But this negative fact, of course in no way diminishes the force of the occurrences just mentioned, if there be good ground for the belief that in those instances the deaths of persons who had not been to Tooting were dependent on the arrival of the children. Before the circumstances are further examined, the fact must be mentioned, that one of the attendants at the Royal Free Hospital, who was attacked with Cholera, died at the Holborn Union Workhouse, and that the disease at the same time broke out in the latter establishment.

It is an important circumstance, that in not one of these five different localities in which the communication of the disease seemed to take place, can the result be ascribed to the epidemic prevalence of the disease in the locality. The five workhouses or asylums had till then been entirely free from the epidemic, and even the subdistricts in which they were situated almost equally so; for the only deaths registered as due to Cholera in the previous three months were a single one, in December, in the Camden Town subdistrict, in which the St. Pancras Workhouse stands, one in October in the

Gray's Inn Lane subdistrict, in which the Free Hospital is situated, and one in November in Hackney; in the entire districts of Holborn and of the Isle of Thanet there had been no deaths from Cholera. Moreover, in four instances, those of Hackney, Gray's Inn Lane subdistrict, Holborn, and the Isle of Thanet, the establishments to which the infected children had been taken, or with which they had had intercourse, were the only localities affected even in January. In the Camden Town subdistrict three deaths occurred in one other locality about the same time, but later than the first of the ten deaths in the workhouse.

Nor was there in any part of the metropolis north of the Thames an increase in the mortality from Cholera during January, 1849. On the contrary, only nine of the 26 districts experienced any mortality from the epidemic during the four weeks ending the 27th of January; four of these had fewer deaths than in the preceding month, and the other five consisted of the four districts in which children brought from Tooting had died, together with the Holborn district, where the entire mortality occurred in the workhouse, inmates of which had had intercourse with the Tooting children.

All these facts concurrently point to the conclusion that the material cause of Cholera was in some way or other transported with the children from the original focus at Tooting to the several establishments referred to. Only two facts appear to be in any way opposed to it. One is, that the man who died in the Holborn Union, after having been in communication with the children in the Royal Free Hospital, was not the first patient who died of Cholera in the former establishment. Another man, who had not been to the Royal Free Hospital, died on the night of the 13th, while the man in question died on the 14th. Both were taken ill on the same day, the 13th. But the man from the hospital had slept in the bed opposite to the other man for two nights previously; and, on the theory that infection may be conveyed in clothes, he may still have been the source of the infection from which the persons in the Union-house suffered. The contagion theory is alone affected by the facts here stated. The other objection is, that the woman, who died in the St. Pancras Workhouse, lived in a different part of the building and had no communication with the sick children. This has less force than the former one. For it does not refute even the belief in the operation of a contagious virus emanating from the sick children; since such a virus might be carried from one part of the workhouse to another; it merely weakens the positive evidence derived from this case, it does not refute it. A third objection already alluded to may be, that in several of the asylums or workhouses to which the children were removed from Tooting no communication of the disease ensued. But this last objection is at once seen to be groundless, when the paramount influence of the condition of the atmosphere over the spread of Cholera is considered. Unless an impure state of air, or, at any rate, local conditions capable of producing it exist, the disease does not extend.

The evidence, then, that the infection of Cholera was transmitted in several directions and for distances of many miles, by means of the children dispersed from the school at Tooting, appears indisputable; and establishes the possibility of the conveyance of Cholera over land in a manner as convincing as the facts relating to the origin of the outbreak at Staten Island, New York, showed that the epidemic might be communicated to the inhabitants of a seaport by the arrival of an infected ship.

In the foregoing statement of the evidence derived from particular facts in favour of the propagation of Cholera from place to place by means of human intercourse, but little reference has been made to the different views which may be entertained respecting the mode in which human intercourse effects this result. But the facts which remain for examination must be considered chiefly in their bearing on *the question, whether the cause of Cholera is a virus reproduced in the bodies of the sick,* or a poison which undergoes its increase entirely in the atmosphere, or, at all events, out of the human organism.

Many of the grounds on which the strictly contagious nature

of Cholera is usually maintained merely tend to show that the disease is communicable by human intercourse. Such are all those general features of the epidemic which accord best with the view that the cause of the disease is a poison only partially distributed over the surface of the country, and conveyed to different spots at different times,—all the facts relative to the origin of the disease in towns or public institutions immediately on the arrival of infected persons, —the asserted efficacy of quarantine and sanitary "cordons" in some instances,—the escape of unfrequented places near foci of the disease,—and, lastly, the gradual rise of the epidemic in towns. These arguments lend no special support to the theory that the Cholera poison is a product of the disease itself. Two other facts which afford presumptive evidence of a connection between the different cases of the disease,—of their dependance one upon another,— are their usually occurring, in a house or in a ward of a public institution, in succession rather than simultaneously, and the relation which, as a general rule, subsists between the duration of the epidemic in a town or public institution and the number of the population. These facts are more readily explained by the doctrine of contagion than by any other theory. But it has already been shown that they are reconcilable with the view that the poison is not reproduced in the human body; and the presumptive evidence furnished by them is certainly much less cogent than the many weighty reasons which exist for believing that the cause of the disease is increased in the atmosphere.

The special direct evidence alleged in favour of the contagious nature of Cholera consists of three classes of facts. The first is, that in a vast majority of the instances in which the introduction of the disease into a town or smaller community has been traced to human intercourse, the seeming vehicle of the infection has been a person or persons actually infected with the disease. The second is, that persons who have washed or handled the clothes, linen, or bedding of Cholera patients, have frequently themselves become affected. The third class of facts is constituted by the attacks of the disease experienced by nurses and other attendants of the sick.

The evidence of the first kind is clearly not conclusive. There are several reasons why much more attention would be paid to those instances in which the persons first attacked in any place had recently come from a possible source of infection, than to the cases in which, just previous to an outbreak, a person had arrived from an infected locality, and had possibly conveyed infection, though not himself under the influence of the disease. In the first place, the illness of the new comer would draw attention to the fact of his having been in an infected locality, which otherwise might remain unknown. Secondly, the idea of contagion is usually associated with that of the portability of the disease; so that many observers would regard the illness of the agent in the transmission of the disease essential to the result. Lastly, the illness of the person who may be supposed to have conveyed infection is undoubtedly an important addition to the evidence, since it establishes the fact of his having really been in contact with the cause of the disease, which might otherwise be questioned, even though he had come from a town, or even from a public establishment, in which it prevailed. On account of their wanting this additional evidence afforded by the illness of the new comer, several cases which otherwise would have been regarded as striking instances of the transmission of Cholera, for example, those of the Birmingham Workhouse and the Tooting School (Nos. 32 and 36 in Table XV.), have been omitted from the list, given at page 158; and if all such cases were recorded, they would probably outnumber those in which the origin of the disease has seemed due to the arrival of persons really suffering from Cholera. It is, at all events, certain, that the cases in which, just before the outbreak, there had been intercourse with infected localities by means of persons, who did not themselves suffer, must have been of frequent occurrence; and the fact of such cases not being frequently recorded is no proof that the infection cannot be conveyed under such conditions.

*The communication of Cholera to washerwomen and others
by the clothes, linen, and bedding* of those who have died
of the disease, has frequently been asserted. In order to
learn whether the actual experience of the medical profession confirmed the current belief in this matter, it was
made the subject of one of the queries issued under the
authority of the Cholera Committee. Eighty-four communications were received in relation to the modes of diffusion
of Cholera. In thirty-five, seeming instances of infection
by means of clothes, linen, or bedding, were stated in general
terms, or with more or less of detail; and in sixteen others
the occurrence of such cases was either asserted or admitted,
though the writers in several instances demurred to the inference generally drawn from the facts. In six communications it was stated that no such facts had been met with;
and in eight others it was shown that sometimes, under circumstances in which the communication of Cholera in this
manner, if possible, would be expected, no such result ensued. In this mere numerical analysis the preponderance
of positive facts appears very decided, even though it be
assumed that the silence of the remaining twenty-three communications in regard to this question should be taken in
a negative sense. But when the information thus obtained
is further analysed, it is found to afford very scanty evidence
of a satisfactory kind in favour of the theory of contagion.

In eleven out of the thirty-five instances adduced no details are given, and there is reason to believe that the cases
had not been investigated. In seven of the remaining
twenty-four, the persons who had been attacked with Cholera, after washing or handling the clothes or bedding, lived
in the same house with the patient or patients to whom the
infected articles belonged, or had passed many hours in the
house during the patient's illness. They had, therefore, been
exposed to any local cause of Cholera which might exist in
the house, and in such cases no special influence can be
attributed to infected clothes or bedding, unless it is shown
that the persons who were employed in washing, or in otherwise handling them in their foul condition, suffered from the

disease in much larger proportion than inmates of the same house not so employed. Single cases occurring under such circumstances are of no weight as evidence ; and, of the seven instances referred to, there are only three in which more than one person was attacked. At St. Luke's Hospital three laundrymaids were attacked, but Dr. Sutherland records their illness only as severe diarrhœa. At the Wakefield Prison 7 out of the 27 prisoners attacked with Cholera, and 4 out of the 16 fatally attacked, were engaged in washing clothes, but the men thus employed being 25 in number, they did not suffer in much larger proportion than the whole body of prisoners, of whom there were only 127. In the Wandsworth Union Workhouse five laundresses were seized with Cholera, and two of them died. Only eight deaths from the epidemic occurred in this workhouse at the same time (the months of December and January, 1848–1849) ; so that the women employed in washing the linen probably suffered in a much larger proportion than other inmates of the house. But, when it is remembered that Cholera is commonly felt more severely in one part of a large establishment than in others, and that there is no reason why the part occupied by the laundresses in a prison or workhouse should not be thus visited, it will be seen that there is nothing conclusive as to the operation of contagion in these facts.

In seventeen instances, of which more or less complete details have been furnished, the clothes or bedding of patients, who had died of Cholera, were removed to distant houses, and the first of the persons subsequently attacked had not, as far as appears, been in the houses whence the supposed vehicles of infection were brought. But here again, in several instances, there is much ground for doubt. In some instances Cholera already prevailed in the localities in which the reception of the foul clothes or bedding seemed to give rise to the disease. In others, the attacks experienced were not fatal, and their nature may, therefore, be questioned. So that, in fact, there are only seven instances in which the evidence seems fairly to establish a connection between the clothes, linen, or bedding, and the cases of Cholera which subsequently occurred in the houses into which they were received. The cases referred to are those related by Dr. Brown of Sunderland, Mr. Ray of Sydenham, Mr. Horton of Bromsgrove, Dr. Lochée of Canterbury, Dr. Beadle of Tewkesbury, and Dr. Smith of Lasswade (Nos. 1, 2, 6, 7, 8, 9, and 12 in Table XVII.).

In these instances, and perhaps in some of the others in which the evidence is less satisfactory, there are grounds for believing that the disease was propagated from one place to another by means of clothes or bedding. But, this being granted, it does not necessarily follow that the infectious property of the clothes was due to their impregnation with emanations or discharges from the bodies of the sick. There is indeed reason to doubt whether the discharges have such a property. For if the discharges from the patients had the power of communicating the disease, the strongest evidence of it would be expected in the persons of washerwomen engaged in cleasing the foul linen and bedding of Cholera Hospitals, or of other establishments, in which a very large number of cases of Cholera had occurred within a short space of time; and it is precisely from such sources that the strongest evidence against the infectious power of the foul linen and bedding has been furnished. The women who washed the vast accumulation of foul linen at Drouet's School, which Mr. Kite describes to have been only very partially moistened with chloride of lime, those who washed the numerous bundles of foul bed-linen sent from the Oxford Cholera Hospital to the Hospital Workhouse, and the women employed by the Sanitary Committee of Leeds, according to Mr. Bearpark's statement, to wash the foul linen of Cholera patients, all escaped without any serious attack of the epidemic. Those at the Oxford Hospital had diarrhœa, but Mr. Allen remarks that this was at the time a general complaint among persons not specially exposed to any known risk of infection. Testimony to the same effect is given by Dr. Parkes, Dr. Dick, Dr. Reid, Dr. Wilson, and Dr. Rae, with respect to the washerwomen employed in washing the foul linen of Cholera patients at University College Hospital, at the Fever Hospital, Bedford, at the St. Giles's Workhouse, at Haslar Hospital, Portsmouth, and at the Royal Naval Hospital, Plymouth. (See Table XVII. in the Appendix.) Lastly, of 30 women employed in the laundry at Millbank Prison, only one suffered; and she had been engaged in ironing, not in washing the linen; while of 100 women otherwise employed, 8 were attacked and died.

The bedding and linen used by Cholera patients in hospitals has therefore, at least very frequently, exerted no infectious power on those who washed them; and the communication of the disease by clothes and linen which has seemed well established in other cases must have been due to special circumstances. To explain the contradictory character of the results several hypotheses might be offered. It might be supposed that the discharges or emanations from the sick have only occasionally a poisonous property,—that in some instances they have been rendered inert by disinfecting agents,—that they are received or imbibed by persons brought into contact with them only under certain external conditions,—that their effects are produced only when a certain susceptibility exists,—or, lastly, that the poisonous matter with which the clothes sometimes seem to be infected is derived from some other source than the bodies of the sick. It does not appear possible at present to determine by direct evidence which of these hypotheses is the more correct one. The first, however, has at all events very little à priori probability in its favour.

Lastly, those arguments in favour of the contagious nature of Cholera must be examined which are founded on the *results of nursing and otherwise attending on persons affected with the disease.* The facts observed in private houses may be divided into two classes, those in which the patients were nursed in their own dwellings, and those in which they had been removed to other houses, not yet visited by the epidemic. To the former class belong

a large number of the facts communicated to the Cholera
Committee, both those where several members of a family
were attacked in succession after attending on earlier victims
of the disease in the same house, and those where nurses
had gone to the houses of persons sick with Cholera, had
nursed them there, and were themselves afterwards seized.
Incidents of this kind are consistent with a belief in the
contagion of Cholera, but are of no weight as independent
proofs that the disease is in the strict sense contagious,
or even that it is in any way communicable; since the persons attacked after nursing the sick had been exposed to the
atmosphere of a locality which probably was infected, as
well as to the proximity of an infected person. The facts
relative to the effects of nursing persons in houses remote
from those in which they probably were infected, are somewhat better fitted to establish the position that Cholera may
be imparted by the sick to the healthy; and they are by no
means deficient in numbers. Nearly all the instances of the
seeming introduction of the disease into towns and public
establishments by human intercourse (cited in Table XV. in
the Appendix) may be regarded as belonging to this category; and several of the earlier cases given in Table XVIII.
are further examples of the same kind. But reasons have
already been stated for at least hesitation in admitting that
such facts, though they be instances of the communication of
Cholera by one person to another, are therefore proofs of the
contagious property of the disease.

The available evidence with regard to the effects of
nursing and attending on Cholera patients in hospitals and
other public establishments, requires more particular examination. Here, again, a distinction must be drawn between
those cases in which the patients were nursed in the
establishments where they took the disease, and those in
which they had been removed to hospitals until then
free from the ravages of the epidemic. It is obvious
that the attacks of nurses in the former circumstances
would be of no import, unless they were proportion-

ably much more numerous than the attacks of persons in the same establishments not equally exposed to contact with the sick. The comparison, too, ought to be made with persons of the same class, for it will presently be seen that different classes of individuals living in the same buildings are not by any means equally liable to be attacked with the disease. It is difficult to find instances in which satisfactory data for such a comparison exist, especially if, in order to avoid the errors likely to arise from different observers applying the term Cholera to attacks of various degrees of severity, the fatal cases alone are taken into the account. In the majority, however, of the eight instances numbered 7, 8, 9, 10, 11, 13, 14, and 15, in Table XVIII., there is ground for, at least, suspecting that the attendants on the Cholera patients did suffer from the disease in consequence of their being thus employed; and in two cases the evidence of this appears very strong, though not conclusive. In the Woolwich Hulks 9 out of the 30 convicts who died had attended on the sick in the Hospital Ship, and two hired nurses were attacked and one of them died. For the explanation of these facts, if the belief in contagion be rejected, it seems necessary to assume that the part of the Hospital Ship in which the Cholera patients were treated had, owing to some local cause, become the chief focus of the disease. The same assumption, too, would be necessary in the case of the Wandsworth Workhouse, where, during the winter visitation, three out of eight persons fatally attacked had been engaged in nursing other Cholera patients. And in the absence of facts showing that this assumption is well founded, it must be conceded that these are instances of the seeming communication of the disease more readily explicable, by the theory of contagion, than on any other principle.

Now, in the two instances just noticed, the nurses who suffered, and the patients whom they had attended, were for the most part persons previously in the same state of health, taking similar food, and living in the same circumstances.

N

In the instances next to be referred to this was not the case,
and the results were very different. In 17 public lunatic
asylums, in which Cholera showed itself, there were 311
deaths amongst 3639 patients *. While out of 408 persons
residing in these asylums in the capacities of officers, attendants, or nurses, only 6 died, and of those 6 only 3 were
nurses. From some cause or other, therefore, the attendants
in these asylums suffered in much smaller proportion than
the insane inmates. Two of these establishments deserve
especial remark. In the West York Lunatic Asylum at
Wakefield, where 98 out of 633 patients died, only one nurse

* The data for the subjoined table are derived from the official returns received by the Commissioners in Lunacy. The number of attendants and resident officers in Althorpe House Asylum, was not given in
the return from that establishment, but has been estimated from a comparison of the numbers in other asylums. The two officers who died in
the Wrekenton Asylum were the superintendent and his son-in-law.

Names of Asylums.	Number of insane patients.	Attacks and deaths from Cholera amongst the insane.		Number of attendants and resident officers.	Attacks and deaths from Cholera amongst the officers and attendants.	
		Attacks.	Deaths.		Attacks.	Deaths.
Peckham House	489	78	43	40	5	
Grove Hall, Bow	407	26	11	32		
London House, Hackney	28	2	2	9		
Althorpe House, Battersea	44	8	6	9		
Bethnal House	567	60	54	71	2	2
Camberwell House	332	23	18	28		
St. Marylebone Infirmary	73	4	4	12		
St. Luke's Hospital	210	11	5	29	2	
Cowper House, Old Brompton	37	4	3	14		
Hoxton Prison	395	39	21	44	1	
Kingsland Asylum, near Shrewsbury	84	13	11	14		
Vernon House, Bretton Ferry	151	9	8	21		
Hull, Bow Asylum	73	9	4	12	1	
Bristol Asylum	79	12	5	12		
Wrekenton Asylum, near Gateshead	37	23	18	9	5	2
West York Asylum, Wakefield	633	133	98	51	2	2
Total	3639	454	311	407	18	6

was fatally attacked out of 51 attendants and other resident officers, and she was the chief nurse in the female Cholera wards during the height of the epidemic. But the second officer who in this asylum died was the clerk, who most probably had had no intercourse with the sick. In the Bethnal House Asylum 54 patients out of 567 perished by Cholera, and the number of attendants was 71, of whom 2 died. Both were nurses, but only one of them appears to have been in attendance on patients affected with Cholera. These facts show, then, in the first place, that if Cholera is contagious, and if its contagious virus finds its victims through the medium of the air, which all alike must breathe, its power is far greater over persons in the condition of the insane than it is over their attendants, who are usually strong and well-fed persons. But the same facts prove that, whatever is the cause of the disease, it may be escaped or resisted by one class of persons, while those of another class in the same building suffer. In this respect they are valuable, for they suggest great caution in inferring the absence of contagion, or other infectious power, from the mere fact of the attendants on the sick escaping the attacks of the disease. A susceptibility of the disease similar to that manifested by the insane, and, it may be remarked, by soldiers fatigued by long marches, is observed in convicts under long sentences of imprisonment, in whom the nervous powers even more than the nutritive functions are depressed. Thus, in Millbank Prison, during the entire epidemic of 1848–49, 48 convicts died, the average number in the prison during the period being 1107; while only 2 deaths occurred among the officers and the members of their families resident in the prison, the number of whom amounted to 195. The prisoners, therefore, suffered in a proportion fourfold greater than the officers and their families.

In Millbank Prison, as in the Lunatic Asylums, the number of deaths among the officers and attendants is too small to afford satisfactory data for estimating the risk incurred in attendance on Cholera patients. But the evidence these

institutions afford, scanty and inconclusive as it is, must
not be overlooked.   The attendants engaged on the sick
certainly suffered in larger proportion than those not so
employed.   The exact number of persons brought into contact with the patients struck with Cholera in the lunatic
asylums is not known ; but there can be no doubt that the
two or three deaths formed a much larger proportion amongst
the attendants thus employed than the three or four deaths
among those officers and attendants, who had little or no
intercourse with the patients labouring under the disease.
In Millbank Prison 20 persons were daily brought into more
or less close contact with the prisoners affected with the
epidemic, and one of them died.   Of the remaining 175
persons in the prison who were not prisoners, and of whom
few at any time entered the infirmaries, also one died, a
proportion more than eight times less.

The rarity of attacks of Cholera amongst the nurses and
medical officers in the hospitals into which persons labouring
under the disease are received as patients, is universally
admitted.   But the experience of all hospitals with regard to
this point is by no means the same.   The communications
received by the Cholera Committee afford, indeed, examples
of the most contradictory character.

The evidence in several instances specially reported on
is apparently most decided as to the safety of nurses attending on patients under such circumstances.   Thus, it results
from the evidence of Dr. Kidd and Mr. Allen of Oxford,
that the nurses at the Cholera Hospital in that city, although
they suffered from diarrhœa, were in no case attacked
with Cholera, while of 25 policemen of the city who were
not brought into relation with the sick at the hospital,
one suffered severely from the epidemic ; and Dr. Hawkins
and Dr. Basham testify that at the Middlesex and Westminster Hospitals, into which many Cholera patients were
admitted (36 dying in the former and 37 in the latter),
no nurse, pupil, or medical officer was attacked.   In the
London Hospital, where 40 of the patients admitted for

attacks of Cholera died, no case of the disease arose in the Hospital among the ordinary patients or among the nurses even of the Cholera wards. In St. George's Hospital, again, according to Dr. Barclay, the Medical Registrar, there was no case among the nurses or persons who were brought into contact with patients suffering under the disease; and " none in those wards in which Cholera patients had at any time been placed." Of five cases that occurred in this hospital, one was a nurse " whose duties kept her entirely out of the way of Cholera patients," and two of the others were surgical patients. Lastly, Dr. Parkes states that at University College Hospital, although many patients suffering from Cholera were admitted and 31 died, not one of the six nurses who attended on them was attacked; and the single patient admitted for another disease, but seized with Cholera in the Hospital, though in an adjoining ward, was not known to have had direct communication with the Cholera patients.

But in several other instances the attendants on the Cholera patients were attacked in large proportion. Thus, with regard to the Cholera Hospitals at Liverpool, it is said by Dr. Wilkinson and Dr. Burgess that *many* of the nurses and of the messengers employed to convey the patients to the hospital died, and it is more precisely stated by Mr. Taylor that of 30 healthy inmates of the workhouse who took the offices of nurses and messengers at the various Cholera Hospitals nine died. Of the Torbay Infirmary, a small institution, into which during the epidemic only Cholera patients were admitted, Mr. Jolley reports, that the matron and two nurses died, and that two other nurses had severe attacks of the epidemic. Again, Mr. Merry, of Hemel Hempstead, says, " The two nurses employed to attend the Cholera patients removed to the Union House were seized most violently, and one died in a few hours."

The foregoing instances, owing to the absence of details, and the nature of the circumstances, would admit of the explanation that the nurses and other attendants suffered from Cholera, not in consequence of communication with the sick,

but owing to the hospitals themselves having become foci of
the disease.   But in the cases which remain to be noticed,
it is quite clear, not only that the persons in contact with the
Cholera patients, or in their neighbourhood, were attacked
either exclusively or in much larger proportion than other
persons in the same establishments not similarly situated,
but also that their attacks were the consequences of the
admission of those Cholera patients; and the number, as
well as the character of these cases, are such as to remove
all reasonable ground for regarding the occurrences to be
detailed as the results of accident.

In the first place, the important testimony of Dr. Peacock
relative to the effects of nursing the infected children brought
from the school at Tooting to the Royal Free Hospital, must
be once more referred to.   From 20 to 25 persons, who had
not been at Tooting, had free intercourse with the children
during the first fortnight; about 14 nurses and 5 male
attendants sleeping in the wards with them every night.
Twelve of these attendants were attacked with severe diarrhœa, four passed into the state of Cholera, and two died.
All the other attendants suffered in a less degree from
diarrhœa.   At the same time there were 50 or 60 persons
in another part of the building, none of whom suffered
from any similar form of affection.

The facts observed at St. Bartholomew's Hospital, and
fully detailed by Dr. Burrows, likewise corroborate the belief that the attendants on the sick are more liable to take
the disease than persons otherwise employed, though they
likewise show that the collecting the patients in special
wards is not necessarily attended with any considerable danger.   One of the ordinary nurses of the Cholera wards was
seized with the disease and died, and two head nurses or
sisters of the Cholera wards had severe diarrhœa; while the
sisters and nurses of other wards, about tenfold more numerous, were not infected in the same way.   Only one of
the patients admitted for other diseases died of Cholera,
and this one was a woman who, having poisoned herself with

oxalic acid, had been placed by mistake in the Cholera department, and remained there two or three days; was then removed to another part of the hospital, and shortly afterwards died there with symptoms of Cholera. Here, then, in all probability, two deaths, and almost certainly one, must be referred to communication with the sick. But when it is remembered that during the epidemic 478 cases of confirmed Cholera were received into the hospital, 198 of which proved fatal, and that all these patients were treated in one comparatively small wing of the building, it must be admitted that no great power of infection was here manifested.

The evidence of the communication of the disease was of a more decided character in St. Thomas's Hospital and King's College Hospital. There were received into St. Thomas's Hospital 147 persons labouring under Cholera, 66 of whom died; and nine persons were attacked in the Hospital. Dr. J.R. Bennett states that all these persons were treated in special wards which did not communicate with any others; that of the nine attacked in the Hospital, six were patients admitted for other diseases, who could have had no communication, except accidentally, with the Cholera patients; that three were nurses, of whom one had served in a ward in a distant part of the Hospital, but the others had been solely occupied with Cholera patients; and that a fourth nurse, who had been for some weeks in the Cholera wards, and had left because she was no longer wanted, returned in a day or two as a patient with Cholera, and died. Into King's College Hospital only 123 cases of reputed Cholera were received, 40 of which were fatal; yet two Cholera nurses, and two patients who had been admitted for surgical complaints some time previously and who lay in a ward adjoining and communicating with the Cholera ward, were attacked and died; and a fifth person, a woman attending her child ill with Cholera, was attacked, but recovered. All these cases occurred within the space of a fortnight, before the epidemic had reached its height, and when only 86

Cholera patients had been admitted into the hospital *.   No
further cases of the disease arose after the patients were
placed in wards which did not communicate directly with
any others.

From the evidence which has now been detailed, it appears indisputable that in some hospitals into which Cholera
patients were received, the disease was communicated to the
attendants and other persons, while in other hospitals no
such communication of the disease occurred. The causes
on which these different results depended are an important
subject of inquiry; and before the bearing of the facts on
the question of contagion is taken into consideration, the
different explanations that might be offered of the apparently contradictory experience of different hospitals may
be briefly noticed.

The different states of susceptibility of different persons,
with regard to the disease, is obviously one cause that probably had a share in determining whether the nurses became
affected or not; but the facts certainly cannot be altogether
explained on that principle. The number of nurses and
other persons affected, even within a few days, in some
hospitals, and the escape of large numbers of persons of
the same class, though exposed throughout the epidemic
in other hospitals, or in the same hospitals at a different
time, seem to show that the cause was not in operation
equally in the two series of places, nor equally at different
times in the same places.

Another view that might be taken is, that the different
modes in which the Cholera patients were disposed in different hospitals occasioned the variety and the results.
And some countenance is certainly afforded to this view by
the fact that among those metropolitan hospitals, the ex-

* See a Clinical Lecture on Cholera by Dr. Budd, Medical Times,
October 20th, 1849, and Mr. Farr's Report on Cholera in England,
p. 18.

perience of which has been ascertained *, there are three in
which the Cholera patients were distributed through the
general wards; and in these hospitals no nurse who attended
on the patients affected with Cholera was attacked. The
information, too, which has been received respecting the St.
Giles's workhouse and the Wandsworth workhouse, favour
the same view.

In the St. Giles's Workhouse only one person employed
about the sick, of whom 109 died of Cholera, was attacked
during the epidemic of 1849, while in 1832 ten of the attendants died. In that year, Dr. Reid remarks, the Cholera patients were collected together in a Cholera Hospital; while in
the late epidemic they were distributed through the different
wards. An observation of the like kind was made at the

* The subjoined table is sufficiently explained by the remarks on the
different metropolitan hospitals in the text. The particulars relative to
other hospitals or infirmaries will be found in Table XVIII. in the
Appendix.

Name of Hospital.	Average number of In-patients.	Number of deaths of Cholera patients admitted.	Number of deaths from Cholera among other patients.	Number of deaths from Cholera among nurses.	How the Cholera patients were disposed.
St. Bartholomew's Hospital.	500	198	1	1	In special wards.
Guy's Hospital......	490	......	8	1	Cholera patients were not received.
St. Thomas's Hospital.	430	66	6	8	In special wards.
London Hospital ...	330	40	none.	none.	In special wards.
Middlesex Hospital.	300	30	none.	none.	Distributed among other patients.
St. George's Hospital.	300	11	2 surgical. 1 medical.	1	Distributed among other patients.
University College Hospital.	110	31	1	none.	In special wards.
Westminster Hospital.	150	37	none.	none.	Distributed among other patients.
King's College Hospital.	96	46	2	2	In special wards.

Wandsworth Union Workhouse; for there during the winter outbreak (1848-49) the patients were collected in special wards, and several nurses were attacked and died, but not a single nurse or attendant suffered in the subsequent summer when the patients were distributed through different parts of the building. It is, however, certainly not the mere collection of Cholera patients in special wards which constitutes the source of danger, nor is the distribution of them even the chief precaution to be taken with the view of averting the risk of infection.

For, on the one hand, the nurses of the Oxford Cholera Hospital, and those employed in attending the Cholera patients in two metropolitan hospitals, in which special wards were set apart for them, namely, the London Hospital and University College Hospital, enjoyed entire immunity from attacks, at all events from fatal attacks; and the experience of other hospitals shows that the risk of infection was by no means proportioned to the number of patients collected together; while. on the other hand, the instances are very numerous in which the communication of Cholera by single patients, labouring under the disease, is supported by evidence which it is scarcely reasonable to doubt. It would seem, therefore, that some external conditions may, on the one hand, prevent the communication of the disease to the attendants, when several patients labouring under it are collected together, and may, on the other hand, promote its communication from single patients. What these conditions are can scarcely be matter of doubt, if the conclusions drawn from the great features of the epidemic in the earlier part of this Report were just. If the state of the air really exerts elsewhere a paramount influence over the extension of the disease, it must operate in hospitals likewise; and inasmuch as these establishments present marked differences of site, as to level, general sanitary condition of the neighbourhood, and density of the surrounding population, differences also in the cubical capacity of the wards in relation to the number of the patients received, and differences in the provisions for effecting adequate ventilation, and for disposing of matters which, if long exposed, would render the air foul, it may, on the assumption that the air has the influence referred to, be safely concluded that these differences in the conditions of the hospitals have had a share in producing the apparently contradictory results which have been detailed. The poison of Cholera, whatever its source, would be especially likely to find victims among the nurses and other persons exposed to it, where want of cleanliness and ventilation, and crowding of the inmates, tended to produce that state of air which is presumed to promote its increase and power of action.

The question next to be considered is, whether the facts which have been detailed with reference to hospitals, lunatic asylums, and a few other public establishments, favour the theory of contagion, which supposes that the poison of Cholera is an emanation from the bodies of the sick. Some of the facts certainly have this tendency, namely, the larger proportion of attacks among the attendants on the Cholera patients than among other persons in hulks, prisons, workhouses, and lunatic asylums, into which patients labouring under the disease were not admitted from without; and the large number of instances in which nurses have taken the disease in hospitals in which the Cholera patients were placed together in special wards, while no communication of the disease has appeared to take place where the patients were dispersed among the patients in the general wards. But if the sick labouring under Cholera give forth into the air around them a poisonous matter, it seems difficult to account for the rare occurrence of infection among the nurses and others brought near them in hospitals, since the contagious Typhus, which has less power of diffusing itself with great rapidity through a city, is often communicated by a single patient to several other persons in the same ward. This infrequent occurrence of infection in hospitals would be more plausibly accounted for by the hypothesis that the poison emanating from the sick is not conveyed by the air into the lungs of the persons around, but is occasionally swallowed by them, owing to accidental circumstances, which are most apt to co-exist with want of cleanliness. This hypothesis, however, as will be shown more fully at a future page, would not agree with some of the more general facts relating to the epidemic.

Some facts favouring the belief that the communication of Cholera is dependent on accidental circumstances, find a satisfactory explanation in another theory. The occurrence, for example, within the space of a few days, of two or three cases of the disease among the nurses or others brought into proximity to the sick in a public hospital, where both before and subsequently no evidence of infection presented itself, would be intelligible, if the cause of Cholera were a matter reproduced altogether in the air, and not emitted from the human body, though capable of being conveyed by sick as well as by healthy persons, probably in their clothes, from one place to another. For a portion of such a poisonous matter might be introduced with the patients into the hospital wards, and then, if the air were not pure, would increase there for a time, and infect one or more persons, but would not continue to exist in an active state, unless the ventilation were very defective; though the same accidental introduction of the poison might happen more than once. In hospitals, on the other hand, in which, owing to a favourable site and good internal arrangements, the air was pure, or nearly so, the poison, though thus accidentally introduced from time to time, might never have the power to produce any effect on the nurses and other inmates. This theory has the advantage of being the one which accords best with the more general facts in the history of the epidemic. But if it should hereafter prove to be the rule that the risk of infection is greater when Cholera patients are collected together in special wards than when they are dispersed in many wards, other conditions, such as space and ventilation, being the same, this theory will not afford a satisfactory explanation of such facts; and it will be necessary to admit here the operation of an influence derived from the sick themselves.

It is scarcely necessary to remark that the almost complete immunity of medical men, who are attacked even less frequently than nurses, is intelligible, even though the disease be contagious, since they are exposed to contact with the sick only during a certain number of hours of the day, and generally enjoy a state of health which renders them in a great measure insusceptible of the disease. In the instances where they have suffered, they have usually undergone great fatigue, while they have been much exposed to the atmosphere of infected localities. The same considerations would, of course, afford an explanation both of their general immunity and of the exceptions to this rule, whatever theories of the disease were adopted.

If the results of the examination, instituted in the foregoing pages into the direct evidence of the contagion of Cholera, be now reviewed, it will be found that, although several arguments in favour of that theory of the cause of the disease have been met with, they are not by any means conclusive. The arguments referred to are chiefly those founded on the fact that, where the origin of the Cholera in towns, institutions, and private houses, has been traced to newly-arrived persons, these persons were generally themselves first affected with the disease,—on the greater liability of the nurses than of other persons to be attacked, in establishments visited by the epidemic,—and on the more frequent occurrence of infection in hospitals when the Cholera patients received into them have been collected in special wards. The facts relative to the seeming communication of the disease to washerwomen and other persons by infected clothes, can scarcely be said to afford any decided support to the theory of contagion.

It may be that more extended observations will prove that all these classes of facts are usually due to a contagious property of the disease. But even then the evidence will only show that the human body forms one nidus for the

reproduction of the poison; that contagion bears a small part
in the propagation of the epidemic; that comparatively few
persons are susceptible of its influence; and that by proper
sanitary precautions it may be almost entirely disarmed of
its power.

The question, whether contagion is an occasional cause
of the propagation of the disease, is therefore left in
doubt. The fact, however, that the disease is communicated by human intercourse, which had already been
deduced from facts of a more general nature, has here been
amply confirmed. And the impression left on the mind
is, that very probably the share borne by human intercourse in the dissemination of the disease is larger than the
general statistical facts relative to the rise and spread of
the epidemic in this country in 1848–49 seemed to indicate.

XI. Human intercourse, however, is certainly only one
cause of the propagation of the disease. The general
features of the epidemic of 1849, and special facts also,
have afforded satisfactory evidence, that some other agent
is engaged in its diffusion. The probability that this other
agent is the wind has already been inferred; but it has not
yet been supported by direct evidence. It is, indeed, difficult to offer any; for no systematic attempt has been made
to determine by observation whether the advance of the
disease is effected or favoured by the wind.

Such scattered observations of the kind as have been met
with may, however, here be adduced, with perhaps the advantage of directing attention to a part of the subject which
much needs investigation.

The following facts observed at Madras are given by
Mr. Scot in support of the view that the infectious prin-
ciple of Cholera may be conveyed by the air:—" His
Majesty's 54th Regiment landed at Madras on the 10th of
May from the H.C. ships *William Fairlie* and *Thomas
Coutts*, in a remarkably healthy state, after a voyage of
48 days, from the Cape of. Good Hope, and marched

into quarters in Fort St. George. Cholera appeared amongst
the men within three days after their landing. In the former
ship, while at anchor in the roads, Cholera made its appearance on or about the 18th of May; they had 65 cases, and
of these 12 proved fatal. The disease did not appear in
the *Coutts* till a fortnight afterwards: they had only 23
cases, of which 6 were fatal. Several circumstances connected with the appearance of the disease on board these
ships deserve to be noticed. No case of Cholera occurred
in either ship while out at sea. The *Fairlie* lay at anchor
so far to the southward as to be directly to leeward of the
fort, and this was during the prevalence of the strong south-
west winds: the disease was at that period established in the
54th Regiment, in the garrison there. The men who worked
upon deck, and those who slept on the landward side of
the ship, were found to be decidedly the most obnoxious to
the attacks of Cholera. The ship afterwards took up a position farther north, and about a quarter of a mile directly
to windward of the *Coutts:* although Cholera had then
existed in the former ship for nearly a fortnight, one solitary
case only had as yet appeared on board the latter ship; this
case was in a sailor who slept on deck in a state of intoxication during the night. Thus situated, the wind blew
directly over the *Fairlie* to the *Coutts*, and the disease at
this juncture appeared in the *Coutts:* all the men attacked,
with one exception, slept on the side of the ship next to the
Fairlie; this side, however, was likewise the landward side."[*]

The passage next to be quoted is intended by Dr. Parkes
only as an illustration of the influence of meteorological
phenomena generally in the extension of the epidemic. But
the agency of the wind, as a means of conveying the cause
of the disease, is implied. Dr. Parkes[†] says, "At Madras
the disease is heard of at a station 90 miles off; a few days

[*] Report on the Epidemic Cholera, in the Presidency of Fort St.
George, by William Scot, Surgeon and Secretary to the Medical Board,
London, 1849, pp. 198–201.

[†] Researches into the Pathology and Treatment of Asiatic or Algide
Cholera, by E. A. Parkes, M.D., London, 1847, p. 174.

afterwards it appears in Madras itself." . . . . "And a wind blows directly from the station, in which the disease had shortly before been prevalent."

In England, where the atmospheric currents are so frequently changing, it is very difficult to determine the relation borne by their direction to the course taken by the epidemic. But it is worthy of observation, that during the three weeks preceding the outbreak of Cholera in the autumn of 1848, the direction of the wind was such as might have conveyed an infected atmosphere from those parts of the north of Europe in which the Cholera then prevailed. The subjoined Table is an abstract from the Meteorological Tables prepared at the Royal Observatory, and published by the Registrar-General.

Weeks ending.	General direction.	Amount of horizontal movement of air.
16th September	Variable. N. and N.N.E. predominant.	490 miles.
23rd „	Generally calm. S.W. on two days. S. by E. and S.S.E. on two days.	440 miles.
30th „	N.E.	837 miles.
7th October ..	S.E. and S.W. and S.	985 miles.

At Sunderland, the more specific observation was made by Dr. Brown, that the house in which " the first case on shore occurred was situated at some distance, nearly a mile from where the infected ships lay, but exactly in the direction in which the prevailing easterly winds would convey any effluvia from the vessels, without interjacent obstacles to its reaching the town."

Again, in a letter quoted by the Commissioners of Health in Ireland, Dr. Biggs says, "On Saturday last, the 7th instant, a strong wind set in from the north-east, of a keenly-piercing nature. This wind blew in a direct line to Armagh from Belfast, where Cholera is now prevalent, and on that evening a girl aged twelve years, when in the female school of the workhouse, was suddenly attacked with malignant Cholera, which proved fatal in fourteen hours. This girl was an inmate of the house for nearly two months, and had had no communication whatever with any infected person or place; I may mention that about the same time a man was suddenly attacked with this disease about a quarter of a mile from the workhouse, on the Belfast road, and has since died. On Sunday evening five persons were suddenly seized with Cholera in the workhouse."

Lastly, in the case of Millbank Prison, it was thought, during the prevalence of the epidemic in London, that there was a connection between the direction of the wind and the renewed outbreaks of the disease in the prison. Cholera certainly reappeared in the prison most frequently when the wind was blowing from the east and consequently over the southern districts of London, where the epidemic was then fiercely raging.

All such observations as these, relating to places on shore, so long as they are few in number, are open to the objection that the coincidence of the outbreak with the particular direction of the wind may have been accidental. At present they are very few: and the belief that the Cholera poison is wafted from place to place by the wind, rests almost entirely on the ground of inference; although it is an inference scarcely admitting of question, if the theory which regards the cause of Cholera as a poisonous matter existing and increasing in the air, but not diffused through it in the manner of gas, is the correct one. For it has been shown that in a large number of instances the appearance of the disease in a town, and the mode of its first extension through it, as well as the origin of the disease in many public institutions, cannot be explained by human intercourse; and human intercourse being excluded, no adequate means for the dissemination of such a poison remains except atmospheric currents. If, too, that theory be correct, other observations not yet noticed may be regarded as proofs that

o

the poison of Cholera is conveyed by the wind; such, for example, as those on which Dr. Bryson founds his remark that Cholera appeared in several ships of the Mediterranean squadron before they had any communication with the shore, and were still at the distance of several miles from an infected locality.

It does not, however, follow from the theory in question, that the Cholera poison should retain its properties when carried by the winds over distances of very many miles. On the contrary, it is more probable that, as a general rule, it would in a long transit be dissipated and destroyed by the purer air with which it would generally be brought into relation; and several of the general features of the epidemic or classes of facts examined in the preceding pages, favour this view.

The information with regard to the share borne by human intercourse in the dissemination of Cholera through England, examined at page 162, tends to show that the influence of atmospheric currents is chiefly exerted in spreading the disease through the different parts of towns, and over parts of a country of limited extent. The history of the invasion of fresh islands and continents by the epidemic leads to the conclusion that Cholera is at all events not dependent on the agency of the wind for enabling it to cross seas; while the remarkable manner in which it often is confined to the course of rivers in passing through an extensive country, and the comparatively slow rate of its progress under all circumstances, are further reasons for believing that the Cholera poison is not, except in very rare instances, carried long distances by the winds without the loss of its morbific properties.

Stronger evidence, therefore, than is afforded by any of the observations quoted above would be needed to establish as a fact that the Cholera poison had been conveyed by the wind for the longer distances there indicated; though the admission may even now be made that its transference by this means over wide spaces probably has happened occasionally, and more frequently, perhaps, in climates such as that of India than in regions where the air is usually cooler and less charged with moisture.

XII. In the course of the remarks suggested by the general features of a Cholera epidemic, no reference was made to the different modes in which the cause of the disease might act on the human body. All the statistical and general facts examined were found eminently consistent with the view, that the agent producing the disease is a matter which exists and increases exclusively in the air or on surfaces exposed to that medium; and such a morbific matter would, of course, be apt to enter the lungs with the breath, and likewise to be swallowed either with the food, on the surface of which it had been deposited, or with the fluids of the mouth which had collected it from the air during the act of breathing. But whether the one or the other channel is that by which the poisonous effects are produced, seemed thus far to be a question of little importance. In more recent pages, however, where particular facts relative to the communication of Cholera were under review, the possible introduction of the poison into the system through the alimentary canal has been referred to as one assumption on which the apparently capricious manifestations of the infectious power of the epidemic in different public establishments might be explained; and a theory which is entirely based on this assumption must now be examined.

The theory referred to,—that which Dr. Snow has propounded, and in support of which he has adduced some startling facts,—gives a new form to the doctrine of contagion, and makes the solid and liquid *ingesta*, instead of the air, the vehicles by which the contagion is imparted to the human system. It supposes that the poison being swallowed acts directly on the mucous membrane of the intestines and excites the flux from its surface; that the poisonous matter is at the same time reproduced in the intestinal canal, and passes out much increased with the discharges; and

lastly, that it then in various ways, but chiefly by those discharges becoming mixed with the drinking-water in rivers or wells, reaches the alimentary canals of other persons, in whom the like disease and accompanying reproduction of the poison ensue.

At the first glance this theory has the aspect of great improbability ; but one fact which it assumes, namely, that the matters which have passed through the alimentary canal exist in some kinds of water used for drinking and for culinary purposes, has been clearly proved by Dr. Brittain, and Dr. Swayne. The theory is supported, too, by other evidence of an unexpected and striking kind, and cannot be passed by without some examination of the grounds on which it is based.

The following are the principal arguments urged in its favour : first, all those usually adduced to show that the diffusion of Cholera is brought about by human intercourse, and, in particular, by contagion ; secondly, those pathological features of the disease which establish the importance of the drain from the intestinal mucous membrane as the source of at least the majority of the characteristic morbid phenomena ; thirdly, the probability that, in the dark and dirty dwellings of the poor and other places where Cholera chiefly spreads, portions of the colourless and almost inodorous discharges of the sick are conveyed into the stomachs of the persons living around them ; fourthly, the appearance of Cholera in those who have recently eaten food brought from infected houses, or have handled the soiled bedding of Cholera patients ; fifthly, the extension of the disease among the inhabitants of groups of houses which were supplied with water from wells, tanks, or cisterns, into which privies, cesspools, or sewers had leaked or overflowed ; and sixthly, evidence tending, or intended to show that the great prevalence of the epidemic in some towns may be due to the fact of the water used by the inhabitants having been rendered foul by the contents of sewers.

The arguments of the first kind have, of course, no special

relation to this theory. The inferences in favour of the propagation of Cholera by human intercourse, which have been drawn from the facts examined in this Report, are, with few exceptions, equally tenable, whether the cause of the disease be supposed to increase in the body or in the air, and to act on the body through the lungs or through the alimentary canal. Some of the objections to which the theory of contagion is liable on the supposition that the communication takes place through the medium of the air, are, indeed, not applicable to this theory. Thus, in some cases, contaminated water might serve to convey the disease to persons not in contact with, nor even in proximity to, the first patients. It will be seen hereafter, however, that this explanation does not satisfactorily meet all cases of the kind referred to.

It is not within the scope of this Report to discuss the arguments derived from the pathology of the disease, but it may be remarked that, notwithstanding their undoubted consistency with the theory, they are in themselves by no means proofs of its truth; since a poison may, through the medium of the blood, affect parts of the body very distant from that part at which it entered the system.

The arguments of the third kind, based chiefly on the want of personal cleanliness in the lower ranks of society, which have furnished the most numerous victims of the epidemic, and on the peculiar character of the intestinal and gastric discharges in Cholera, need more particular notice. There is no doubt that in the houses of the poor, and even in some public institutions, the hands of the nurses and others about the sick must often be soiled with the discharges; and it is not unlikely that occasionally, from want of cleanly habits, portions of these discharges may unconsciously be swallowed by them with their food. The escape of medical practitioners and other persons of the middle and higher classes who visit infected houses, may be explained by their habitual attention to cleanliness, as well as by their rarely taking food or drink in the places where the

disease prevails. The foul state of mines and the practice
of miners to take food in the mines, would likewise, if this
theory were admitted, explain the great mortality experienced in the mining districts. On the other hand, however, it must be noticed, that the women and children who
do not work in the mines were attacked there in as large
numbers as the men; while the attendants on the lunatics,
in several asylums in which the insane patients suffered
severely, almost entirely escaped; and neither of these facts
is quite satisfactorily accounted for by the theory in question.

The instances of the supposed communication of the disease by contaminated food hitherto published, are very few
and altogether unsatisfactory; and the communications received by the Cholera Committee do not confirm the belief
that the disease is imparted by means of the clothes and
bedding of the sick, to persons handling or washing them.
It may be, however, that washerwomen usually are protected
by reason of their hands being necessarily kept clean, or
that the poison is destroyed by the hot and alkaline fluid in
which the clothes are immersed.

Several of the instances adduced in proof of the association of local outbreaks of Cholera, affecting groups of houses,
with a contaminated state of the water supplied to those particular houses, are doubtless remarkable. And if it could
only be shown that the Cholera discharges are poisonous,
these occurrences might be accepted as evidence of the
poison being distributed with the water used for drinking.
But the facts fall far short of being themselves proofs of the
poisonous nature of the discharges, while there is no great
improbability in the supposition that the association of the
contaminated state of the water, in these instances, with outbreaks of Cholera, was a mere coincidence. In the dwellings
of the poor, such an ill construction of the drains and water-
pipes, cesspools and cisterns, as would permit of the admixture of their contents, seems not to be very infrequent; and
the communication of the disease from house to house might

be explained either by reference to the frequent intercourse subsisting between the persons dwelling in them, or on the supposition that the poison was conveyed from one house to another by the air. In one instance cited, however, that of Albion Terrace, Wandsworth, the houses were not of that class in which the frequent intercourse of the inhabitants would be a likely means of propagating the disease. This, then, is an instance in which the only alternative seems to be between the communication of the disease by the water, and infection by the atmosphere.

The replies to the queries issued by the Cholera Committee with reference to the water supply of the localities visited by Cholera, are in some instances consistent with the view that the local extension of the disease may be connected with the contamination of the water by the discharges of the first patients. In Willow Place, Hammersmith, where seven deaths occurred, the water, according to Mr. Horton, was evidently contaminated by neighbouring cesspools, which were at 3 feet distance from the wells. In Mill Square, Hoxton, where there were several deaths, the water, Mr. Hawthorne says, was "taken from a well sunk a few yards off a cesspool; the soil around was infiltrated by refuse, and the water very bad." Dr. Plomley gives a similar account of the water drunk by the hop-pickers at East Farleigh, in Kent, of whom 46 died out of 1000, the first case being that of a man who had arrived the evening before, and who had been suffering from diarrhœa during the previous day. Lastly, the water of the Walsall Workhouse was, according to Dr. Burton, more or less contaminated by soakage from cesspools.

But the information received by the Committee respecting the water supply of other localities, in which Cholera was very rife, is equally adverse to the view that attributes so great an influence to the drinking-water.

Mr. Frost states that the water used by the inhabitants of the Potteries, the locality most severely visited at Notting-Hill, was drawn "from a pump, near which there is no

sewer," and was "not likely to be contaminated in any way."
The water used at the group of six cottages at Long Handboro' is described by Mr. Shurlock as "Pure." And in
several public establishments severely visited by Cholera, no
source of contamination of the water was detected. Mr.
Kite states that the water for Drouet's school was "drawn
from artesian wells, and was not contaminated." The water
used at the Wakefield Lunatic Asylum is described by Dr.
Wright as "quite pure," "from a well 30 yards deep, aided
by drifts from other springs in the ground to the north.
None of these springs are near the sewers, and the drifts are
far below (?) their level." The water of the Hertford County
Prison, likewise, is said by Dr. Davies to be "extremely
sweet and pure, from springs in the chalk, pumped from
wells within the prison walls."

These facts are not, however, fatal objections to the
theory; for in the examples of groups of houses supplied
with apparently good water, which are few, it is possible
that some source of contamination may have been overlooked.
And in the cases of public establishments, it is likewise
possible, though highly improbable, that the extension of
the disease from ward to ward has been due to the conveyance of portions of the discharges from one ward to another,
and from the sick to the healthy, in consequence of the
intercourse maintained between the different inmates.

The last argument adduced in support of the theory under
consideration, is that the prevalence of Cholera throughout
large towns has been proportioned, in many cases, to the
degree in which the water drunk was contaminated with the
outpourings of sewers.

Exeter and Hull serve as the chief examples. Hull was,
in 1832, supplied, though scantily, with pure water from
springs distant three miles from the town; and in that year
it suffered but slightly from Cholera, only 300 deaths occurring, and those chiefly among inhabitants of the poorer class.
In 1849, the supply of water was more abundant, but it was
drawn from the river Hull at a point nearly four miles above

the confluence of the Hull with the Humber, and quite within reach of the sewage from the town of Hull, which is, in fact, poured into the former river, and must be carried by each tide some distance up the river, past the works of the water company; and in this year the number of deaths was 1178.

Exeter, in the year 1832, was most imperfectly supplied with water, by private wells, an ancient conduit, and water-works of very limited power: so that much of the water used was obtained by dipping from the river and adjacent streams; and the two principal sources of the supply of this kind were contaminated by the contents of one of the main sewers. The epidemic of that year was fatal to 347 persons in Exeter. The supply of water has, since 1832, been derived from the river at a point two miles above the town, and out of reach of the influence of the sewage or the tide; and the mortality during the year 1849 amounted to only 44 deaths, many of which were the deaths of persons infected before their arrival.

Now, it is quite obvious that many more instances of this kind would be necessary to establish that the relation between the character of the water and the mortality from Cholera was that of cause and effect; and the facts communicated to the Cholera Committee on the subject do not countenance such a view. With regard to Hull itself, it is remarked by Dr. Sandwith that "the Cholera broke out in two public institutions, the Retreat and the Infirmary, with precisely similar results, although the former is supplied with water from the Derringham Spring, and the latter from the river Hull. The number of inmates in the Retreat was 90, and in the Infirmary 73. In each there were 9 cases of the disease, and 4 deaths." The character of the water is described more or less precisely in the cases of six other towns, which, in the year 1848, suffered a mortality from Cholera exceeding 100 in 10,000 inhabitants, and in all the six it is said not to have been contaminated. In Bridgenorth, Dr. Strange states, "The water used for drinking was spring water." The same was the case at Hedon, according to Dr. Sandwith; and likewise at Dowlais, where the water, although very scanty, is described by Mr. White as being "of the purest description, caught immediately as it issues from the rock at some distance from any infected place." The source of the water distributed at Plymouth and Leeds is not specified; but Mr. Eccles, with regard to the former place, and Mr. Bearpark with regard to the latter, state that it was pure, and express their belief that it cannot have been contaminated. At Ilford, again, where the mortality from Cholera was 59 in a population of 4500, Dr. Chambers describes the water as derived from springs, and pure, except in the instance of one group of houses.

Of three other towns, respecting which information has been received, and the mortality of which ranged from 45 to 56 deaths per 10,000 inhabitants, namely, Swansea, Wakefield, and Sunderland, the first does not derive its supply from one general source, which, being contaminated, could have served to distribute the poison*; but the cases of Sunderland and Wakefield are especially important. At Sunderland, Dr. Brown states, "The water is pumped from a depth of nearly forty fathoms out of the sand, which underlies the superficial stratum of magnesian limestone." "It is pure and sparkling," and "is transmitted through the town by 24 miles of iron pipes." In Sunderland, then, Dr. Brown remarks, "Water, contaminated by passage through infected places, or from sewers, drains, or cesspools, can have had nothing to do with the diffusion of Cholera." The town of Wakefield generally, as well as the prisons there, which have been mentioned in this Report, are alike supplied with

---

* Its chief supply, according to Dr. G. G. Bird, is drawn from public and private springs, from wells and pumps, and from the Swansea Waterworks. The water of the wells and pumps is rendered foul by privies. The water of the waterworks is brought from springs on high land some miles from the town, and the part of the town to which it was distributed suffered least from Cholera. But this was also the part of which the sanitary condition was generally most favourable to health.

water by the waterworks, which derive it from the river Calder, about four miles from the town. Now, in the month of January, 1849, Cholera prevailed with severity in the old prison, 16 convicts dying there, and the river water must have been then contaminated by the discharges of the Cholera patients; yet only 3 fatal cases occurred at that time in the town. In the subsequent summer the disease prevailed with much severity in several parts of Wakefield; the river, again, must have become contaminated, but the disease did not reappear in the prison.

These facts, if there were no other grounds for doubt, would afford reason for great caution in admitting the conclusions drawn by Dr. Snow from the facts relating to Exeter and Hull. The majority of them prove that the disease can spread through towns without the aid of contaminated water; and the case of Wakefield even throws doubt on the power of contaminated water to produce the disease.

Two other instances remain to be noticed, which tend even more directly to weaken the inference drawn from the increased mortality from Cholera in Hull in 1849, compared with that experienced in the year 1832. In Wigan and in Portsmouth the excess in 1849 was far greater than it was in Hull; yet in neither of these towns can it be ascribed to an alteration of the water supply. At Wigan, according to information received from Mr. Daglish, the water drunk by the inhabitants is derived in part from springs and wells in the town, but chiefly from landsprings at a high level two miles from the town. The water itself is impure; but there can be no admixture with the sewerage; and the supply has been increased, and its distribution extended, since 1832.

At Portsmouth there can, of course, be no admixture of the contents of the sewers with the water used for drinking at its sources. The sewers empty themselves into the harbour; and the main supply of water, according to Mr. Garrington and Mr. Slight, comes from springs in the neighbourhood of the Tarlington Waterworks, situated on the slope of Portsdown Hill, six or seven miles distant; much, likewise, being drawn from a few public pumps and numerous private wells. The water of these wells is contaminated by percolation from cesspools and from the surface. The water from the waterworks is hard, and the whole supply is insufficient. But neither as regards the sources, nor as regards the quality of the water, has any essential alteration taken place since 1832.

In both these towns, then, the excessive mortality from Cholera in 1849 must have had some other cause than the admixture of the sewerage matters with the water drunk by the inhabitants ; and this cause has probably been the increased density of the population with a consequent deterioration of the atmosphere, and more constant and closer communication amongst the inhabitants. And in the case of Portsmouth, there seems to have been the additional influence of a more general state of the atmosphere favourable to an increase of the disease. For Gosport, situated at the opposite side of the harbour, suffered a rate of mortality from Cholera which, by comparison with the mortality in 1832, was equally excessive. If, then, such were the probable causes of the increased mortality in these towns, there seems no reason to seek a special cause for the same result in the case of Hull, which had undergone as great an increase in population, and, in site and sanitary condition, presented so much that was fitted to favour an excessive virulence of the epidemic

* The data for this table are derived from Mr. Farr's Report, and from the paper of Dr. Merriman, in the 27th vol. of the Med. Chir. Transactions.

Place or District.	1832.		1849.	
	Population, 1831.	Deaths from Cholera.	Population, 1851.	Deaths from Cholera.
Hull	28,591	300	50,552	1178
Wigan	20,774	30	77,545	563
Portsmouth . . .	46,282	86	72,676	568
Gosport	6,184	5	16,908	196

Of the slight mortality in Exeter in the year 1849, on the other hand, a sufficient explanation is found in the circumstance of its being situated in a tract of country in which the epidemic was very late in exerting its influence (see page 91), and in which its effects were everywhere very slight except in the two coast towns of Brixham and Torquay. (See Map II.)

The inferences which have been drawn with regard to the share borne by the Thames water in the diffusion of Cholera, must now be examined. London is supplied with water of various degrees of purity; and when the districts of London are arranged in three classes—the first consisting of those supplied from the Thames between Battersea and Waterloo Bridges, where the water is foul from the contents of the sewers being carried upwards by the tide; the second of those supplied by the river Lea, the New River, and the Ravensbourne, which are also more or less foul; and the third of those supplied from the Thames at Kew and Hammersmith, a point to which the contents of the great London sewers are not carried,—it is found that, in the first class of districts, the deaths from Cholera in 1849, for every 10,000 inhabitants, ranged from 28 to 205; while in the second class it ranged from 19 to 96; and in the third class from 8 to 38.

It is by no means certain that the purity of the water distributed to the three classes of districts corresponds with these three degrees of mortality from Cholera; but even if this were established, it would not thereby be proved that the degree of mortality was dependent on the state of the water. For the elevation of the different classes of districts varied in nearly the same ratio; the average elevation varying, in the first class, from 2 feet below high-water mark to 22 feet above that level; in the second, from 2 feet to 88 feet; and in the third, from 12 to 100 feet above the same level; and it is a well-established fact that differences of elevation usually have associated with them corresponding differences in the mortality produced by the epidemic.

To determine the relation subsisting between the water and the mortality from Cholera more precisely, it is necessary to compare them in the cases of the several districts taken separately. The subjoined table * gives these data,

* The data for the subjoined Table are, of course, derived from the published Returns of the Registrar General. Those districts supplied by more than one Water Company are omitted.

Water Company, and Source of Supply.	Districts.	Mortality from Cholera in 10,000 Inhabitants.	Elevation above High Water, in Feet.
Southwark and Kent— Thames at Battersea, Ravensbourne, ditches, and wells.	Rotherhithe	205	0
Southwark — Thames at Battersea.	St. Olave	181	2
	Bermondsey	161	0
	Wandsworth............	100	22
Lambeth and Southwark — Thames at Battersea and Thames Ditton.	St. George's Southwark	164	0
	St. Saviour	153	2
	Newington	144	2
	Lambeth	120	3
	Camberwell	97	4
East London — River Lea, at Lea Bridge.	Bethnal Green	90	36
	Poplar	71	10
	Whitechapel.............	64	28
	Stepney.................	47	16
	St. George's in the East	42	15
Chelsea — Thames at Battersea—filtered.	Westminster............	68	2
	Chelsea	46	12
	Belgrave	28	19
Kent — Ravensbourne, in Kent.	Greenwich..............	75	8
	Lewisham	30	28
New River — Chadwell Spring, Herts ; River Lea, near Hertford and Tottenham ; and wells in Middlesex and Herts.	West London	96	28
	St. Giles.................	53	68
	East London............	45	42
	London, City..........	38	38
	St. Martin..............	37	36
	Strand	35	50
	Holborn.................	35	53
	St. Luke	34	49
	Islington	22	88
	Clerkenwell	19	53
West Middlesex — Thames at Barnes.	Marylebone	17	100
Grand Junction — Thames at Kew.	Paddington	8	76
	Hanover Square, and May Fair	8	149

together with the elevations of the districts, and shows at once, that although in the smaller groups of districts supplied by the different water companies, the mortality from Cholera throughout them presents a general relation to the source of the water supply, yet the individual districts in each group differ one from another very widely in the degrees of mortality they suffered; while the relative levels of the districts in each group still present a general correspondence with their rates of mortality. The great difference in the mortality from Cholera between the several parts of an area deriving its water supply from one company, is well seen in the cases of the districts supplied by the Chelsea and Southwark Water Companies respectively; and in relation to these, as examples, the question may be asked, How did it happen, if the character of the water has a great influence on the mortality from Cholera, that in the Belgrave district only 28 persons in 10,000 died, and in the Westminster district, also supplied by the Chelsea Company, 68 persons in 10,000; and, again, that in the Wandsworth district the mortality was only 100, and in the district of St. Olave 181 in 10,000 inhabitants, both these districts receiving their water supply from the Southwark Company? In the former instance, it is clear that differences in elevation, and in the amount of poverty, were the conditions which most probably caused the unequal mortality. In the latter, the result must be ascribed to the differences in elevation and in the density of the population. Now, varieties in these conditions could not have affected the state of the water itself, and two of them, elevation and density of population, would have little if any direct influence on the liability of the inhabitants to be affected by impure water; while, if it be assumed that the mortality from Cholera is dependent on the state of the air, it is easy to understand how great poverty and density of population may compensate for the absence of a low level, and, *vice versâ*, how this may supply the want of the two other conditions.

We shall see presently additional reasons for believing

that, even if the theory of Dr. Snow were generally correct, the influence of the character of the water must be very inconsiderable.

Some other facts, however, adduced in support of the view, that the purity or impurity of the water has a great influence, must now be noticed. The absence of Cholera in some large public establishments having independent supplies of water from Artesian or ordinary wells, is contrasted with the severity of it in others in which the water used is taken from the Thames. It is shown, for example, that in Bethlehem Hospital, which is situated in one of the districts most severely visited by the epidemic, not a single case of the disease occurred among 400 inmates; and that in the Queen's Prison, similarly situated, only one death occurred. Both these establishments derive their water for drinking and cooking from deep wells. It may be added, that in the Horsemonger Lane Gaol, which has also a good well within the prison walls, there was only one case, that of a man admitted into the prison, according to Mr. Wintour Harris, only a week previously. It is certainly remarkable that Bethlehem Hospital was the only large lunatic asylum in the metropolis that escaped, and the only one supplied with spring water; and that the prisons in the unhealthy southern districts were spared, while two in Westminster, a less severely visited part of London, but supplied with Thames water, namely, the Millbank Prison and the Tothill Fields House of Correction, suffered intensely, 48 deaths occurring in the former among 1106 prisoners, and 13 in the latter amongst 800. The water supply of Millbank Prison is taken direct from the river just below Vauxhall Bridge, though it is filtered for drinking through sand and charcoal. The Tothill Fields Prison is supplied by the Chelsea Water-works Company.

These at first sight appear strong facts. But it must be borne in mind that Bethlehem Hospital, though on the borders of a densely-populated and low district, is surrounded by wide open spaces—that it includes within its boundary wall 15 acres of ground—that this space is occupied by only 400 persons, which gives the proportion of only 26 persons to an acre, while in the entire district of St. George's, Southwark, in which it stands, there are 181 to an acre—that the building itself is in all its parts spacious, well-ventilated, clean, and by no means crowded, while the patients are abundantly fed—so that, in fact, this institution afforded no local cause or condition for the development or action of the poison there.   In the case of the Queen's Prison, of which the population numbers about 300, it must be remembered that the inmates, being debtors, not only have sufficient food, but are allowed also a limited quantity of fermented liquor ; and in the instance of the Horse-monger-Lane Gaol, the comparatively small number of in-mates, namely, 228, and the short periods of their deten-tion, compared with the longer terms of imprisonment in the Millbank and Tothill Fields Prisons, must be borne in mind.   But, independently of these considerations, there are other reasons for doubting the conclusions drawn from the nearly entire escape of the establishments in question. In numerous instances, institutions supplied with pure spring water, as the Wakefield Asylum, the Hull Asylum, and the Wrekenton Asylum, near Gateshead, were severely attacked by Cholera; and large establishments supplied with contaminated river water have been spared by the disease at times when the surrounding population was suffering.   The Wakefield Prisons have already been cited as examples of the last fact. The London House Asylum at Hackney, supplied by the New River Company, likewise had no case of Cholera in the summer of 1849, and the Grove Hall Asylum, Bow, supplied by the East London Company from the river Lea, had only one case then, although the disease had appeared in both simultaneously, and in the latter with great severity, evidently from some other cause than the character of the water supply, between November, 1848, and February, 1849, when the water supplied to them could have been scarcely at all polluted by the discharges of persons sick elsewhere.

The same difficulty, therefore, which the total escape of

P

Bethlehem Hospital and the two prisons in Southwark presents in relation to the theory of the distribution of the poison through the air, occurs in the cases last referred to, if the theory of the distribution by means of the drinking water be adopted.

Thus, then, it appears that of the arguments by which this theory is supported, only two, besides that founded on the pathology of the disease, have a wide basis in facts, namely, the first and the third of those enumerated at page 194. The two arguments referred to might be used in favour of any theory which should regard the cause of Cholera as a poison partially distributed—not diffused as a gas—through the air, having a connection of some kind or other with poverty and dirt, and capable of being conveyed from place to place by human means. Those arguments, on the other hand, which have a special reference to the reproduction or increase of the poison in the alimentary canal, and to its diffusion through towns or groups of houses by means of the admixture of the intestinal discharges with food, and especially with the water taken as drink, are exceedingly defective in facts of a conclusive nature, and are in a great measure controverted by the evidence contributed by the correspondents of the Cholera Committee. It remains to show the apparent incompatibility of the theory with some of the best-established general features of Cholera epidemics.

There is, in the first place, great difficulty in reconciling it with the obvious influence of season on the rise and subsidence of the epidemic in large towns. In a city like London, supplied with water for drinking from a large river, the temperature of which varies very closely with the temperature of the air, it might be argued that the poison being able to exist only in water of a certain degree of warmth, the diffusion of the disease in this way can take place only in the summer season, when the temperature of the river water at night is above 60° Fahr. But this argument would be inapplicable in the cases of towns supplied from sources which cannot be contaminated by admixture with the contents of the sewers; and here the influence of season in the diffusion of the disease must be ascribed to a direct action of the atmosphere, or of imponderable agents operating through it on the poisonous matter in the course of its transmission from person to person, or from spot to spot, by whatever means its transmission may be effected.

Another and strong objection to the theory is afforded by those great variations in the intensity of the epidemic in London and Paris, unattended by, and therefore not referable to, variations of temperature, which have been described and illustrated at pages 34 and 35. The phenomena referred to seem to be fatal to the view that the river water distributed through these cities was the medium by which the cause of the disease was diffused. For no such alteration, apart from changes of temperature, can be conceived to have taken place in the water of the Thames and Seine as would suddenly destroy the poisonous organic matters poured into them. Those exceptional cases, too, in which Cholera has become widely diffused through towns in the coldest season of the year, as at Glasgow, Dumfries, and Paisley, in the winter of 1848-49, cannot be explained by the view that the cause of the disease is diffused through the drinking water, if, in order to bring the usual relations of the disease to the seasons into accordance with the theory, it is assumed that a certain temperature of the water is essential.

Again, the extraordinarily rapid extension and increase of the epidemic at its commencement in some instances, as at Paris in 1832, when it destroyed 7000 persons within the first 18 days, and in the smaller town of New Orleans, in 1848, where it was within the same space of time fatal to 800 persons, is likewise inconsistent with the belief that the cause of Cholera, being reproduced only in the bodies of the sick, is distributed chiefly by the water drunk and by human intercourse, and is in every case taken with some ingesta into the stomach. With regard to the share supposed to be borne by water, the inconsistency with the

P 2

theory is the greater in the case of Paris in 1832, since in that instance the rapid diffusion took place when the mean temperature was much below 60° Fahr.

Nor can the rise of the epidemic in London in October, 1848, be with more probability referred to the agency of the water supply. It will be recollected that the first two cases occurred at Horsleydown, on the 22nd and the 30th of September, and that 26 persons, living for the most part near the banks of the river, but as widely apart as Woolwich and Chelsea, and some of them inhabitants of Harp Court, Fleet Street, and others of Spitalfields, were attacked by the disease within a week from the latter date. It has been shown by Dr. Parkes that the infection of these 26 persons cannot be traced to communication with the first two patients: and it can surely not be ascribed to the discharges of those two patients having been conveyed to the different localities by the water of the Thames. The water drunk at Spitalfields, it may be remarked, was derived, not from the Thames itself, but from the Lea River at Lea Bridge.

The dissemination of Cholera through the country receives no elucidation from this theory. At all events, the extension of the disease from town to town cannot be due to the contamination of the water of rivers by the discharges of the sick, inasmuch as the epidemic, in most instances, ascended rivers instead of following the course of the water downwards; and human intercourse, having been found incapable of explaining all the facts, the aid of atmospheric currents has seemed necessary to effect the diffusion of the poison. Hence in the theory under examination it has been assumed that the discharges of the patients becoming dry under certain circumstances, the poisonous matter is wafted about in the form of dust. But when it is considered that in all probability a very small quantity of the watery discharges of Cholera patients ever enter the atmosphere in that state, it seems impossible to admit that the diffusion of the disease in the course of a few days through a wide tract of country, or even through a large city, can be ascribed to the action of a portion of the virus thus transmitted from place to place. In such cases, if the agency of human intercourse is inadmissible, the dissemination of Cholera cannot be accounted for by the mere scattering of any poison supposed to increase exclusively in the human body; the poison, whatever its source, must in such cases have undergone increase in the air itself.

It seems needless to adduce further proofs from the history of Cholera of the insufficiency of the theory proposed by Dr. Snow. It may be remarked, however, that the proportions in which the two sexes and persons of different ages succumbed to the epidemic, are strikingly inconsistent with the main assumptions of which it is constructed. If the disease be contracted by swallowing portions of the discharges of those already labouring under the disease, with which the hands have been soiled, or by drinking water contaminated with those discharges, women, who are by far the most frequent and constant attendants on the sick, ought to have suffered much more than men; and adult men, inasmuch as they drink comparatively little of unmixed water, would have experienced likewise less mortality from the epidemic than young persons and children of either sex, who would be more liable to imbibe the poison in that way.

This theory, as a whole, then, is untenable. It has, however, directed attention to circumstances which may be hereafter shown to bear a part in the production or increase of this as well as other epidemics; and the inquiries it suggests must not be neglected when the causes and mode of propagation of such diseases are again made the subject of investigation.

It is not probable that in the case of Cholera the influence of water will ever be shown to consist in its serving as a vehicle for a poison generated in the bodies of those who had suffered from the disease. But it may be proved that the poisonous matters which produce Cholera, as well as other epidemic diseases, are capable of increasing in foul water as well as in foul air. At all events, it is scarcely probable that water containing putrid matters in a state of solution or of suspension can be habitually swallowed without at least the risk of injury to the health. This subject needs and is likely henceforth to receive more systematic investigation. Already, indeed, since the last epidemic of Cholera in London, one mode, in which a large surface of water contaminated with the foul outpourings of sewers may largely contribute to the unhealthiness of a city, has been set forth with scientific precision by Mr. Farr. With the aid of calculations, made by Mr. Glaisher, he has shown that in the summer season as much probably as 4,000,000 gallons of water rises daily in the form of vapour from the surface of the Thames at London, carrying with it into the atmosphere some portion of the putrid contents of the river.

CONCLUSIONS.

At the commencement of this Report an outline was given of six different theories, embodying the chief varieties of opinion relative to the cause and mode of diffusion of Asiatic Cholera; and it was proposed to examine the more important facts in the history of the epidemic, in order to determine, if possible, which theory is supported by the largest amount of evidence. The task indicated has now been, however imperfectly, fulfilled, and it remains to set forth the results of the inquiry.

1. The theory that the cause of the disease is a general state of the atmosphere—a general "atmospheric influence," or "epidemic constitution"—has been found untenable. The wide extent which the epidemic soon attained in England in 1848, the obvious dependence of its increase in the summer of 1849, and of its decrease and subsequent disappearance in the autumn and winter of that year, on some influence exerted throughout the country, and the association of the disease, where it was very rife, with those characters of site and those defects of sanitary provisions,

which have been termed "localising conditions,"—these three general facts constitute the sole support of the theory in question. Other facts, as general and as well established, are irreconcilable with it. The duration of the epidemic for many months in a country and even in a single city is obviously inconsistent with the belief that the cause is an influence belonging to the moving body of the atmosphere; and if the atmospheric influence is regarded as independent of the moving air, though acting through it—some "electrical state" or "telluric influence"—the following features of the epidemic are still difficulties little less than insuperable in the way of adopting this theory : first, the very partial distribution of the epidemic, even among places presenting equally the so-called "localising conditions;" second, the outbreak of the disease at different times, in several parts of a comparatively limited tract of country, in the several parts of the same town, or even of the same building ; third, the cessation of the disease, also at different times in different localities ; fourth, its lingering in a few spots when the general conditions favouring it have obviously ceased ; fifth, its extension from centres in different parts of the country ; and, sixth, the evident connection in many cases subsisting between the successive outbreaks in neighbouring places, and especially in different parts of a town or of a public establishment, where the occurrence of the first outbreak of the series has evidently been the condition determining those which followed. Still more difficult would it be to explain satisfactorily by this theory, in any form which might be given to it, the comparatively slow and step-by-step progress of the epidemic in a determinate course over a continent ; its slower progress in winter than in summer ; its frequent arrest in the winter ; its often affecting a mere narrow tract of country, leaving unscathed the regions on either side ; its extension through a country in different directions at the same time ; its march for months together against the direction of the wind ; the rapidity with which it has crossed the Atlantic Ocean, contrasted in a striking manner with its slow

progress on land; the constancy with which, in invading an
island or fresh continent, it has appeared at the largest seaports before extending inland; the great leaps it sometimes
seems to make over entire countries in passing from one seaport to another; and, lastly, many facts to be noticed presently, which clearly connect its extension with the intercourse and locomotion of mankind.

2. The persistence of the epidemic for a certain time, even
in localities of small extent, and its very partial distribution
in a country, a town, and even parts of towns, are two facts
which at once suggest the inference that the cause of the
disease is a material substance, and that it is only partially
distributed.   This inference is confirmed by the characters
above referred to, as those presented by the epidemic in its
progress over a country, and by the fact that, within a limited
area, many spots have remained free from it, which exactly
resembled the localities attacked in respect of the supposed
localising conditions.   It is certain, however, that Cholera
is so far connected with the conditions of low site and defective sanitary provisions, that it is never very rife, except
where they are present in a marked degree.   Now, all these
conditions alike tend to produce a damp and impure state
of the air in the places where they exist; while the variations of the intensity of the epidemic, attending variations of
season and temperature, and the slighter effects of other
known meteorological changes, are most easily explicable by
referring them to the increase or decrease of moisture and
impurities in the air, which necessarily result from a rise or
fall of temperature, and from a stagnant or rapidly-moving
atmosphere respectively. The natural inference is, therefore,
that the matter which is the cause of Cholera, increases and
finds the conditions for its action, under the influence of foul
or damp air with the aid of some degree of warmth; and
this being premised, other facts become intelligible, namely,
the persistence of the disease in the winter, for the most
part in the interior of large establishments, where there is
warmth, together with that impurity of air produced by the

accumulation of many human beings within a limited space; the preference manifested by the disease throughout an epidemic for low and densely-populated districts, especially the tracts of countries about the mouths of rivers, and for crowded towns and dirty and ill-ventilated parts of towns, or single dwellings of the same character even in elevated situations; and likewise its appearing at the commencement of an epidemic, as a general rule, first in places of the character described, since in those places the impure and damp air would be found earliest and in greatest abundance.

The increase of the epidemic at its climax results chiefly from the increased number· of individual localities then affected; and since this increase in the number of separate outbreaks takes place, as a general rule, most rapidly at that season when a high temperature, and other meteorological conditions, tend to increase the impurity of the air, and in those districts where local conditions affect the state of the air in the same way, it may be inferred that, while the increase and action of the cause of the disease depend on the state of the air in small localities, its transmission from spot to spot is facilitated by the state of the atmosphere over larger areas. This view is, of course, corroborated by the more rapid extension of the epidemic over the continent of Europe in the summer season; by its extension, especially along low tracts of country bordering rivers, while it avoids mountainous regions; and by the fact that in this country it was very late in attacking some districts lying far inland, and on a high level, though they were densely populated, and eventually, owing to their defective local sanitary conditions, were visited severely. The state of the atmosphere which thus favours the transmission of the cause of Cholera from one country to another, and that opposite state which, at other times, and in other places, prevents its transmission, thus arresting the progress of an epidemic, or in a country or town where it already exists, causing it to become extinct, are in part known only by their effects. The former state is generally associated with a high temperature, the latter with a low or falling temperature; but there occur very remarkable variations in the intensity of the epidemic not referable to temperature, which show that some unknown conditions of atmosphere, though not the cause of Cholera, exert a powerful influence over it, either by acting directly on the material cause of the disease, or by affecting other matters in the air, which enable it to exist or increase.

It may further be inferred from the very local and persistent character of the outbreaks of Cholera, that its cause is not a gaseous, diffusible substance, but rather matter in the form of solid or liquid particles capable of attaching themselves to surfaces of other bodies.

3 The results arrived at with reference to the means by which this Cholera poison is conveyed from place to place, have next to be noticed.

A large body of evidence renders it certain that human intercourse has, at least, a share in the propagation of the disease, and that it under some circumstances is the most important, if not the sole means of effecting its diffusion.

The progressive advance of the epidemic along great lines of human traffic, the rate of its progress varying according to the activity and means of human intercourse in different countries, but in no case surpassing the rate at which men travel; and its appearing first at the sea-ports of any island or continent, which it is newly invading,—are evidence only of the presumptive kind. A nearer approach to actual proof is made in the facts that in India the disease has travelled for some hundreds of miles, and during several months, in the teeth of the monsoon, and is, therefore, at least, in some cases, independent of the influence of the wind; and that it has continued to prevail in ships during voyages of many weeks after they had left the infected ports, and also among bodies of troops for several weeks, while they marched through districts, till then healthy.

Evidence of a more direct kind is afforded by the circumstance that the origin of the disease in the seaports of the British Isles and America has, in a large proportion of cases, been immediately preceded by the arrival of ships from infected ports, and of ships actually bringing persons already affected with Cholera. In several instances, too, the first patients attacked in these ports had had communication, more or less immediate, with sick persons brought in the ships; and in some cases the facts have been such as to admit of no other explanation than that the disease was imported by the infected ships.

The information collected relative to the origin of the disease in different towns, parts of towns, and public establishments in England, also leaves no reasonable room for doubt that the disease is propagated by human intercourse on land as well as by sea; and the published works, giving accounts of recent epidemics in France, Germany, and America, support the same view.

The facts, however, by no means sanction the belief that Cholera is always propagated in this way. On the contrary, it is certain that the extension of the disease over large towns, if not over larger areas, may take place independently of communication between the sick and the healthy. This is proved by the frequent outbreak of the disease within public establishments, such as prisons and lunatic asylums, in almost every case without a source of infection being traced, and likewise by the rapidity with which the arrival of an infected ship, or the occurrence of the first indigenous case in a large city, is followed by the appearance of the disease in various and distant parts of the city; the extension of the epidemic having, in some of these cases, been so rapid that several hundreds, or even thousands, of persons have perished in the course of between two and three weeks.

In the cases where human intercourse cannot have been the means of diffusing Cholera, the agent most likely to have conveyed the poison from one spot to another is the wind. The poison of Cholera being so dependent on the states of air for its existence, increase, and power of action, and having the capability of passing from place to place, must,

it would seem, not only be exposed to the air, but, even
though it be in part attached to the surfaces of bodies,
must, in part, also float in the air. The statistical facts,
showing the extension of the disease from centres, and
the successive attacks of different localities, though they
might be owing to the transmission of the cause of the
disease by human intercourse, are quite in accordance
with the view that the poison is scattered by varying
atmospheric currents from the foci in which it had been
developed and increased; while the extension of the disease through a large city with the rapidity above mentioned
is, indeed, explicable by no other agency, if the cause of the
disease be a substance of the nature supposed. There are,
however, few direct observations which tend to confirm this
view, by showing a correspondence between the position of
a place newly attacked with regard to an existing focus of
the disease and the direction of the wind at the time or just
previously; and of the few observations which exist the
majority are unsatisfactory. The belief, then, in the influence
of the wind rests wholly on negative evidence and inference.

If, however, the atmospheric currents, as is most probable,
share with human intercourse the office of disseminating
Cholera, their part would seem, from the facts communicated
to the Cholera Committee, as well as from theoretical considerations, to be rather the diffusion of the disease over
limited areas—its transmission from some spots to others
near at hand—than its conveyance to distant places, which is
probably effected, in a majority of cases, by the locomotion of men. But the proportion of instances in which the
introduction of the epidemic into towns, parts of towns, and
individual houses or public establishments has been due to
the one or the other mode of diffusion, cannot at present be
determined.

4. The propagation of the disease by human intercourse
does not prove its contagious nature. If the poison of
Cholera increases in, or under the influence of, damp and
impure air, and is likewise capable of attaching itself to the

surfaces of bodies, to the walls of rooms and to furniture, it will also be collected by the clothes of persons living in infected dwellings, will be carried by them from place to place, and, wherever it meets with the conditions favourable to its increase and action, will produce fresh outbreaks of the epidemic. That its propagation in such a mode as this is at least more frequent than its communication by virtue of true contagion is to be inferred, from the impossibility of tracing communication between the first and subsequent cases at the commencement of the epidemic in a large city ; from the apparent impossibility that any direct communication can have taken place in many of these cases ; still more decidedly from the great rapidity with which the disease sometimes spreads at once through the whole population of a city ; from the influence of season and temperature, and of the characters of localities on the rate of the diffusion of the epidemic ; and from the occasional alternations of its intensity during its prevalence in a town. The ultimate cessation of the epidemic throughout a country, and even a continent, the restriction of its course in crossing a continent to a tract of comparatively limited extent, furnish, perhaps, still stronger objections to the theory of contagion ; for not only are they, like most of those before mentioned, characters which diseases known to be in the strict sense contagious do not present, but they suggest the belief that the propagation of the disease cannot be maintained by any matter emanating from the bodies of the sick.

Some facts, which constitute presumptive arguments, of more or less force, in favour of the dependence of the epidemic on contagion, namely, the relation, as a general rule, borne by the numbers of the population of a town, and even of a public establishment, to the duration of the epidemic there, the successive attack of the different inmates of a house, or of the ward of a lunatic asylum, the ultimate cessation of the disease after a limited number of days in each house or ward, and the fact that, in the cases where the introduction of the disease into a locality has been traced to human intercourse, the supposed vehicle of the infection has usually been a person already suffering from the disease, or clothes or bedding which had been used by the sick in other places,—all these facts have been found susceptible of explanation in other ways; though the explanations offered have in some instances been necessarily of a conjectural nature.

With reference to two other arguments, which, if established, would only prove that Cholera is in some cases contagious, the evidence examined has been found contradictory. The frequent communication of the disease by the clothes or bedding of the sick to the persons who handle or wash them, under circumstances rendering other sources of infection than emanations received from the bodies of the sick improbable, appears to be by no means proved. The preponderance of evidence is, in fact, opposed to its occurrence. On the other hand, the evidence respecting the especial liability of nurses and others attending on the sick to suffer from Cholera, though conflicting, is, in some instances, of such a character as to preclude the absolute rejection of the view that the disease has a contagious property, even though it does not usually spread by virtue of contagion.

5. The question, whether the poison of Cholera enters the body through the lungs or through the alimentary canal, has not been conclusively solved; but no sufficient reasons have been found for adopting the theory that the poison is swallowed with the food or drink, is reproduced in the alimentary canal, and being discharged with the secretions of the stomach and intestinal canal, propagates the disease by finding access in the same vehicles to the stomachs of other persons. This theory has been found especially inconsistent with the great mass of evidence which establishes the influence of the different conditions of the atmosphere, and with nearly all those facts which would be equally opposed to any view which regards the human body as the exclusive nidus for the reproduction

of the morbific matter. So much, indeed, of the theory as attributes the extension of the disease among the inhabitants of groups of houses or of towns to the contamination of the water used for drinking or culinary purposes, undoubtedly explains very readily some facts in the history of the epidemic in London; but even this part of the theory is found to be supported by very scanty evidence, and to be contradicted by other facts, which, if they do not prove that the character of the water drunk is altogether destitute of influence with reference to the diffusion of Cholera, at least show that its power and effects are very inconsiderable in comparison with those of other conditions.

Of the six theories, then, mentioned at pages 4 and 5 of this Report, that alone is supported by a large amount of evidence which regards the cause of Cholera as a matter increasing by some process, whether chemical or organic, in impure or damp air, and assumes that, although, of course, diffused with the air, it is also distributed and diffused by means of human intercourse.

This theory explains much that would otherwise seem capricious in the course of Cholera; and it elucidates the relation subsisting between Cholera and other epidemic diseases. Severe epidemics of Cholera have sometimes been immediately preceded in the same countries or cities by the prevalence of fevers, or of diarrhœa and dysentery; and this has been made an argument in support of the vague notion of an "epidemic constitution." For it has been supposed that this epidemic influence, in the course of its development, gives rise at one time to fever or diarrhœa, and at another time to Cholera. It has been imagined, therefore, that the prevalent diarrhœa preceding Cholera resulted from the slighter action of the peculiar atmospheric influence which subsequently produced the more formidable epidemic. But it is not by any means a general rule that an increasing prevalence of diarrhœa, or of any other epidemic disease, precedes the appearance of Cholera; and the occasional association of Cholera with such diseases is capable of being otherwise explained. The fact in question, and the similarity of the local conditions favouring Cholera, and epidemic diseases generally, together with other facts examined in this Report, seem to agree best with the view that these several diseases are caused by different poisons, all of which find their means of increase in similar states of the atmosphere, though there probably are modifications of the atmospheric conditions more essential or more favourable to some of these diseases than to others.

In the statement that the theory above indicated is the only one supported by a large amount of evidence, it is not implied that this theory is adopted to the exclusion of all others. For the possibility that Cholera is occasionally communicated by a virus produced in, and emanating from, the sick, has already been admitted; and other questions relative to the means by which the cause of the disease is disseminated and its introduction into the human body effected, have been left open for further inquiry.

PREVENTIVE MEASURES.

The ultimate object of an inquiry into the subjects treated of in this Report is, of course, the discovery of the means by which the onward progress of Cholera may be stayed, its increase and diffusion moderated, and individuals protected from its attacks. The partial attainment of this object is all that at present can be hoped for; but the principles by which endeavours to attain it thus partially should be guided, are for the most part free from doubt.

From among the great features of a Cholera epidemic three stand forth as of paramount importance: one, the undoubted influence of locality and of the sanitary condition of towns and dwellings on the degree of severity with which the epidemic visits them; a second, the equally certain influence of season and temperature, together with some unknown condition of the atmosphere on the general prevalence, and rate of extension of the epidemic; and a third, the share taken by human intercourse in determining not only the progress of the epidemic, and the direction of its advance, across a continent, but also its extension from continent to continent, and most probably its communication from one town to another in the same country, and from one locality to another in the same town.

This third great feature of the disease is less generally admitted than the two others; but the question here is not whether the evidence is so complete as to compel belief, but simply whether it amounts to so great a degree of probability that it cannot wisely be neglected in the consideration of the measures to be taken for the prevention, arrest, or mitigation of a destructive pestilence.

Now, with regard to the *first* of these features of the epidemic, there cannot be a doubt with regard to the course of action which it calls for, as the duty and interest of every portion of the community. The more fortunate classes are, it is true, exposed to proportionably little danger, since they are often able to leave the neighbourhood of spots in which the disease is raging, and usually dwell in the more elevated, open, and airy parts of towns, and in more spacious and cleanly and less crowded houses.

But it is also true that the power of the disease through a town is increased in proportion to the degree in which the conditions of insalubrity referred to are present in various parts of it; and not merely the poor, who live in the spots where moisture and foul air feed the cause of the disease, but all the inhabitants, are exposed by the existence of these evils to a greater risk of becoming its victims. And further, it is certain that the more intensely the epidemic prevails in a large town, the more does the whole district for miles around suffer, and the more danger is there of its being propagated to other districts. By improving the drainage of low parts of the town, opening close courts, thinning the buildings in the more crowded parts, putting a stop to the burial of the dead in large cities, keeping even the smallest streets constantly free from filth, covering drains and sewers, and abolishing cesspools, and other sources of foulness in the air and soil; by improving the dwellings of the poor in respect of ventilation, giving them the means of maintaining a due warmth in their rooms without excluding the external air, promoting the general substitution of good water-closets for open privies, inculcating cleanly habits among the poor, and affording them that most important requisite, an abundant and constant supply of good water, by means of which they may attain cleanliness;—by adopting these measures, it cannot be doubted that the public authorities would not only lessen the ravages of the disease amongst the people dwelling in the localities thus improved, but also greatly weaken the force of the epidemic over a far wider space. All these things should be done before the pestilence comes, and in the time of its presence it would further be wise to enforce cleanliness and ventilation even in the interior of houses by a *house-to-house inspection*.

These principles seem now to be more generally understood, and happily are being more widely acted upon, than at any former period. But as public functionaries are apt to direct their efforts too exclusively to the removing evidences of dirt, and to think all must be well where the eye finds cleanliness, it may not be superfluous to call especial attention to the fact, that mere overcrowding and want of ventilation has in several instances enabled Cholera to exert its worst effects. This want of ventilation is especially common in workhouses and other pauper establishments, and in public lodging-houses, in which the number of inmates ought to be strictly limited, and in a time of pestilence reduced.

The consideration of the *second* great feature of the epidemic, teaches that the efforts to restrain and overcome it, though less obviously needed, might be more successful in the cold than in the hot season. In the winter the diffusion of the disease takes place slowly and with difficulty, human intercourse being probably, in certain states of the atmosphere, the sole means by which its propagation from place to place is effected. Hence the disease at this time gradually becomes limited to a few isolated spots; its cause exists for the most part only in the interior of inhabited buildings, and in these it ought to be attacked. Wherever cases of Cholera occur during the winter, those measures of purification, which at all times would be proper, should be put in force with the more energy, from the consideration that during this season they are likely to be attended with greater success.

Free ventilation is, perhaps, the most efficient means of destroying the Cholera poison, especially in winter, for there is reason to believe that in fresh cold air the poisonous matter soon becomes inert. The removal of all obvious dirt, and the thorough cleansing of every surface of wall, floor, or ceiling, with the unsparing application of lime and of disinfecting liquids, the washing of furniture, and the exposure of it to the open air, the destruction of foul clothes, even of those worn by inmates of the house who are yet healthy, as well as those which belonged to the sick,—all these measures might reasonably be enforced during the winter, since at that season so great a result as the entire eradication of the pestilence might possibly be attained. This result, however, can be hoped for only from the systematic adoption of such measures in all infected parts of the country simultaneously. For, if the disease be allowed to maintain itself in a single district throughout the winter and the early months of the spring, it will most probably increase there, and soon spread widely, in spite of all efforts to restrain it, in the ensuing summer; the renewed warmth and other qualities of the air more frequently attendant on a high than on a low temperature enabling the poison then to maintain its morbific power, or even to increase, in its passage through the atmosphere.

May not other means of preventing the extension of the epidemic, whether in the winter or in the summer season, be suggested by the facts relative to the share borne by human intercourse in its diffusion?

If the march of the epidemic is dependent mainly on human intercourse, and if foul ships and barges, bodies of troops, dirty vagrants, and foul clothes are the means by which the infection is most frequently carried from one country to another, and from one town to another, surely some measures might be devised which would be at the same time effectual in checking the propagation and extension of the disease, and consistent with the other great interests of society.

Quarantine can no longer be adopted as the means of preventing the entrance of Cholera into England; for it is incompatible with the present state of commercial intercourse, and with the well-being of a commercial country. Moreover, quarantine has undoubtedly often failed of its object, partly from its being evaded by the crews of infected ships; partly, perhaps, from the ships being placed so near to habitations on shore, that the infected air of the ship would be carried to them by atmospheric currents; and in some cases, probably, because clothes still containing infectious matter were conveyed on shore during, or subsequent to, the period of quarantine.

For similar reasons sanitary cordons around towns are now impracticable, and have at former periods often, though apparently not always, failed to prevent the diffusion of Cholera.

But if the ordinary regulations of quarantine and sanitary cordons are relinquished, it is the more desirable to adopt other measures which shall oppose some obstacle to the importation of Cholera, and to its propagation from one town to another in this country.

It cannot be doubted that ships are more or less fitted to convey the disease or its cause, from port to port, in proportion to their want of cleanliness, defective ventilation, and over-crowded state, and that if these evils, of which the two former are so flagrant in the smaller trading vessels, and the two latter in ships carrying passengers, could be removed, the danger of the importation of Cholera would be greatly lessened. While, therefore, it is much to be desired, on general grounds, that measures should be adopted for inculcating and enforcing attention to cleanliness and free ventilation in the whole mercantile marine, the especial application of measures of this kind to ships coming from ports where Cholera prevails, as far as may be practicable, is imperatively called for. A close inspection of all such vessels should be made on their arrival in port; and it would not be unreasonable to require that, in consideration of the restrictions of quarantine being abrogated, there should be brought with each ship coming from an infected port an official certificate of its having been inspected, and found cleanly and not overcrowded, and the crew healthy at the time of its sailing.

On the arrival of ships having persons ill of Cholera on board, or having had deaths from that disease during the voyage, more active measures must be adopted; and the best that have been recommended seem to be, the removal of the sick to a hospital ship, moored at a distance from the other shipping in the harbour, or to a special hospital in an isolated and airy situation on shore; 2, permission to the rest of the crew to land after exchanging their dress for fresh clothes provided from the shore; 3, the thorough exposure of all articles of dress and baggage to the air and disinfecting agents before they are removed from the ship; and 4, the thorough cleansing of the ship itself, with the free use of disinfecting agents in every part of it, but especially in the parts occupied by the crew and passengers, or their baggage.

If, notwithstanding such precautions as these, Cholera find its way into the country, then the low lodging-houses frequented by vagrants and the vagrant-wards of workhouses should be narrowly watched. For these especially are the places in which the disease is fostered, and whence it seems to be distributed widely to other localities. In these establishments, then, the most scrupulous cleanliness and free ventilation should be mantained, and even the personal cleanliness of the inmates, as far as possible, enforced.

When Cholera appears in the places referred to, or within dwellings of the poor, intercourse with the surrounding popu-

lation of course cannot be interdicted.   But still, it is possible
to adopt measures which would not only check the extension of
the disease among the inhabitants of the infected houses, but
greatly diminish the risk of its propagation to other localities.
Of these, the most important is the provision of spacious and
well-ventilated buildings in airy dry sites, for the reception
of the inhabitants of the infected spot, while their dwellings
are cleansed and disinfected.   These "Houses of Refuge," it
cannot be doubted, have saved many lives from destruction
by Cholera, both in this country and on the Continent.   No
considerable town should be without one ; and several should
be prepared in the environs of the larger cities.

The " Houses of Refuge " would receive the healthy, but
for those already labouring under Cholera other asylums
must be found.

There has been much difference of opinion respecting the
desirableness of establishing Cholera Hospitals.   But it surely
cannot be disputed that those struck with Cholera amongst
the poor, ought to be carried to some Hospital, if they are at
all in a fit state to be removed.   They cannot be properly treated
in their homes, and the mere change to a purer air offers them
a better chance of recovery.   Moreover, in the rooms in
which the poor are struck with Cholera, those who nurse
them, and in a less degree those who visit them, are exposed
to danger, probably not from contagion, but in most cases
from the pestiferous atmosphere of the locality; while, if the
sick are placed in the spacious and well-ventilated ward of a
Hospital, nearly all danger from approaching them is at an
end.   Wherever, therefore, General Hospitals do not exist,
or cannot afford sufficient space, Cholera Hospitals should
be established.

The buildings selected for the purpose should, if possible,
be situated in the least crowded parts of the towns or districts
in which they are needed. They should have spacious rooms,
with provisions for permitting the free circulation of air
through them ; and, during their occupation, the most strict
attention should be paid to their ventilation and cleanli-

ness: otherwise they may prove an injury rather than a benefit.

In the General Hospitals, too, the same conditions of ample space, free ventilation, and scrupulous cleanliness, are the essential requisites. If they are provided, it is probably a matter of little moment whether the Cholera patients are placed together in special wards or dispersed among the ordinary patients in the general wards of these establishments.

Whether the sick be removed to Cholera Hospitals, or to the wards of General Hospitals, it should equally be an object of care to prevent the accidental introduction of infection together with the patients, and with this object it is desirable that the clothes brought with the patients should be removed from them in a special receiving-room, and at once be either destroyed, or subjected to a disinfecting process. And even in the case of the healthy removed from infected dwellings to Houses of Refuge, care should be taken that foul clothes be not carried with them, and that the clothes they wear should as soon as possible undergo an efficient cleansing.

The propriety of adopting measures founded on the belief that human intercourse aids in the dissemination of Cholera, has been urged upon those who may still doubt the propagation of the disease in that way. And, on the same principle, other precautions, suggested by the view that the discharges from the stomach and intestines contain the Cholera poison, must here be recommended, although the theory based on that view has been found generally untenable, and, at most, susceptible of very partial application. The precautions referred to are, the immersion of the soiled linen of the patients, and subsequently of their bedding, in water to which some disinfecting liquid has been added; care that neither the food nor the drinking water can in any way be contaminated by the discharges of the patients, and especial care on the part of nurses and others about the sick to wash their hands before taking food; to which may be added, as a measure more feasible in Hospitals than in the dwellings of the poor, the placing a small quantity of a chemical decomposing liquid in all the vessels into which the discharges of the patients are received.

One other method of combating the pestilence has been proposed and partially carried into effect; namely, the house-to-house visitation of infected districts, with the view of discovering and treating all cases of diarrhœa, some of which may be presumed to be cases of Cholera in an early stage. This measure, however, is based on principles which do not properly belong to the subject of this Report. It would, therefore, be out of place here to inquire into the amount of success with which it has been attended.

APPENDIX.

TABLE I.

RACTS of COMMUNICATIONS received by the Cholera Committee relative to the Characters of Site and Sanitary Condition of various Places.

a.—Places which suffered a high rate of Mortality from Cholera.

e of place. Reporter.	Number of deaths from Cholera.	Character of Site.	Sanitary Condition.
nl Union se. Whitfield.)	9 from Cholera 4 „ Diarrhœa Reg.-Gen.	Low and damp, much of the land about it in a state of waste.	
ought ital. Blachall.)	125 (30 cases occurred on board).	Moored in the Thames, at Greenwich.	
rish Hulks Dubba.)	In 1848, 20. In 1849, 30. (Population 800.)	Moored in the Thames, near to marshes.	
g Pauper ool. r. Kite.)	140. (Number of inmates about 1000.)	Low.	Supply of water constant and abundant. Cleanliness much attended to. Drainage indifferent, drains close to building. Population dense and numerous. Ventilation imperfect.
se at South- Middlesex. Buxham.)	6 deaths (in 13 cottages).	Open, but a brickfield, and bounded on north side by a loop of the Paddington Canal.	No impurities on surface or other apparent cause, except impurity of water, taken chiefly from the Paddington canal, and great crowding of the cottages. Thirteen people, seven adults and six children, sleeping in a room 20 feet by 7 feet. Cholera ceased on tents being erected.
am and Ro- mer. Stratton in eport to Sir Burnett.)	126 deaths. (Pop. 37,616.)	Rochester and Chatham, immediately on the banks of the Medway, but low; a portion of either below high-water mark. The greater part of Chatham in the bottom of a hollow or valley, which is ventilated only when the wind is blowing in one particular direction.	The drainage and sewerage chiefly, or altogether, on surface. Every house has its open privy or cesspool. In various parts are stagnant ditches, containing large deposits of all manner of filth from the overflowing of privies and slaughter-houses. Dungheaps, commons, extensive marshes around or opposite.
d Parish ... Stratton.)	41 deaths. (Pop. about 8000)	The lower part of Strood, a long narrow street, bounded on either side by flat marshy ground below high-water mark, and in part a swamp, receiving the surface drainage of the town.	

Name of place, and of Reporter.	Number of deaths from Cholera.	Character of Site.	Sanitary Condition.
Canterbury ...... (Mr. Reid to Prov. Med. and Surg. Assoc.)	70. (Pop. 15,435.)	In a valley, a mile wide, open to the N.E. and S.W. Hills on either side of moderate height. Soil chiefly alluvial. Lower part liable to occasional inundations from the river, which occurred in the winter of 1848–1849. Meadows frequently covered with water in wet seasons.	The poor chiefly agricultural labourers. Cottages dirty. Drainage bad. Cesspools general. Water partly good, from springs; that of lower classes chiefly from wells or pumps, or directly from the river.
Margate Infirmary. (Mr. Field.)	9 deaths. (220 patients.)	Remarkably healthy. On chalk cliff close to the sea, a half mile west of Margate.	
Ilford .... (Dr. T. K. Chambers.)	57. (Pop. 4800.)	...	Sewerage formerly very imperfect. A drain through village gave out very offensive smells through gully holes. These trapped about time of outbreak of Cholera.
Southampton .... (Dr. Oke.)	240. (Pop. 34,098.)	Open and airy, where upper classes reside, and they not attacked. Charlotte Row, where the disease was violent, in a high situation detached from the town.	
Stonehouse Barracks. Royal Marines. (Dr. Millar to Sir W. Burnett.)	...	On sea level, on a peninsula running southwards between Stonehouse Pool and Millbay, with Bunker's Hill on the north. Houses on the west side of barracks. Millbay on the east.	On the west hemmed in by a dirty lane, in which the drains are bad, ashpits open, privies very defective. Population low and crowded, and in which Cholera was generally present. On south bounded by a sewer. On east Millbay, into which sewers empty themselves, and in which the waters are left in a measure at rest, and foul matters allowed to subside, forming a fetid mud. Ventilation of men's rooms in barracks defective.
Torton Barracks, Gosport. (Dr. Wilson.)	...	Occupy a low level, said to be a reclaimed marsh, somewhat swampy around. Close to the river is an arm of the sea, which is dry at low water.	Supply of water excellent. Means of ventilation and cleanliness abundant.

Name of Place and of Reporter.	Number of Deaths from Cholera.	Character of Site.	
Crosscombe, a village, near Wells. (Dr. Boyd.)	23.	A deep valley, sheltered on north, south, and partly on west by high hills, streams running through it.	
Dowlais .... (Mr. White.)	...	On the side of a hill, 800 feet above the level of the sea; the inclination of hill towards a ravine, down which flows a torrent in winter; dry in summer.	No artificial drainage. No supply of water except from scanty springs. Construction and arrangement of houses not favourable to ventilation. Population dense. Exterior of houses very filthy.
Tewkesbury...... (Dr. Viner Beadle.)	54. (Pop. 7644.)	Lies low. Entire soil alluvial. Subsoil blue lias. All the lower parts flooded several times during the winter. Water surrounding it, and extending for miles in some directions.	Mortality high, 29 in 1000. The poor live wretchedly in confined and ill-ventilated alleys, with few privies, pumps, or drains. Abominations reeking through the alleys the prevailing characteristic.
Walsall.......... .. (Dr. Burton.)	133. (Pop. 16,056.) Reg.-Gen.	Upon a limestone crop, 100 feet above a rivulet, which flows through lower part of town.	
Walsall Workhouse. (Dr. Burton.)	28.	On ascent above the town near top of a ridge. Open country around.	Exhalations from sewer through privies and untrapped drains. Rooms well-ventilated and not crowded. The number of cases of Cholera diminished after the drains were trapped.
Boston Workhouse. (Mr. Coupland.)	19.	The town on level ground, with large drains carrying off the neighbouring waters. Some parts very low and filthy.	Well-ventilated, clean, with a good dietary. The water is rain-water, but good, clear, and abundant.
Wakefield Old Prison. (Mr. Dunn and Mr. Milner.)	19. (Pop. 127.)	On a low plot of ground near a brook. Soil clay. The Old Prison on the lower portion of the ground, which is very flat and little raised above the level of the water.	Old Prison. No means of warming and ventilating it. Outlet of drains defective, always containing water, which soaked into soil on which the prison stands. Air damp. Cells cold and damp. Day-rooms crowded, privies opening into them in an objectionable state. Drains run under the building.
Wakefield Lunatic Asylum. (Dr. Wright.)	106. (Pop. 620.)	Elevated but sheltered. Soil heavy, and damp; subsoil clayey.	Dysentery frequently prevalent. General mortality high.

	Number of Deaths from Cholera.	Character of Site.	Sanitary Condition.
...land .... Brown.)	368. (Pop. 66,500.)	... ...	Water supply abundant, but great overcrowding, especially in Sunderland parish, where there is one inhabitant to three square yards. Mortality from Cholera in 1832, and from measles in 1834, greatest in Sunderland. Population crowded in ill-ventilated lanes, alleys, and small courts.
Lye Waste, village near urbridge. Norris, to vincial Med. Surg. Asso-ion.)	73 or 74. (Pop. 800 or 900.)	A soft clay soil.	Many of the cottages built of clay, rooms small, crowded, and ill-ventilated. Very little drainage. Habits uncleanly. Constant decomposition of animal and vegetable matters.
...n Harbour. . Brown.)	(Pop. 3000.)	A considerable part built on a cliff above the seashore and the harbour. Soil clay, of no great depth; below this, magnesian limestone, through which water percolates with great facility; by no means a damp place, and generally very healthy.	Its elevation secures free ventilation. Lanes and streets not narrow. Sewerage and drainage excellent. Few nuisances.
...and y, all villages. . Grieve, in report of Dr. uce to Sir W. rnett.)	During first 14 days, 13.	Low and damp, except a small portion of Cairnbulg, which lies a little higher.	Very bad, low, and damp. Water in stagnant pools. Dunghills near doors, consisting of fish refuse, with seaweed, and dirty water from the houses.
...an, Peter-d. . Robb and . Jamieson Dr. Bruce's port.)	16.	On a high level, along the verge of precipitous rocks, thoroughly pervaded by every moderate breeze.	Neither drainage nor sewerage. All the filth collected in heaps near the doors.—Dr. Jamieson. Habits and mode of living not conducive to health. Majority poor and improvident, meanly fed and clothed. Dwellings filthy, overcrowded, and ill ventilated.
...Brent ...... r. King.)	11. (Pop. 1303.)	On southern edge of Dartmoor, high, warm. No considerable deposit of fæcal or decaying vegetable matter can take place. One of the healthiest places in South Devon.	

b.—Places in which few or no Deaths from Cholera occurred.

Name of Place, and of Reporter.	Number of Deaths from Cholera.	Character of Site.	Sanitary Condition.
Deptford Dock Yard. (Dr. Bruce to Sir W. Burnett.)	2 cases amongst the labourers. 1 case amongst marines. — Dr. Bruce. 800 men employed in dockyard; 250 marines	Low, close to the Thames.	
Ashford .... (Mr. Whitfeld.)	1 death.—Reg.-Gen. (Pop. of district, 5874.)	High, and exposed to every change in the wind.	Town surveyed in reference to its sanitary condition, and many improvements made and nuisances removed.
Farnham .... (Mr. Sloman to Prov. Med. and Surg. Association.)	1 doubtful case in this town. 4 deaths at 1½ mile distant from it. (Pop. of district, 8438.)	... ...	Generally very healthy, though some localities in very unhealthy condition.
Reading district.. (Dr. Bradshaw.)	The town peculiarly bare of cases of Cholera, in most trying months singularly healthy. 17 in district. (Pop. 19,521.)	Built on a bog, surrounded by water meadows. Thames on one side, a canal on the other. Atmosphere remarkably humid.	By no means in a sanitary state as to drainage and the like.
St. Albans ...... (Dr. Lipscombe.)	8. (Pop. 10,430.)	Open, airy, with facilities for drainage.	
Teignmouth ...... (Dr. Walker.)	No cases, nor anywhere along course of the river. 2 in district. (Pop. 8766.)	Old red sandstone. Free ventilation up and down the valley of the Teign, between the sea and Dartmoor.	Drainage tolerably good.
Frome .... (Dr. Harrison.)	No case, though 3 fatal cases within 6 miles. (Pop. 12,500.)	Elevated, on rapid declivity of hill. North-eastern aspect.	Good water by wells and springs. Drainage moderately good. Houses mostly dry and wholesome, and not crowded with inhabitants. Streets generally of sufficient width. Accumulation of filth, &c. prevented.
Cheltenham ...... (Dr. Abercrombie.) (Dr. Smith.)	6. (Pop. 31,411.)	No large river or other piece of water near.—Dr. Abercrombie.	Well drained. Plenty of light pure air and water.—Dr. Smith.

	Number of Deaths from Cholera.	Character of Site.	Sanitary Condition.
Hasland.)	No death. 2 deaths in district.— Reg.-Gen. (Pop. 12,273.)	Very low. Numerous stagnant drains in its immediate neighbourhood. River impounded by hills so as to be above level of the surrounding lands. Frequent and long-continued floods.	The most favourable conditions for the attack of Cholera. No sewers. Much filth on surface. Slaughter-houses, pigsties, &c.
	No death. 1 death in district.— Reg.-Gen. (Pop. 11,751.)	The site of Stamford is on limestone, with a small river running through it. Open from east to west. A good descent from all the streets into the valley. Country unenclosed to the north.	
on,........... Fernside.)	Only 26 deaths, and 3 or 4 of these included with questionable propriety. 29 deaths in district.— Reg.-Gen. (Pop. 50,887.)	On an eminence, its elevation and exposure unfavourable to miasmatic accumulation. On north bank of Ribble, 12 miles from its mouth.	Water abundant. Less crowding in houses than in most large towns. Evil o very imperfect drainage in some degree counteracted by soil—sand. Rate of mortality 26 to 30 in 1000 annually, chiefly amongst children.
and, York-Blagborough.)	One case fatal— (Pop. 6968.)	... ...	Abundant water. Privies well cleared. All offensive matters removed, and the interior of houses whitewashed where necessary as soon as the epidemic threatened.

Places in which the Mortality from Cholera was near the average proportion for England and Wales, or is not ascertained.

	Number of Deaths from Cholera.	Character of Site.	Sanitary Condition.
ney Union rkhouse. r. Hovell.)	...	High and well drained.	
tone .... Plomley.)	38. (Pop. 18,000.)	... ...	Thousands of open cesspools and privies. Defective drainage. Insufficient supply of water.
	36. (Pop. 11,693.)	Low and marshy, scarcely 4 feet above the level of the river Ouse.	

Name of Place, and of Reporter.	Number of Deaths from Cholera.	Character of Site.	Sanitary Condition.
Stonehouse Millbay Barracks.	...	On east side of Millbay, 80 yards from the mud, and on high ground.	Eighty yards removed from the sewage mud, with a good fall for the drains. Sleeping rooms for the men large. They enjoyed a high state of exemption from Cholera as compared with Stonehouse barracks.
Exeter .... (Dr. Shapter.)	43. (Pop. 31,000.)	Good.	The larger proportion of cases occurred in the lower parts of the city, near the streams, which there traverse it. Out of 92 cases, 55 lived close by the mill-stream, into which one of the large city sewers empties itself, and which runs through the lowest part, producing dampness.
Oxford .... (Dr. Kidd.)	75. (Pop. 30,000.)	... ...	Dividing the city into two parts, an eastern and a western,—only one case (an intemperate man) occurred in the former, and all the rest, about 70 (deaths?) in the latter. This western district has a swampy soil, with scarcely any fall for drainage. This part is on clay, and is traversed by the minor streams and subdivisions of the Isis, into which the cesspools and privies are emptied; these streams are not always in a flowing state, but are sometimes dammed up by large collections of offensive matter.
Northampton ... (Mr. Bryan to Prov. Med. and Surg. Association.)	49. (Pop. 20,000 or 30,000.)	Principal part of town in an elevated position, one portion, the South-quarter, lying low, with meadows near it, which are inundated at several parts of the year. On the south-western side of the town flows the river Nen.	The "South-quarter" abounds in close, ill-ventilated courts, of which the greater number open at one end upon a foul wide ditch, and the meadows. Drainage in other parts tolerably good. Water good, from springs. The water supplied by the company was somewhat foul in 1849.
Abergavenny ... (Mr. Foote to Prov. Med. and Surg. Association.)	9 (from Diarrhœa 13). (Pop. 7256.)	Some parts situated favourably for health. Many parts built on low marshy ground.	In best parts, streets broad, but drainage only imperfect. In low parts no cleansing or drainage. Bad ventilation. Destitution.

TABLE II.

CHARACTER of the Localities most severely visited by Cholera in various Towns and other Places.

Place and Reporter.	Local Circumstances.
Wandsworth .... (Mr. Howell.)	Every case of Cholera (in Mr. Howell's practice) traced to local causes, such as impure air, imperfect drainage, or poisoned water, or the three combined.
Kensington .... (Mr. Guazzaroni.)	The great majority of cases in over-crowded badly-ventilated houses, where the drainage and supply of water was indifferent.
Waltham Green .... (Messrs. Rowe and Rowland.)	The disease was most prevalent where deficient ventilation, foul and bad water, poverty and dirt, existed. Cases of two men attacked after emptying a night-soil cart.
Hammersmith .... (Mr. Barrows.)	In two instances foul drains, in one Typhus, had prevailed a few months previous.
Marylebone; Lisson Grove Dispensary District. (Dr. M'Intyre and Dr. Miller.)	Many cases in these places noted either for damp or refuse filth, confined ventilation from faulty building, or houses imperfectly drained, or small tenements crowded with inmates.—Dr M'Intyre. Foul and ill-ventilated spots. Bad ventilation the leading feature, damp in some, ill ventilation in others. —Dr. Miller.
St. Giles' and Bloomsbury Parishes. (Dr. Reid.)	The virulence of the epidemic was concentrated in certain unclean, undrained, densely-populated, and comfortless localities. In 36 common lodging-houses.
Somers Town, St. Pancras (Mr. Eastcott.)	The worst cases in the dirtiest neighbourhoods. Squalor, confined foul air, and, above all, the crowding many persons together are predisposing causes.
Clapton Workhouse ...... (Mr. De Berdt Hovell.)	Defective ventilation, and, to a certain extent, damp. Wards crowded, and not high pitched. No cases of Cholera or Diarrhœa since the ventilation has been improved and the wards less crowded.
Buxton...................... (Mr. Hawthorn.)	In all the places the elevation is favourable, but there is no drainage; the water is bad, population dense, ventilation and cleanliness very defective. No case traced to a clean neighbourhood.
St. John's Wood .... (Mr. Tracy.)	In stables, associated with Typhus and Scarlet Fever.

Place and Reporter.	Local Circumstances.
Holloway .... (Dr. Wilkinson.)	In chief seats of Cholera, houses damp, ventilation very bad, cleanliness much neglected. Density of population in one or two streets very great.
Hackney Road, Bethnal Green, District No. 4. (Mr. Vest.)	In almost every case ventilation imperfect; effluvium from overflowing or uncovered privies; in many a drain beneath the sleeping-room. Many cases in Cul-de-Sacs; in places having drains from slaughter-houses or similar nuisances.
Hackney .... (Mr. Clarke.)	A spot known as Homerton New Town, bounded on the west by a colour factory, pouring out a fetid smoke, and on the south by the main parish sewer.
Hackney Road .... (Mr. Byles.)	All cases not traced to contagion were connected with deficient ventilation, and damp and foul air.
Islington .... (Dr. Semple.)	Malaria from bad drainage, and bad ventilation a general cause.
Shoreditch, Haggerstone District. (Mr. Hooper.)	Generally very unfavourable as regards ventilation, drainage, cleanliness, and, in many instances, no apparent cause except deficient ventilation.
Kingsland .... (Mr. Burchell.)	"There can be no doubt that damp, foul air, with bad ventilation, are favourable to the production of Cholera. I had numerous cases where such were the probable causes."
St. Olave's Union .... (Mr. Corner to Dr. King.)	*St. Olive's Parish.*—In the four streets which suffered most there is want of cleanliness, bad drainage, water, and ventilation. *St. John's Parish.*—Of seven streets, three are badly drained; in two, putrid effluvia from sewers or drains; one is dirty, one badly ventilated; in another, houses small and dirty; in two, water bad. One street is clean, but unhealthy from unknown cause. Another is a reputable street, but has a covered sewer at the back. In five out of the seven, the obvious circumstances are unfavourable.
Bermondsey .... (Mr. Jas. Paull.)	The great bulk of cases near the filthy tidal ditches, and near their entrance into the Thames.
Officers of Customs ...... (Dr. M'William.)	The Water Guard were attacked in by far the larger proportion, and those most who were exposed in merchant ships to deficient ventilation, want of all comfort, bad cooking, and irregular meals, Thames water taken up alongside of vessel, and emanations from banks of river.

Place and Reporter.	Local Circumstances.
Lewisham.................... (Mr. Haycraft.)	Cholera prevailed chiefly in two localities deficient in drainage and abounding in nuisances of every description.
Deptford .... (Dr. Bruce to Sir W. Burnett.)	The town pre-eminent for want of drainage and consequent accumulations of filth, and large proportion of labouring classes; the worst and most numerous cases were in the worst localities. Several fatal cases in one house immediately after some filthy cesspools had been cleaned out and a large quantity of their contents allowed to run over the street. Five fatal cases in a vagrant-beggars' lodging-house. Worst cases occurred wherever there were filthy exhalations and crowding.
Greenwich Hospital...... (Dr. Baith and Mr. M'Ternan to Sir W. Burnett.)	A drain of many years' accumulation was opened and emitted a pestilential stench. The mortality in that part of the establishment was great in comparison with other localities.
Woolwich Town .... (Mr. M'Donald.)	Most of cases observed by Mr. M'Donald in lodging-houses badly ventilated.
Chelmsford .... (Dr. Badeley.)	The houses were dirty and ill-ventilated, with a horrible stench from rabbits kept in the room where second case occurred.
Southend .... (Mr. Warwick.)	In no case was there any local cause to which the outbreak could be attributed.
Sheerness.................... (Mr. Cross and Mr. Smith to Sir W. Burnett.)	The majority of the cases in parts of Mile Town and Blue Town most remarkable for bad drainage, filth, crowding, and every other sanitary defect. A case on board Admiral's Tender attributed to its lying off the mouth of principal town sewer.
Brompton, Chatham, Marine Barracks. (Dr. Stratton.)	The Royal Marine Barracks are commodious and tolerably well ventilated. A good supply of water. Privies and dust-holes defective but improved. The proportion of cases in the lower or basement story was double the proportion in other parts of the Barracks; no other cause than position to account for this. The back row of rooms on this story is on a level with the ground.
Chatham .... (Dr. Stratton to Sir W. Burnett.)	The disease chiefly confined to the narrow lanes and alleys, which are crowded and deficient in cleanliness, and where Fever is always more or less prevalent, yet many of the very worst entirely escaped.
Maidstone .... (Dr. Plomley.)	Of the 30 residents who died of Cholera, 28 lived in localities with no drainage or very imperfect drainage, with no supply, or a very imperfect supply, of water. The cesspools and privies in most instances open and situated very near to the dwellings. In some cases the privies formed part of their living rooms.

Place and Reporter.	Local Circumstances.
Canterbury .... (Dr. Lochée.)	The majority of the cases were in a part of the city close to the river, where cases of insalubrity abounded.
Brighton .... (Dr. Ormerod and Dr. Cowie.)	In all the cases some unfavourable circumstances, as deficient ventilation, bad drainage, foul cesspools, accumulation of dung and refuse.—Dr. Cowie. Third, fifth, and sixth cases in dirty, ill-drained, or filthy and damp close street.—Dr. Ormerod.
Hastings .... (Dr. Mackness.)	The cases generally appeared in densely-populated badly-drained parts of the town.
Reading .... (Mr. Vines and Mr. Workman to Dr. Bradshaw.)	Of four cases attended by Mr. J. W. Workman two occurred in localities well ventilated and not densely populated. Nearly all the cases in the neighbourhood of cesspool, drain, or some such source of contamination.—Mr. Vines.
Bedford .... (Dr. Dick, and Mr. Yates & Dr. Evans.)	Ventilation and cleanliness in most of the places very bad. But Cholera did not prevail in the parts visited by Fever. One side of a street or part of a row of houses attacked, the other left free.
Winchester .... (Dr. White.)	All the cases, with one exception, occurred near the streams of river Itchen, in densely-crowded courts abounding in nuisances, the streams dammed up for the purpose of obtaining water power.
Portsmouth .... (Mr. Henderson and Mr. North to Sir W. Burnett.)	In neighbourhood of affected houses effluvium from defective cleanliness often perceived, but the disease visited houses which were situated in comparatively comfortable circumstances, and left uninjured those in the most unfavourable condition.—Mr. North. In nearly every instance where our inquiries were made, collections of vegetable and animal matter in a state of decomposition were in close approximation to the dwellings; open privies, stagnant ditches, or collections of water, crowded close neighbourhood, and bad ventilation were also obvious.—Mr. Henderson.
Southampton .... (Dr. Oke.)	Diarrhœa and Cholera most prevalent and fatal in those habitations where no attention was paid to cleanliness by the occupants, and no sewerage had been provided. Cholera broke out with fearful virulence in an assemblage of houses (Charlotte Place) in a high situation, but where the streets are narrow and dirty, houses small, pauper tenements, and without sewers. (Population 800; 40 deaths!)
Exeter .... (Dr. Shapter.)	Houses of by far the larger proportion dirty and ill-ventilated; in fact, presenting those conditions which usually predispose to malignant and fatal disease.

Place and Reporter.	Local Circumstances.
Stonehouse .... (Mr. Perry, in a Report to Dr. Milroy.)	Mr. Perry, who treated 200 cases, says " in the great majority the attack was referrible to foul air in their dwellings, or to their being employed in cleansing drains and gully-holes, or to intercourse with sick."
Torpoint .... (Dr. McClure, in a Report to Dr. Milroy.)	The disease confined to the lower classes, and to the more wretched, filthy, and worst-ventilated districts.
Plymouth .... (Dr. Rae to Sir W. Burnett.) (Mr. Eccles to Dr. Milroy.) (Dr. Yonge and Dr. Moore.)	It has prevailed fearfully in some localities in connection with crowded dirty rooms, bad air, low living, vice, and wretchedness.—Dr. Rae. The worst cases in the narrowest and dirtiest streets. —Dr. Moore. Where the worst nuisances, foul ash-pits, deficient drainage, filthy privies, and cesspools existed, there it was found that Cholera was at hand (a plan given). In the same locality, chiefly Typhoid Fever, Scarlatina, epidemic Catarrh, Diarrhœa, &c., prevail, and are more obstinate.
Torquay .... (Dr. Black, Mr. Stewart, and Mr. Jolley.)	All the cases in a locality of which the drainage is very bad.—Dr. Black. Places badly drained and ill ventilated.—Mr. Stewart and Mr. Jolly.
Oxford .... (Dr. Kidd, Mr. T. Allen.)	Speedwell Street was remarkable for violence and concentration of the Cholera outbreak, and for its apparent freedom from those unfavourable circumstances which are usually observed in the haunts of the disease ; but the western district, in which nearly all the cases occurred, was badly drained, and the inhabitants inattentive to domestic cleanliness ; it, in this and other respects, contrasting with the eastern district. In the streams running through the western district are accumulations of matter, choking them up, and exhaling fetid odours. One of the streams nearly dry with pools of sewer matters. Privies and pigsties numerous.
Swansea .... (Dr. G. G. Bird and Mr. Michael.)	Close crowded courts, streets where drainage was absolutely or almost entirely wanting. Offal of every description in the streets. Gutters filled with stagnant water. Houses dirty, and crowded with small apertures for light and air. Sleeping-rooms with no provision for ventilation. Such were almost universally the places in which the cases of Cholera occurred.
Wells .... (Mr. Livett.)	The individual habitations all more or less confined and ill ventilated, but nothing of a general nature in the neighbourhood likely to have caused the disease.

Place and Reporter.	Local Circumstances.
Gloucester .... (Mr. Hicks.)	Principal localities, " Sweet-briars," badly drained.
Tewkesbury............... (Dr. Viner Beadle.)	Most fatal in ill-ventilated, ill-drained, and lowest parts, with no privies or drains save the common gutter (instances are given).
Holyhead .... (Rev. C. Williams and Mr. Walthew.)	Great severity of disease, limited to a rather narrow spot, on a very low level. No other apparent local cause.
Bridgenorth .... (Dr. Strange.)	In almost every case some special circumstances as to filth, bad drainage, &c. In several are open gratings of a drain before the door or window.
Stockport .... (Dr. Rayner.)	The greater comparative mortality in certain situations shows that intemperance, impure air, low, damp situations, accumulations of filth and decomposing animal and vegetable matters, predispose to the epidemic, and add to severity of the disease.
Manchester .... (Dr. Pincoff.)	Localities tolerably well drained, but as bad as possible as regards supply of water, density of population, ventilation, and cleanliness.
Chorlton upon Medlock.. (Dr. Pincoff.)	Elevation, drainage, supply of water, and density of population favourable, though in two or three of the infected localities the cleanliness was deficient.
Bolton .... (Dr. Black, Mr. Snape, and Mr. Livy.)	All parts of the town became affected, and frequently the (apparently) most healthy places.—Dr. Black. Deficient ventilation, damp, and foul air have appeared to exert little influence.—Mr. Snape. All the cases under my observation, with two exceptions, in midst of bad drainage, insufficient ventilation, and filth.—Mr. Livy.
Liverpool .... (Dr. Dickinson, Dr. Burgess, and Mr. Taylor.) The Workhouse	The disease confined for most part to the worst-ventilated, low, and ill-ventilated (drained?) courts. The worst-ventilated, damp, and overcrowded lodging-houses sometimes alone attacked. The establishment cleanly and well ventilated.
Preston..................... (Dr. Fearnside.)	In many instances (some cited) the local causes were such as must have predisposed to Cholera.
Lancaster .... (Mr. J. J. Harrison.)	Streets generally confined, ill drained, and dirty, in which fatal cases occurred. Some lines of streets in the best localities escaped, though no large portion of the town was exempt.

Place and Reporter.	Local Circumstances.
Boston .... (Mr. Clegg.)	Cases in the town confined to the filthiest parts.
Hull .... (Dr. Sandwith.)	Limited to ill-drained localities at first, but on its acquiring greater malignancy, not one street in the town unvisited by it.
Hedon .... (Dr. Sandwith.)	Several cases in different parts of the town at a distance from the drains.
Wakefield.................. (Mr. Statter and Dr. Wright.)	The part where Cholera was most prevalent and fatal was a low, close, dirty street, of bad repute in all respects, full of depôts of filth and manure, without any sewerage, and with few surface drains. After these streets were cleansed the disease subsided. With one or two exceptions, all persons attacked lived in cottages. No instance in which the residence of those attacked was in perfectly healthy situation, though thousands of people in similar and less favourable localities escaped.
Wakefield Prison .... (Messrs. Dunn and Milner.)	Cases confined to the Old Prison. Diarrhœa there in larger proportion than in other parts of the establishment (see sanitary condition and site).
Wakefield Town .... (Mr. Statter.)	In a village three miles from the town eight deaths occurred amongst 150 inhabitants, in eight or nine days; here animal and vegetable rubbish abounded, and when these were removed no more Cholera occurred.
Wakefield Lunatic Asylum. (Dr. Wright.)	The greatest proportions of victims to Cholera (amongst the women) was in No. 1, 14, and 13 Wards, the two former very clean and orderly wards, and the last not particularly the reverse. In Male Wards, Cholera was most rife in Wards 3, 1, and 4, and in the basement story of men's eastern wing of old building; No. 3 is one of the receiving wards for dirty and refractory patients. It is on the ground floor. In the three other wards the chief appearance of ammoniacal vapour was detected. No. 4 was used as a Cholera Hospital at that time. No proportionate manifestation of noxious exhalation was remarked in other wards fatally visited by Cholera, and as many perished in No. 5 and in No. 6, where the ventilation is unexceptionable as in No. 1.
Rotherham .... (Dr. Shearman.)	Nowhere but in places notoriously filthy, ill ventilated, and not drained.
Sunderland .... (Dr. Brown.)	The disease spread, as a general rule, more in the dirtier localities, but dirt is not essential to the diffusion of the disease.

TABLE III.—State of the Wind and the Mortality from Cholera in Paris from the 19th of March to the 30th of September, 1849.

Months.	Days of Month.	No. of days with each state of wind.	Prevailing direction of the wind.	Average daily No. of deaths from Cholera.
March ...	19th to 27th	9	North and north-east, strong wind on 20th and 23rd.	41·3
March ... April ...	28th to 9th ......}	13	South, south-west, and south-east	81·2
,,	10th to 12th	◡	North-west, strong wind on 11th	74·6
,,	13th to 15th	3	South-south-west, south, and south-south-east	83
,,	16th to 18th		North and north-west . .	79·6
,,	19th	1	South-east, strong wind . .	63
,,	20th and 21st	2	North-east	60·5
,,	22nd to 29th	⌒	South and south-west .	51·5
April ... May	30th to 2nd ......{	3	North-east	77
,,	3rd to 5th		South-east	104·3
,,	6th to 12th	,	Variable	169·1
,,	13th to 23rd	11	South and south-west, strong wind on 14th (north-west on 19th).	157·3
,,	24th		North-east	127
,,	25th to 29th		South, south-east, and south-west	103·8
,,	30th		East, north-east . .	124
,,	31st	▲	South, south-east . .	151
June......	1st to 3rd	3	South and south-west .	259·6
,,	4th	1	East	454
,,	5th and 6th	2	South and south-west .	560
,,	7th to 11th	5	North, north-west, and west .	640·6
,,	12th to 15th	⁖	North, north-east, and east .	367·5
,,	16th and 17th	2	West and west-north-west . .	214
,,	18th	ˋ	South-south-east . .	189
,,	19th to 22nd	.	South-west and west-north-west .	122·2

TABLE III.—*continued*.

Months.	Days of Month.	No. of days with each state of wind.	Prevailing direction of the wind.	Average daily No. of deaths from Cholera.
June...	23rd to 25th	3	South and south-east . . .	74
„	26th to 28th		West and north-west . . .	55
„	29th	1	South-east	47
June... July...	30th and 1st ...... }	2	North	42
„	2nd to 5th		South-west and west, strong wind on 3rd.	26·2
„	6th and 7th	2	South-east	30
„	8th	1	South-south-west	28
„	9th	1	West-north-west	18
„	10th to 16th		North-east and east, strong wind on the 12th, 13th, and 14th.	32·4
July... August	17th to 2nd ...... }	17	West and south-west, strong wind on the 18th, 19th, and 25th.	28
„	3rd	1	West-north-west	27
„	4th and 5th	2	East	22
„	6th	1	North-north-west	21
„	7th	.	East-north-east	33
„	8th to 18th	11	South and west, and south-west, strong wind on 13th.	51·5
„	19th	.	North-north-west	53
„	20th to 25th	6	North and north-east, west on 24th	47·1
„	26th to 31st	^	South and south-west . . .	45
Sept...	1st to 6th	6	Variable, south-east, south-west, north-east, and south.	70·1
„	7th to 9th	3	Variable, north, and north-east, and north-west.	63·6
„	10th to 14th	5	South and south-west . . .	45·2
„	15th to 22nd	8	East and north-east (on 19th north-north-west).	26
„	23rd to 27th	5	South-east	10
„	28th to 30th	3	Variable, west, south, and south-west, strong wind on 30th.	7

TABLE IV.—Showing the Monthly Mortality from Cholera, and the average

Months.	London. 1832.		London. 1849.		Paris. 1832.		Paris. 1849.		Liverpool. 1849.		Berlin. 1831.	
	Mean monthly temperature.	Deaths from Cholera.	Mean monthly temperature.	Deaths from Cholera.	Mean monthly temperature.	Deaths from Cholera.	Mean monthly temperature.	Deaths from Cholera.	Mean monthly temperature.	Deaths from Cholera.	Mean monthly temperature.	Deaths from
January ...	36·5	...	40·1	292	34·70	-	41·54	?	40·5	5	40·35	...
February..	39·0	57	43·2	180	38·12		43·70	?	44·0	7	33·35	...
March......	41·0	880	42·5	40	42·08	~0	43·16	573	43·2	18	39·06	...
April	52·0	335	43·2	9	51·24	12733	47·66	1929	43·8	19	52·45	...
May	55·5	50	54·0	24	55·76	811	59·90	4509	53·8	96	54·45	...
June	61·0	194	57·9	279	63·14	868	65·12	8669	57·1	424	60·35	...
July	60·5	1363	62·1	2555	67·10	2573	64·94	865	59·9	1085	67·30	...
August ...	63·5	1198	62·9	5368	69·44	969	65·12	1382	60·1	1575	65·61	2
September.	58·0	670	58·8	5031	59·90	357	60·98	1142	57·2	874	55·87	577
October ...	55·5	336	51·1	337	52·34	~2	53·62	115	48·8	62	53·29	562
November.	45·5	27	44·1	20	42·06		43·84	?	45·9	2	37·55	133
December .	42·0		39·1	2	39·74		39·20		39·9	6	34·92	14

...ature in the corresponding months in several Epidemics in several Cities and Towns.

		1849.		Cologne. 1849.		Stockholm. 1834.		Malmö.		St. Petersburg.	Deaths from Cholera.		Moscow.	
Mean monthly temperature.	Deaths from Cholera.	Mean monthly temperature.	Deaths from Cholera.	Mean monthly temperature.	Deaths from Cholera.	Mean monthly temperature.	Deaths from Cholera.	Mean monthly temperature.	Deaths from Cholera.	Mean monthly temperature.	1848	1849	Mean monthly temperature.	Deaths from Cholera.
32·02	...	48·58	...	33·89	...	25·55	...	...	...	14·68	...	487	...	...
32·52	...	36·99	...	41·51	...	32·59	...	...	...	18·61	...	206	...	...
32·71	...	42·55	...	39·87	...	33·69	...	...	...	25·13	...	358	...	...
42·76	...	52·61	...	47·43	...	38·84	...	...	...	36·63	...	554	...	...
39·67	...	56·43	...	58·61	...	49·71	...	...	...	47·79	...	710	...	...
41·61	...	66·57	...	63·21	...	58·29	...	58·19	...	59·18	...	673	...	...
45·30	...	65·59	2	66·07	92	67·94	...	61·03	...	63·13	...	1	64·1	...
67·03	942	68·14	261	61·86	259	61·16	169	61·01	193	60·62	...	1	62·6	...
56·28	1167	56·77	878	58·98	610	52·01	3416	51·32	151	51·01	...	1	54·7	101
50·02	141	51·69	360	50·74	203	43·57	52	42·58	34	41·34	175	...	41·9	2989
40·03	16	39·45	39	39·85	10	33·38	7	36·17	...	30·40	666	...	29·3	1295
32·90	...	...	...	33·08	...	30·04	21	...	...	22·60	580	...	18·95	1

TABLE V.—Showing the number of Deaths registered as caused by Cholera in England, the Metropolis, and the several Counties, and equivalent Registration Divisions of England, during each month, from July, 1848, to April, 1849.

	July.	August.	September.	October.	November.	December.	January.	February.	March.	April.	7 Months October to April.
ENGLAND	...	...	...	325	336	400	658	371	302	107	
London	66	64	31	122	217	139	292	180	40	9	969
Middlesex (exclusive of the Metropolitan districts.)	3	8	3	16	9	1	8	2	1	...	37
Surrey	...	...	1	3	...	...	3	2	...	1	9
Kent	6	7	4	6	6	10	9	1	1	2	35
Sussex	1	4	2	1	1	1	...	1	...	...	4
Hampshire	4	3	6	5	3	5	2	4	4	...	24
Berkshire	...	1	1	1	2	5	6	...	...	...	14
Hertfordshire	...	2	2	2	3	10	23	6	8	...	63
Buckinghamshire	1	1	4	1	17	30	3	2	1	...	54
Oxfordshire	...	...	1	1	2	...	...	...	...	...	3
Northamptonshire	3	4	2	...	1	2	...	1	2	1	7
Huntingdonshire	1	1	...	1	...	1	...	1	...	...	3
Bedfordshire	1	1	1	4	1	2	1	...	...	1	9
Cambridgeshire	...	5	3	8	8	20	5	1	2	...	44
Essex	2	1	2	4	1	6	7	5	2	...	25
Suffolk	1	2	1	4	3	3	5	1	...	1	17
Norfolk	...	2	6	6	2	5	38	9	1	1	63
Wiltshire	1	...	1	2	1	1	1	2	...	...	7
Dorsetshire	...	...	...	1	...	...	1	...	...	...	2
Devonshire	4	4	8	6	2	4	3	1	3	3	22
Cornwall	1	2	10	2	4	1	1	1	...	1	10
Somersetshire	1	...	1	...	2	2	...	...	1	1	6
Gloucestershire	...	5	...	2	1	2	4	1	1	1	12
Herefordshire	...	1	...	...	...	...	...	...	...	...	...
Shropshire	1	1	2	...	...	...	3	3	1	2	9
Staffordshire	2	7	5	2	5	3	1	...	...	1	12
Worcestershire	...	2	1	5	...	...	...	1	...	...	6
Warwickshire	3	9	8	2	5	5	5	1	1	2	21
Leicestershire	6	6	2	...	...	3	1	...	1	1	6
Rutlandshire	...	...	...	1	...	...	...	...	...	...	1
Lincolnshire	5	2	2	3	14	8	1	3	...	1	30
Nottinghamshire	2	1	...	4	2	1	1	1	3	...	12
Derbyshire	2	1	...	3	...	1	1	...	2	...	7
Cheshire	3	8	4	13	2	...	1	1	...	1	18
Lancashire	49	33	27	22	10	20	15	12	28	29	136
West Riding	18	20	23	18	16	19	48	13	8	7	129
East Riding	3	3	7	30	5	1	13	4	1	3	57
North Riding	2	4	2	1	1	2	1	...	...	...	5
Durham	3	7	6	11	16	21	50	67	149	16	330
Northumberland	...	2	1	5	18	42	62	31	38	18	214
Cumberland	4	3	3	1	2	6	35	7	2	3	56
Westmoreland	...	...	...	...	...	...	...	...	...	...	...
Monmouthshire	1	2	...	...	...	...	1	...	...	...	1
South Wales	3	1	3	5	1	4	2	5	1	1	19
North Wales	...	2	1	1	3	4	2	...	...	...	10

LE VI.—Showing the Number of Deaths registered as caused by Cholera in gland, London, and the several Counties during each month from May, 1849, to cember, 1849, and the proportional mortality from Cholera during the year 1849.

	May.	June.	July.	August.	September.	October.	November.	December.	Eight months.	Population, Census 1851.	Deaths from Cholera per 10,000 persons in each county during the entire year 1849.
	327	9046	7879	15,572	20,379	4684	844	163	51,805	17,961,768	30
on	24	279	2555	5368	5031	337	20	2	13616	2,362,236	72
lesex	2	3	99	134	135	21	3	...	397	150,606	29
y	...	4	35	167	91	12	1	...	250	202,521	14
	5	15	165	507	440	68	...	...	1195	485,021	27
x	...	18	46	71	194	22	1	2	354	336,844	12
pshire	2	8	668	360	170	20	3	...	1229	405,370	35
shire	...	4	16	66	32	25	1	...	144	170,065	8
	...	1	9	61	123	64	23	5	286	167,298	20
inghamshire	2	1	5	81	51	30	...	...	170	163,723	13
dahire	...	1	2	21	63	27	1	...	115	170,439	7
	...	3	1	6	36	66	24	...	136	212,380	7
	3	...	...	2	2	2	2	3	14	64,183	3
	...	...	1	7	28	24	11	...	71	124,478	6
ridgeshire	1	1	3	40	146	51	17	...	259	185,405	16
hire	...	5	127	108	57	12	2	4	315	254,221	13
	...	13	19	26	47	11	2	...	118	184,207	7
	4	74	274	943	819	221	15	2	2352	567,098	7
wall	...	3	70	360	342	94	21	1	831	355,558	4
	28	32	34	165	287	192	168	21	927	443,916	8
	1	5	33	151	324	41	1	1	557	369,318	18
	1	10	3	17	39	2	1	...	73	337,215	3
	3	...	2	23	90	54	2	...	173	442,714	5
	29	148	286	390	501	94	10	2	1460	458,805	37
	...	...	...	...	1	...	...	...	1	115,489	·1
	...	1	37	133	115	14	...	2	302	229,341	13
	...	5	44	364	1614	560	75	9	2671	608,716	51
	...	2	17	27	198	120	50	17	431	276,926	19
	...	2	15	39	180	41	3	1	281	475,013	7
	...	1	1	5	3	3	2	2	17	230,308	·8
	...	...	...	2	5	...	...	...	7	22,983	4
	4	2	5	206	135	8	6	...	366	407,222	10
inghamshire	1	1	2	22	39	32	19	16	132	270,427	5
yshire	2	3	3	6	17	14	1	...	46	296,084	2
hire	3	46	170	142	225	57	6	2	651	455,725	13
shire	111	574	1453	2544	2745	589	63	14	8098	2,031,236	48
Riding	4	36	68	738	2281	776	143	36	4082	1,325,495	35
Riding	2	2	112	514	1405	82	2	1	2120	257,288	97
h Riding	1	2	3	11	20	5	...	1	43	215,214	3
	20	83	66	189	666	288	35	14	1361	390,997	51
humberland	5	...	13	207	672	303	60	1	1261	303,568	53
berland	1	1	3	97	148	104	18	1	373	195,492	24
moreland	...	...	...	...	...	...	...	...		58,287	2
monthshire	6	74	94	892	172	22	16	...	776	177,130	52
h Wales	63	577	966	1241	575	102	16	3	3543	607,456	67
h Wales	...	6	41	39	113	43	...	...	242	404,328	6

TABLE VII.—Deaths from Cholera and Diarrhœa together in England, London, and the several Counties, in each month of the year 1849.

	January.	February.	March.	April.	May.	June.	July.	August.	September.	October.	November.	December.	The Year.
ENGLAND .	1468	1069	1010	773	1048	2972	9694	19471	25307	6898	1715	755	721908
London . .	446	366	146	99	127	428	3239	6861	6043	632	127	71	18606
Middlesex .	18	10	5	3	7	10	112	175	202	37	9	7	595
Surrey . .	9	7	7	5	5	9	46	132	134	23	8	10	466
Kent . .	38	11	10	14	17	37	201	629	621	115	14	8	1715
Sussex . .	19	14	13	8	10	37	66	190	271	60	10	6	634
Hampshire .	21	18	14	13	16	21	740	445	259	58	15	10	1630
Berkshire .	22	10	9	11	5	13	24	88	56	40	12	8	392
Hertfordshire .	29	13	16	5	8	6	16	71	155	84	36	9	446
Buckinghamsh.	8	11	5	3	5	2	19	92	73	46	6	9	279
Oxfordshire .	9	6	6	5	6	8	6	27	91	38	7	12	221
Northamptonsh.	6	9	9	2	1	15	7	14	56	99	37	...	204
Huntingdonsh.	1	2	1	1	8	2	3	4	10	6	7	12	48
Bedfordshire .	5	3	5	4	7	2	1	18	52	41	16	5	159
Cambridgeshire	12	13	7	10	11	6	13	52	189	72	23	10	418
Essex . .	19	10	11	5	7	17	59	210	412	105	12	8	576
Suffolk . .	20	12	11	17	14	19	18	45	98	25	12	10	296
Norfolk . .	53	21	16	10	13	17	20	55	165	84	15	12	481
Wiltshire .	17	9	10	9	9	15	154	128	89	27	5	16	498
Dorsetshire .	6	1	2	3	2	17	27	38	60	17	5	4	182
Devonshire .	14	15	16	17	23	93	311	1010	908	269	28	18	2732
Cornwall .	9	4	6	5	6	8	81	336	370	110	28	11	974
Somersetshire .	22	16	13	23	46	55	49	226	371	236	189	38	1284
Gloucestershire	17	24	17	24	53	177	318	454	606	141	26	21	1578
Herefordshire .	2	1	2	...	1	3	2	6	4	5	2	1	29
Shropshire .	9	12	12	8	10	10	48	148	133	22	5	9	426
Staffordshire .	43	46	40	39	41	45	86	459	1877	726	125	43	3575
Worcestershire	12	7	9	13	6	10	29	50	262	143	69	30	639
Warwickshire .	35	21	20	38	25	33	64	179	392	146	47	30	1030
Leicestershire .	7	2	12	6	14	8	10	27	40	31	10	4	171
Rutlandshire .	2	...	...	1	...	...	1	3	5	1	...	3	16
Lincolnshire .	17	14	17	15	19	18	20	241	189	38	18	11	617
Nottinghamsh.	8	10	12	4	4	20	19	71	106	64	32	23	375
Derbyshire .	6	6	10	4	7	11	15	21	54	26	4	5	168
Cheshire .	13	14	17	10	22	70	208	225	347	101	23	18	1068
Lancashire .	135	133	181	157	258	790	2049	3414	3569	986	206	96	11974
West Riding .	109	63	49	53	58	96	174	939	2702	1033	260	76	5612
E. R. with York	18	11	6	15	11	11	142	573	1626	138	18	10	2577
North Riding .	8	2	5	4	4	4	6	14	39	10	7	7	110
Durham . .	65	76	169	31	33	96	86	255	777	355	50	29	2022
Northumberland	77	38	45	31	11	8	29	248	752	349	87	4	1677
Cumberland .	43	12	7	6	7	8	19	122	171	119	21	9	544
Westmoreland	1	2	...	4	1	1	2	1	3	2	1	...	18
Monmouthshire	10	8	10	4	19	88	101	403	197	31	27	4	902
South Wales .	23	27	22	28	89	612	1007	1294	639	146	51	17	3955
North Wales .	5	9	10	6	3	15	47	48	136	56	4	6	345

DEVONSHIRE.

Districts.	Sub-Districts.	CHOLERA.										
		1848.			1849.							
		Oct.	Nov.	Dec.	Jan.	Feb.	March.	April.	May.	June.	July.	August.
Axminster . .	Lyme . . .											
	Axminster . .									1		
	Chard-tock .											
	Colyton . .											
Honiton . .	Honiton . .											1
	Ottery St. Mary											
St. Thomas .	East Budleigh .					1						
	Exmouth . .											1
	Woodbury . .											
	Broad Clist .											
	Topsham . .											
	Heavitree . .											1
	St. Thomas .											
	Alphington .											
	Christow . .										1	
	Kenton . .											1
Exeter . .	2 Sub-districts			1	1		1		1			13
Newton Abbot .	Teignmouth .						1					
	Chudleigh . .										1	
	Moreton Hampstead											
	Ashburton .											
	Newton Abbot .											2
	Torquay . .											
Totnes . .	Paington . .											
	Brixham . .											
	Dartmouth .											
	Totnes . .										1	
	Buckfastleigh .											
	Ugborough (South Brent).										5	7
	Harberton .											
Kingsbridge .	Blackauton .											
	Stokenham .											
	West Allington											
	Kingsbridge .	1		1								
	Modbury . .											1
Plympton St. Mary	Yealmpton .								3	52	9	20
	Plympton . .	1								6	11	14
Plymouth . .	2 Sub-districts	3	2	1	1					14	151	294
East Stonehouse .	East Stonehouse .			1	1		1	2			43	78
Stoke Damerel .	Devonport (3 sub-districts).										24	282
	Stoke Damerel (2 sub-districts).										26	151
Tavistock . .	Buckland Monachorum.							1			2	61
	Tavistock . .											6
	Milton Abbot											
	Lifton . .										1	

DEVONSHIRE.

CHOLERA 1849					DIARRHŒA 1849													Sub-Districts.
Sept.	Oct.	Nov.	Dec.	12 months	Jan.	Feb.	March	April	May	June	July	August	Sept.	Oct.	Nov.	Dec.	12 months	
.	.	.	.	.	.	.	.	.	.	.	.	.	.	.	.	.	.	Lyme.
.	.	.	.	1	.	.	.	1	.	1	.	.	.	1	.	.	3	Axminster.
.	.	.	.	.	.	.	.	.	.	.	.	.	.	.	.	.	.	Chardstock.
.	.	.	.	.	.	.	1	.	1	.	.	.	.	.	.	.	2	Colyton.
4	.	.	.	5	.	.	1	.	.	1	2	.	1	.	.	.	5	Honiton.
.	1	.	.	.	.	.	.	.	.	1	.	.	.	.	.	.	1	Ottery St. Mary.
1	.	.	.	2	.	.	.	.	.	.	1	.	.	1	.	.	1	East Budleigh.
.	1	.	.	2	.	.	.	1	1	.	.	1	1	1	2	1	8	Exmouth.
1	.	.	.	1	.	.	.	.	.	1	.	.	.	.	.	.	1	Woodbury.
.	.	.	.	.	.	.	.	.	.	.	.	.	.	.	.	.	.	Broad-Clist.
.	.	.	.	.	.	.	.	.	.	.	.	.	.	.	.	.	.	Topsham.
2	1	.	.	4	.	.	.	.	.	.	.	2	1	1	.	.	4	Heavitree.
4	2	1	.	8	.	.	1	1	.	.	.	1	2	1	.	1	7	St. Thomas.
.	.	.	.	.	.	.	.	.	.	.	.	2	1	2	.	.	4	Alphington.
.	.	.	.	1	1	.	.	.	.	.	.	2	.	.	.	.	3	Christow.
.	2	.	.	3	.	.	.	.	.	.	.	.	.	.	.	.	.	Kenton.
15	15	.	.	47	1	2	.	.	5	1	7	5	12	3	.	.	36	Exeter.
2	1	.	.	3	.	.	1	.	.	1	1	4	1	1	.	.	9	Teignmouth.
1	1	.	.	3	.	.	1	.	.	.	.	.	.	.	.	.	1	Chudleigh.
.	.	.	.	.	.	.	.	.	.	.	.	1	.	.	.	1	2	Moreton Hampstead.
2	.	.	.	2	.	.	.	.	.	.	.	1	1	.	.	1	2	Ashburton.
.	2	1	.	6	.	.	.	.	1	1	.	2	4	2	.	1	11	Newton Abbot.
45	25	.	.	72	1	2	.	1	1	.	1	2	4	1	.	2	15	Torquay.
.	.	.	.	.	.	.	.	.	.	1	.	.	2	.	.	.	4	Paignton.
17	50	7	1	75	.	.	.	.	.	.	.	1	1	4	2	1	8	Brixham.
.	.	.	.	.	.	.	1	.	.	.	1	1	1	2	1	.	7	Dartmouth.
6	12	.	.	20	.	.	.	1	.	.	.	.	.	1	.	.	1	Totnes.
.	.	.	.	.	.	.	.	.	.	.	.	.	1	.	.	1	Buckfastleigh.
.	.	.	.	12	.	.	.	.	.	.	.	.	1	.	.	1	Ugborough.
.	.	.	.	.	.	.	1	.	.	.	.	.	.	.	.	.	1	Harberton.
1	2	.	.	3	.	.	.	.	.	.	.	.	.	.	.	.	.	Blackauton.
.	.	1	.	1	.	.	.	.	.	.	.	.	.	.	.	.	.	Stokenham.
.	.	.	.	.	.	.	1	1	1	.	.	.	.	.	.	.	3	West Allington.
.	.	.	.	2	.	.	.	.	.	.	.	.	.	.	.	.	.	Kingsbridge.
10	3	.	.	13	.	.	.	.	.	.	.	2	2	.	.	.	4	Modbury.
16	7	.	.	105	.	.	.	.	.	.	1	.	3	.	.	.	4	Yealmpton.
11	.	.	.	46	1	.	.	1	.	.	.	.	.	.	.	.	2	Plympton.
364	.	.	.	740	1	.	.	1	3	6	8	8	6	8	4	4	41	Plymouth.
27	.	.	.	172	.	1	.	.	.	1	1	3	3	.	.	.	9	East Stonehouse.
173	7	.	.	486	2	.	2	2	1	1	5	16	11	4	2	1	47	Devonport.
58	8	.	.	324	.	.	.	2	2	.	5	1	5	2	1	.	18	Stoke Damerel.
15	2	.	.	81	2	1	.	.	.	1	1	1	5	1	.	12	Buckland Monachorum.
41	.	.	.	65	.	.	.	.	1	.	1	1	1	.	.	3	Tavistock.
1	.	.	.	8	.	.	.	.	1	.	.	.	.	.	.	1	Milton Abbot.
.	.	1	.	2	.	.	.	.	.	.	.	.	.	.	.	.	Lifton.

TABLE VIII.

DEVONSHIRE.

Districts.	Sub-Districts.	1848.			1849.							
		Oct.	Nov.	Dec.	Jan.	Feb.	March	April	May	June	July	August
Okehampton	Bratton Clovelley	·	·	·	·	·	·	·	·	·	·	·
	Hatherleigh	·	·	·	·	·	·	·	·	·	·	·
	Okehampton	·	·	·	·	·	·	·	·	·	·	·
	Chagford	·	·	·	·	·	·	·	·	1	·	·
	North Tawton	·	·	·	·	·	·	·	·	·	·	·
Crediton	Morchard Bishop	·	·	·	·	·	·	·	·	·	·	·
	Bow	·	·	·	·	·	·	·	·	·	·	·
	Crediton	·	·	·	·	·	·	·	·	·	·	·
	Cheriton Fitzpaine	·	·	·	·	·	·	·	·	·	·	·
Tiverton	Silverton	·	·	·	·	·	·	·	·	·	·	·
	Cullompton	·	·	·	·	·	·	·	·	·	·	·
	Uffculme	·	·	·	·	·	·	·	·	·	·	·
	Tiverton	·	·	·	·	·	·	·	·	·	·	·
	Washfield	·	·	·	·	·	·	·	·	·	·	·
	Bampton	·	·	·	·	·	·	·	·	·	·	·
	Dulverton	·	·	·	·	·	·	·	·	·	·	·
South Molton	Witheridge	·	·	·	·	·	·	·	·	·	·	·
	Chulmleigh	·	·	·	·	·	·	·	·	·	·	·
	South Molton	·	·	·	·	·	·	·	·	·	·	·
Barnstaple	Barnstaple	·	·	·	·	·	·	·	·	1	·	3
	Paracombe	·	·	·	·	·	·	·	·	·	·	·
	Combmartin	·	·	·	·	·	·	·	·	·	·	·
	Ilfracombe	·	·	·	·	·	·	·	·	·	·	·
	Braunton	·	·	·	·	·	·	·	·	·	·	3
	Bishop's Tawton	·	·	·	·	·	·	·	·	·	·	·
Torrington	High Bickington	·	·	·	·	·	·	·	·	·	·	·
	Winkleigh	·	·	·	·	·	·	·	·	·	·	·
	Dolton	·	·	·	·	·	·	·	·	·	·	·
	Shebbear	·	·	·	·	·	·	·	·	·	·	·
	Great Torrington	·	·	·	·	·	·	·	·	·	·	·
Bideford	Bideford	·	·	·	·	·	·	·	·	·	·	·
	Northam	1	·	·	·	·	·	·	·	·	·	·
	Parkham	·	·	·	·	·	·	·	·	·	·	·
	Hartland	·	·	·	·	·	·	·	·	·	·	·
	Bradworthy	·	·	·	·	·	·	·	·	·	·	·
Holsworthy	Milton Damerel	·	·	·	·	·	·	·	·	·	·	·
	Holsworthy	·	·	·	·	·	·	·	·	·	·	·
	Black Torrington	·	·	·	·	·	·	·	·	·	·	·
	Broadwoodwidger	·	·	·	·	·	·	·	·	·	·	2
	Clawton	·	·	·	·	·	·	·	·	·	·	·
Number of deaths from Cholera and from Diarrhœa respectively in each month		6	2	4	3	1	2	3	4	75	274	941
Number of places in which deaths from Cholera occurred during each month		5	1	4	3	1	2	2	3	7	11	19
Number of places in which deaths occurred, whether from Cholera or from Diarrhœa, in each month		·	·	·	10	13	10	14	13	16	18	31

—continued.

DEVONSHIRE.

CHOLERA. 1849.					DIARRHŒA. 1849.													Sub-Districts.
Sept.	Oct.	Nov.	Dec.	12 months.	Jan.	Feb.	March.	April.	May.	June.	July.	August.	Sept.	Oct.	Nov.	Dec.	12 months.	
14	.	.	.	14	.	.	.	.	.	.	.	.	1	.	.	.	1	Bratton Clovelley.
4	.	.	.	4	.	.	.	.	.	.	.	.	.	.	.	.	.	Hatherleigh.
.	.	.	.	.	.	.	.	.	.	.	.	.	.	.	.	.	.	Okehampton.
.	.	.	.	1	.	.	.	.	.	.	1	.	.	.	.	.	1	Chagford.
.	.	.	.	.	.	.	.	.	.	.	.	.	.	.	.	.	.	North Tawton.
.	.	.	.	.	.	.	.	.	.	.	.	.	.	.	.	.	.	Morchard Bishop.
.	.	.	.	.	.	.	.	.	.	.	.	.	.	.	.	.	.	Bow.
.	.	.	.	.	.	.	.	.	.	.	.	.	.	5	.	.	5	Crediton.
.	.	.	.	.	.	.	.	.	.	.	.	4	.	1	.	.	5	Cheriton Fitzp.
1	1	.	.	2	.	.	.	.	.	.	.	1	.	.	.	.	1	Silverton.
.	.	.	.	.	.	1	1	.	1	.	.	.	.	.	.	.	3	Cullompton.
.	.	.	.	.	.	.	.	.	.	.	.	.	.	1	.	1	2	Uffculme.
1	2	.	.	3	.	.	.	.	.	.	.	.	4	.	.	.	4	Tiverton.
.	.	.	.	.	.	.	.	.	.	.	.	.	.	.	.	.	.	Washfield.
.	.	.	.	.	.	.	.	.	.	.	.	.	.	.	.	.	.	Bampton.
.	.	.	.	.	.	.	.	.	.	.	.	.	.	.	.	.	.	Dulverton.
.	.	.	.	.	.	.	.	.	.	.	.	.	.	.	.	.	.	Witheridge.
.	.	.	.	.	.	.	.	.	.	.	.	.	.	.	.	.	.	Chulmleigh.
.	.	.	.	.	.	1	1	1	.	1	1	.	1	.	.	3	9	South Molton.
8	9	1	.	22	1	1	.	1	1	.	.	2	2	1	1	1	11	Barnstaple.
.	.	.	.	.	.	.	.	.	.	.	.	.	.	.	.	.	.	Parracombe.
.	.	.	.	.	.	.	.	.	.	.	.	.	.	.	.	.	.	Combmartin.
20	1	.	.	21	.	.	.	.	.	.	.	1	9	2	.	.	12	Ilfracombe.
6	.	.	.	9	.	1	.	.	.	.	.	.	.	.	.	.	1	Braunton.
.	.	.	.	.	.	.	.	.	.	1	.	.	.	1	.	.	2	Bishop's Tawton.
.	.	.	.	.	.	.	.	.	.	.	.	.	.	.	.	.	.	High Bickington.
.	.	.	.	.	.	.	.	.	.	.	.	.	.	.	.	.	.	Winkleigh.
.	.	.	.	.	.	.	.	.	.	.	.	.	.	.	.	.	.	Dolton.
.	.	.	.	1	.	.	.	.	.	.	.	.	.	.	.	.	.	Shebbear.
.	.	.	.	.	.	.	.	.	.	.	.	.	.	.	.	.	.	Great Torrington.
.	.	.	.	1	.	.	.	.	.	.	.	.	.	.	.	.	.	Bideford.
.	1	.	.	2	1	1	.	.	.	.	.	.	.	.	.	.	2	Northam.
.	.	.	.	.	.	.	.	.	.	.	.	.	.	.	.	.	.	Parkham.
.	.	.	.	.	.	.	.	1	.	.	.	.	.	.	.	.	1	Hartland.
.	.	.	.	.	.	.	.	.	.	.	.	.	.	.	.	.	.	Bradworthy.
.	.	.	.	.	.	.	.	.	.	.	.	.	.	.	.	.	.	Milton Damerel.
.	.	.	.	.	.	.	.	.	.	.	.	.	.	.	.	.	.	Holsworthy.
.	.	.	.	.	.	.	.	.	.	.	.	.	.	.	.	.	.	Black Torrington.
.	.	.	.	2	.	.	.	.	.	.	.	.	.	.	.	.	.	Broadwoodwidger.
.	.	.	.	.	.	.	.	.	.	.	.	.	.	.	.	.	.	Clawton.
	233	11	1		11	14	10	14	15	19	35	65	87	48	12	17		
	26	5	1															
	35	10	12															

TABLE VIII.

Districts.	Sub-Districts.	1848.			1849.									
		Oct.	Nov.	Dec.	Jan.	Feb.	March.	April.	May.	June.	July.	Aug.	Sept.	Oct.
Stratton........	Kilkhampton ..	..	..	..	..	..	..	..	..	.1	..	.1	..	..
	Stratton	..	..	..	..	..	..	..	..	1	..	1	..	..
	Week St. Mary..	..	..	..	..	..	..	..	..	..	..	..	..	..
Camelford	Boscastle	..	..	..	..	..	..	..	..	..	..	..	..	..
	Camelford	..	..	..	..	..	..	..	..	..	..	.1	..	..
Launceston	Altarnun	..	..	..	..	..	..	..	..	..	..	..	..	..
	North Petherwin	..	..	..	..	..	..	..	..	..	..	..	..	..
	St. Stephen	..	..	..	..	..	..	..	..	..	..	..	..	..
	Launceston	..	..	..	..	..	..	..	..	..	..	..	..	..
	Northhill	..	∴	..	..	..	..	..	..	..	..	..	1	..
St. Germans	Antony	..	..	..	..	..	..	..	..	..	2	79	169	9
	St Germans	..	..	..	..	..	..	..	..	..	.1	1	2	..
	Saltash	..	..	..	..	..	..	..	..	..	3	25	14	..
Liskeard........	Callington	..	..	..	..	..	..	..	..	..	..	44	38	6
	Liskeard	..	..	..	..	..	..	..	..	..	1	5	7	4
	Looe	..	..	..	1	..	..	..	..	..	1	9	..	..
	Lerrin	..	..	..	..	..	..	..	..	..	..	.1	..	..
Bodmin	Llanlivery	..	..	..	..	..	..	..	..	..	..	2	..	..
	St. Mabyn......	..	..	2	..	..	..	..	..	..	..	..	..	..
	Bodmin	..	..	..	..	..	..	..	..	..	..	..	..	..
	Egloshale	..	..	..	..	..	..	..	..	..	..	..	..	..
St. Columb	Padstow........	..	..	..	..	..	..	..	..	..	..	..	..	1
	St. Columb	..	..	..	..	..	..	..	..	..	2	..	..	..
	Newlyn	..	..	..	..	..	..	..	..	..	..	..	..	1
St. Austell......	Fowey..........	..	..	..	..	..	..	..	..	..	..	..	1	..
	St. Austell......	..	..	..	..	..	..	..	..	..	1	2	..	.1
	Mevagissey	..	..	..	..	..	..	..	..	..	36	60	4	3
	Grampound	..	..	..	..	..	..	..	..	..	1	..	..	..
Truro	Probus	..	..	..	..	..	..	..	..	..	..	..	..	..
	St. Just	..	..	..	..	..	..	..	..	..	..	1	1	..
	St. Agnes	..	..	..	..	..	..	..	..	..	..	..	..	..
	St. Clement	..	..	..	..	..	..	..	..	..	1	10	12	14
	Kenwyn........	..	..	..	..	..	..	..	..	..	..	2	22	7
	Kea	..	..	..	..	..	..	..	..	..	..	1	5	..
Falmouth	Mylor	..	..	..	..	..	..	..	..	..	..	1	1	1
	Falmouth	..	..	..	..	..	..	..	..	1	1	5	12	1
	Penryn	..	..	..	..	..	..	..	..	..	..	..	6	22
	Constantine	..	..	..	..	..	..	..	..	..	..	1	1	2
Helston........	Wendron	..	..	..	..	..	..	1	..	..	..	2	..	..
	Helston	..	..	..	..	..	..	..	..	..	..	..	..	..
	St. Keverne	..	..	..	..	..	..	..	..	..	..	..	..	..
	Breage	..	..	..	..	..	..	..	..	..	..	1	..	..
	Crowan	..	..	..	..	..	..	..	..	..	..	..	..	..
Redruth........	Gwennap	..	..	..	..	..	..	..	..	..	..	1	19	1
	Redruth........	..	..	..	..	..	..	..	..	..	..	..	29	7
	Illogan	..	..	..	..	..	..	..	..	..	..	..	15	4
	Camborne	..	1	..	..	..	..	..	..	..	1	..	1	4
	Phillack........	1	..	..	..	..	..	..	..	..	2	30	10	..
Penzance	Uny Lelant	..	..	..	..	..	..	..	..	..	..	..	..	..
	St. Ives	..	..	..	..	..	..	..	..	1	..	2	12	1
	Marazion	..	..	..	..	..	..	..	..	..	..	1	..	..
	Penzance	..	..	..	..	..	..	..	..	..	.1	..	..	2
	St. Just in Pen- with.	1	2	..	..	..	..	..	..	..	1	..	..	1
	St. Buryan	..	..	..	..	..	..	..	..	..	..	..	..	..
Scilly Islands ..	Scilly Islands ..	..	..	..	..	..	..	..	..	..	1	2	..	1
Number of deaths from Cholera and from Diarrhœa respectively in each month		2	4	2	..	1	..	1	..	3	79	369	339	98
Number of places in which deaths from Cholera occurred during each month..................		3	2	1	..	1	..	1	..	2	14	22	25	22
Number of places in which deaths occurred, whether from Cholera or from Diarrhœa, in each month		..	..	..	5	3	4	4	6	7	24	29	30	24

—continued.

CHOLERA 1849			DIARRHŒA 1849													Sub-Districts
Nov.	Dec.	13 months	Jan.	Feb.	March	April	May	June	July	Aug.	Sept.	Oct.	Nov.	Dec.	12 months	
..	..	..	..	..	..	..	..	..	..	..	..	..	..	..	..	Kilkhampton.
..	2	..	..	..	..	..	..	..	..	..	..	..	..	..	..	Stratton.
..	..	..	..	..	..	..	..	..	..	..	..	..	..	..	..	Week St. Mary.
..	..	..	1	..	..	..	..	..	1	..	..	..	..	..	1	Boscastle.
..	1	..	1	..	..	..	..	..	1	1	..	..	1	..	4	Camelford.
..	..	..	..	..	..	..	..	..	..	..	..	..	..	..	..	Altarnun.
..	..	..	..	..	..	..	..	..	..	..	..	..	..	..	..	North Petherwin.
..	1	..	..	..	..	..	..	..	1	1	..	..	..	1	3	Launceston.
..	2	..	1	..	..	..	..	..	..	1	..	1	..	..	2	Northhill.
..	199	..	..	..	..	1	1	..	3	6	1	..	..	1	12	Antony.
..	3	..	..	..	..	..	1	..	..	..	..	..	..	..	1	St. Germans.
..	34	..	..	..	..	..	..	2	2	1	..	..	..	..	5	Saltash.
..	102	..	..	..	..	1	..	3	9	4	1	..	..	..	18	Callington.
..	17	..	..	..	..	1	..	..	1	1	..	..	..	..	2	Liskeard.
1	12	..	..	1	..	..	..	..	1	..	..	..	2	..	4	Looe.
..	1	..	..	..	..	..	..	1	..	..	..	..	..	..	1	Lerrin.
..	2	..	..	..	..	..	..	..	1	1	..	..	..	..	2	Lanlivery.
..	2	..	..	..	1	..	..	..	..	..	..	1	..	..	2	St. Mabyn.
..	..	..	..	..	..	..	..	..	..	..	..	..	..	..	..	Bodmin.
..	..	..	..	..	..	..	..	..	..	..	..	..	..	..	..	Egloshale.
..	1	..	..	..	..	..	..	..	..	..	..	..	..	..	..	Padstow.
..	2	..	..	..	..	..	1	..	..	..	..	..	..	1	2	St. Columb.
..	1	..	..	..	..	..	..	..	..	..	..	..	..	1	1	Newlyn.
..	5	..	..	..	..	..	..	..	2	..	1	..	..	..	3	Fowey.
..	1	..	..	..	..	..	..	..	..	1	..	..	..	..	1	St. Austell.
..	128	..	..	..	..	..	..	..	..	2	..	..	..	..	2	Mevagissey.
..	1	..	..	..	..	..	..	..	..	..	..	..	..	..	..	Grampound.
..	..	..	..	..	..	..	..	..	..	..	..	..	..	1	1	Probus.
..	..	..	..	..	..	..	..	..	..	..	..	..	..	1	1	St. Just.
..	7	..	..	..	..	..	..	1	..	1	..	..	2	..	4	St. Agnes.
..	37	..	..	..	..	..	..	..	..	..	..	..	..	..	..	St. Clement.
..	31	..	..	..	..	..	..	..	1	1	1	..	..	1	4	Kenwyn.
..	6	..	..	..	..	..	..	..	..	..	..	..	..	..	..	Kea.
..	7	..	..	..	..	..	..	..	..	..	..	..	..	..	..	Mylor.
..	34	..	..	..	..	1	..	..	..	1	1	1	..	..	4	Falmouth.
..	36	..	..	..	..	1	..	3	..	2	2	1	..	1	7	Penryn.
..	6	..	..	..	..	..	..	..	..	..	..	..	..	..	..	Constantine.
..	6	..	..	..	1	..	..	..	..	..	..	1	..	..	2	Wendron.
..	..	..	..	..	..	..	..	..	..	..	..	..	..	..	..	Helston.
..	..	..	..	..	..	..	..	..	..	..	..	..	..	..	..	St. Keverne.
..	1	..	..	2	3	2	1	..	..	1	..	..	..	..	9	Breage.
..	..	..	..	..	..	..	..	..	..	..	..	..	..	..	..	Crowan.
..	21	..	..	..	..	..	..	..	..	1	1	..	..	..	2	Gwennap.
..	22	..	..	..	..	..	..	..	..	..	..	..	..	..	..	Redruth.
..	20	..	1	..	..	1	..	..	..	..	..	..	..	..	2	Illogan.
..	6	..	..	..	..	..	..	1	1	1	1	..	..	..	4	Camborne.
..	53	..	..	..	..	..	..	1	1	..	..	..	..	..	1	Phillack.
..	..	..	..	..	..	..	1	..	..	..	..	..	..	..	1	Uny Lelant.
..	17	..	2	1	..	..	..	..	..	4	3	3	..	..	13	St. Ives.
..	1	..	..	..	..	..	..	..	..	..	..	..	..	..	..	Marazion.
..	2	..	..	..	..	..	..	..	..	..	..	1	2	1	4	Penzance.
..	6	..	..	..	1	..	..	1	..	4	..	1	..	1	6	St. Just in Penwith.
..	..	..	..	..	..	..	..	1	..	..	..	..	..	..	1	St. Buryan.
..	4	..	..	..	..	..	..	..	..	..	..	..	..	..	..	Scilly Islands.
1			6	4	6	4	6	4	11	34	27	15	7	10		
2																
11																

TABLE IX.—Showing the distribution of Cholera and Diarrhœa over the and the Months during which the

Districts.	Sub-Districts.	1848.			1849.									
		Oct.	Nov.	Dec.	Jan.	Feb.	March.	April.	May.	June.	July.	Aug.	Sept.	Oct.
Ludlow . .	Lentwardine .	..	..	..	..	..	..	..	..	..	..	..	..	..
	Ludlow .	..	..	..	..	..	..	..	..	..	..	..	..	..
	Cainham .	..	..	..	..	..	..	..	..	..	..	..	..	..
	Munslow .	..	..	..	..	..	..	..	..	..	..	..	..	..
	Diddlebury .	..	..	..	..	..	..	..	..	..	..	..	..	..
Clun . .	Clun .	..	..	..	..	..	..	..	..	..	..	..	..	..
	Bishop's Castle	..	..	..	..	..	..	..	..	..	..	..	..	..
	Norbury .	..	..	..	..	..	..	..	..	..	..	..	..	..
	Lydbury .	..	..	..	..	..	..	..	..	..	..	..	..	..
Church Stretton	Church Stretton	..	..	..	..	..	..	..	..	..	..	2	..	..
	Wall .	..	..	..	..	..	..	..	..	..	..	1	..	..
Cleobury Mortimer .	Cleobury Mortimer.	..	..	..	..	..	..	..	..	..	..	1	..	..
	Stoddesden	..	..	..	..	..	..	..	..	..	..	..	..	..
Bridgnorth .	Chetton .	..	..	..	..	..	..	..	..	..	..	..	..	..
	Bridgnorth	..	..	..	..	..	..	..	..	..	1	34	34	..
	Worfield .	..	..	..	1	..	..	..	..	1	..	3	..	..
Shiffnall .	Albrighton	..	..	..	..	..	..	..	..	..	..	..	..	..
	Shiffnall .	..	..	..	..	..	..	..	..	..	..	..	1	..
Madeley .	Dawley .	..	..	..	..	..	..	..	..	..	..	1	1	..
	Madeley .	..	..	..	..	..	..	..	..	..	..	14	17	1
	Broseley .	..	..	..	..	..	..	..	..	..	..	8	4	1
	Much Wenlock	..	..	..	..	..	..	..	..	..	..	..	8	5
Atcham .	Condover .	..	..	..	..	..	..	..	..	..	..	14	1	..
	Pontesbury	..	..	..	..	..	..	..	..	..	..	..	..	..
	Westbury	..	..	..	..	..	..	..	..	..	..	..	..	..
	Alberbury	..	..	..	..	..	..	..	..	..	..	..	..	..
	Montford	..	..	..	..	..	..	..	..	..	..	..	..	..
	Battlefield	..	..	..	..	..	..	..	..	..	..	..	..	..
	Atcham .	..	..	..	..	..	..	..	..	..	..	..	..	..
Shrewsbury	St. Mary .	..	..	..	..	..	..	..	..	..	6	35	20	1
	St. Chad .	..	..	..	..	1	1	..	..	..	28	18	7	..
Oswestry .	Knockin .	..	..	..	..	..	..	..	..	..	..	..	..	..
	Llansilin .	..	..	..	..	..	..	..	..	..	..	..	..	..
	Oswestry .	..	..	..	..	..	..	..	..	..	..	..	1	1
	St. Martin	..	..	..	..	..	..	..	..	..	..	..	1	..
Ellesmere .	Overton .	..	..	..	..	..	..	..	..	..	..	..	..	..
	Hanmer .	..	..	..	..	..	..	..	..	..	..	..	..	..
	Ellesmere .	..	..	..	..	..	..	1	..	..	..	2	..	..
	Baschurch	..	..	..	..	..	..	..	..	..	..	..	..	..
Wem . .	Wem .	..	..	..	..	..	..	..	..	..	..	..	..	..
	Prees .	..	..	..	..	1	..	..	..	..	..	..	..	..
	Whitchurch	..	..	..	..	..	..	1	..	..	..	1	3	..
Market Drayton	Moreton Say	..	..	..	1	..	..	..	..	..	..	..	..	..
	Market Drayton	..	..	..	1	..	..	..	..	..	2	..	9	2
	Hodnet .	..	..	..	..	..	..	..	..	..	..	..	..	..
Wellington .	Ercall Magna	..	..	..	..	..	..	..	..	..	..	..	..	..
	Wellington	..	..	..	..	..	..	..	..	..	..	..	4	..
	Wombridge	..	..	..	..	..	..	..	..	..	..	..	..	3
Newport .	Newport .	..	..	..	..	1	..	..	..	..	..	1	..	..
	Gnosall .	..	..	..	..	..	..	..	..	..	..	..	1	1
Number of deaths from Cholera and from Diarrhœa respectively in each month		..	..	..		3	1	2	..	1	37	133	111	15
Number of places in which deaths from Cholera occurred during each month .		..	..	..		3	1	2	..	1	4	12	15	8
Number of places in which deaths occurred, whether from Cholera or from Diarrhœa, in each month . .		..	..	..		9	7	7	9	9	10	14	20	10

WORCESTERSHIRE, STAFFORDSHIRE, and SHROPSHIRE "Cholera Fields,"
Deaths occurred in each Sub-District.

SHROPSHIRE.																
CHOLERA.			DIARRHŒA.													
1849.			1849.													
Nov.	Dec.	12 months	Jan.	Feb.	March	April	May	June	July	Aug.	Sept.	Oct.	Nov.	Dec.	12 months	Sub-Districts.
..	..	..	..	..	..	1	..	..	..	..	..	..	..	..	..	Leintwardine.
..	..	..	..	..	..	..	..	..	..	..	..	..	..	..	1	Ludlow.
..	..	..	..	..	..	..	..	1	..	..	..	..	1	..	2	Caineham.
..	..	..	..	..	..	..	..	..	..	..	..	..	..	..	..	Munslow.
..	..	..	..	..	..	..	..	..	..	..	..	..	..	..	..	Diddlebury.
..	..	..	..	..	..	..	..	..	..	..	..	..	..	..	..	Clun.
..	..	..	..	..	..	..	..	1	..	..	..	..	..	..	1	Bishop's Castle.
..	..	..	..	..	..	..	..	..	..	..	..	..	..	..	..	Norbury.
..	..	..	..	..	..	..	..	..	..	..	..	..	..	..	..	Lydbury.
..	..	2	..	..	..	..	1	..	..	1	..	..	..	..	2	Church Stretton.
..	..	..	..	..	..	..	..	..	1	..	..	..	..	..	1	Wall.
..	..	1	..	2	1	2	1	..	..	..	..	1	..	..	7	Cleobury Mortimer.
..	..	..	..	..	..	..	..	..	..	..	..	..	..	..	..	Stoddesdon.
..	..	..	..	..	..	..	1	..	..	2	..	..	..	..	2	Chetton.
..	1	76	1	..	..	..	..	..	3	2	..	1	..	..	8	Bridgnorth.
..	..	5	..	1	..	..	..	..	..	..	..	..	..	..	1	Worfield.
..	..	1	..	..	..	..	..	1	1	..	..	..	..	2	Albrighton.
..	..	..	..	..	..	..	..	..	..	..	..	..	..	..	Shiffnall.
..	..	22	..	..	..	..	1	..	2	2	..	..	..	5	Dawley.
..	1	13	..	..	..	..	..	..	1	..	..	1	2	Madeley.
..	..	14	..	1	..	..	..	..	..	..	..	..	..	Broseley.
..	..	13	..	1	..	1	1	..	1	..	..	..	3	Much Wenlock.
..	..	..	..	..	..	..	..	..	..	..	..	..	..	Condover.
..	..	..	..	..	..	..	..	..	..	..	..	..	..	Pontesbury.
..	..	..	..	..	..	..	..	..	..	..	..	1	1	Westbury.
..	..	..	..	..	..	..	..	..	..	..	..	..	..	Alberbury.
..	..	..	..	..	..	..	..	..	..	..	1	..	1	Montford.
..	..	..	..	..	..	1	..	..	..	..	..	..	1	Battlefield.
..	..	62	..	..	..	..	1	2	3	5	3	..	13	Atcham.
..	..	38	2	2	2	1	..	2	2	1	..	..	13	St. Mary.
..	..	..	..	..	..	..	..	1	..	..	1	St. Chad.
..	..	..	..	1	..	..	..	1	..	..	3	Knockin.
..	..	8	..	1	..	1	2	..	1	..	..	3	Llanddfin.
..	..	..	..	..	..	..	..	..	..	..	..	Oswestry.
..	..	..	..	..	..	1	..	..	..	..	1	St. Martin.
..	..	3	..	1	..	..	1	..	1	..	3	Overton.
..	..	..	..	..	..	..	..	..	1	..	Hanmer.
..	..	..	..	..	..	..	..	1	1	2	Ellesmere.
..	..	1	..	..	..	..	..	..	1	1	2	Baschurch.
..	4	5	..	..	..	..	..	..	1	1	Wem.
..	..	14	1	1	1	..	1	..	2	..	1	5	Prees.
..	..	..	..	..	..	..	..	..	..	Whitchurch.
..	..	4	1	..	1	..	1	3	1	..	1	9	Moreton Say.
2	..	5	..	1	1	1	1	2	..	1	1	7	Market Drayton.
..	..	2	1	..	1	1	1	1	..	..	4	Hodnet.
..	..	2	1	..	3	..	..	..	..	3	Ercall Magna.
																Wellington.
																Wombridge.
																Newport.
																Gnosall.
9	9		6	9	11	6	10	9	11	14	19	8	8	7		
1	2		5													
8	8															

STAFFORDSHIRE.

Districts.	Sub-Districts.	CHOLERA.												
		1848.			1849.									
		Oct.	Nov.	Dec.	Jan.	Feb.	March.	April.	May.	June.	July.	Aug.	Sept.	Oct.
Stafford	Stafford	..	..	..	1	..	..	..	..	..	..	..	..	..
	Castle Church	..	..	..	..	..	..	..	..	..	..	..	1	..
	Colwich	..	..	..	..	..	..	..	..	..	..	..	..	..
Stone	Stone	..	1	..	..	..	..	..	..	..	1	1	..	..
	Eccleshall	..	..	..	..	..	..	..	..	..	..	..	1	1
	Trentham	..	..	..	..	..	..	..	..	..	..	..	3	..
Newcastle-under-Lyme	Whitmore	..	..	..	..	..	..	..	..	..	..	..	2	..
	Newcastle-under-Lyme	..	..	..	..	..	..	..	..	1	1	129	94	14
	Audley	..	..	..	..	..	..	..	..	..	..	..	..	..
Wolstanton	Wolstanton	..	..	..	..	..	..	..	..	..	..	1	2	..
	Tunstall	..	..	..	..	..	..	..	..	..	..	5	1	1
	Burslem	..	..	..	..	..	..	..	..	2	32	22	12	1
Stoke-upon-Trent	Hanley	..	..	..	..	..	..	..	..	..	..	8	16	6
	Shelton	..	1	..	..	..	..	1	..	1	1	6	18	16
	Stoke-upon-Trent	..	1	..	..	..	..	..	..	..	..	6	19	3
	Fenton	..	..	..	..	..	..	..	..	..	..	..	..	1
	Longton	..	..	..	..	..	..	..	..	..	..	..	..	1
Leek	Norton	..	..	..	..	..	..	..	..	..	1	1	..	..
	Leek	1	..	..	..	..	..	..	..	..	..	1	1	..
	Leek Frith	..	..	..	..	..	..	..	..	..	..	..	..	..
	Longnor	..	..	..	..	..	..	..	..	..	..	..	..	..
Cheadle	Alton	..	..	..	..	..	..	..	..	..	..	..	..	..
	Ipstones	..	1	..	..	..	..	..	..	..	..	..	..	..
	Dilhorne	..	..	..	..	..	..	..	..	..	..	..	..	..
	Cheadle	..	..	1	..	..	..	..	..	..	..	..	2	..
Uttoxeter	Uttoxeter	..	1	..	..	..	..	..	..	..	..	..	..	..
	Abbot's Bromley	..	..	..	..	..	..	..	..	..	..	..	..	..
	Sudbury	..	..	..	..	..	..	..	..	..	..	..	..	..
Burton-upon-Trent	Tutbury	..	..	..	..	..	..	..	..	..	..	1	..	..
	Repton	..	..	..	..	..	..	..	..	..	..	..	..	..
	Gresley	..	..	..	..	..	..	..	..	..	..	..	..	..
	Burton-upon-Trent	..	..	..	..	..	..	..	..	..	..	..	..	5
Tamworth	Tamworth	..	..	..	..	..	..	..	..	..	..	1	..	..
	Fazeley	..	..	..	..	..	..	..	..	..	..	..	..	..
Lichfield	Lichfield	..	..	..	..	..	..	..	..	..	1	..	1	1
	Yoxall	..	..	..	..	..	..	..	..	..	..	..	..	..
	Rugeley	..	..	..	..	..	..	..	..	..	..	..	3	..
Penkridge	Penkridge	..	..	..	..	..	..	..	..	..	..	1	2	1
	Brewood	..	..	..	..	..	..	..	..	..	..	1	2	..
	Cannock	..	..	..	..	..	..	..	..	..	..	1	..	..
Wolverhampton	Tettenhall	..	..	..	..	..	..	..	..	..	1	1	3	..
	Wombourn	..	..	..	..	..	..	..	..	..	..	1	2	1
	Kinfare	..	..	..	..	..	..	..	..	..	..	..	..	..
	Wolverhampton	..	..	..	..	..	..	..	..	1	..	47	36	48
	Willenhall	..	..	..	..	..	..	..	..	..	..	56	217	8
	Bilston	..	..	..	..	..	..	..	..	..	3	68	475	76
Walsall	Darlaston	..	..	..	..	..	..	..	..	..	1	2	34	7
	Bloxwich	..	..	..	..	..	..	..	..	..	..	..	..	1
	Walsall	..	..	..	..	..	..	..	..	..	..	..	26	105
	Aldridge	..	..	..	..	..	..	..	..	..	..	..	2	1
West Bromwich	Handsworth	..	..	..	..	..	..	..	..	..	..	..	1	..
	Oldbury	..	..	..	..	..	..	..	..	..	..	..	5	6
	W. Bromwich (3)	1	..	..	..	..	..	..	..	..	1	1	9	10
	Wednesbury	..	..	..	..	..	..	..	..	..	..	2	143	67
Dudley	Rowley Regis	..	..	..	..	..	..	..	..	..	..	..	..	6
	Tipton	..	..	1	..	..	..	..	..	..	1	2	66	38
	Sedgeley	..	..	1	..	..	..	..	..	..	..	1	86	87
	Dudley	..	..	..	..	..	..	..	..	..	..	1	21	38
Number of deaths from Cholera and from Diarrhoea respectively in each month		2	5	3	1	..	..	1	..	5	44	307	1623	519
Number of places in which deaths from Cholera occurred during each month		2	5	3	1	..	..	1	..	4	11	24	32	28
Number of places in which deaths occurred, whether from Cholera or from Diarrhoea, in each month					21	23	16	19	21	12	26	21	39	35

| CHOLERA. | | | DIARRHŒA. | | | | | | | | | | | | Sub-Districts. |
| 1849. | | | 1849. | | | | | | | | | | | | |
Nov.	Dec.	12 months	Jan.	Feb.	March	April	May.	June.	July.	Aug.	Sept.	Oct.	Nov.	Dec.	12 months	
..	..	2	..	..	..	..	..	..	..	3	..	..	1	4	Stafford.
..	..	1	..	2	..	..	..	1	..	1	..	1	..	5	Castle Church.
..	..	..	..	2	..	..	1	..	..	1	..	..	..	2	Colwich.
..	..	2	..	..	..	..	..	..	..	..	..	..	..	1	Stone.
..	..	2	..	..	..	..	..	..	..	..	1	..	1	1	Eccleshall.
..	..	3	..	..	..	..	..	..	..	..	..	..	..	1	Trentham.
..	..	..	..	..	..	..	..	..	..	..	..	..	..	..	Whitmore.
..	..	2	..	..	..	..	1	1	..	6	3	5	..	..	18	Newcastle - under-Lyme.
..	..	..	..	..	..	..	1	1	2	1	..	..	..	..	5	Audley.
..	..	2	..	..	..	..	..	..	..	..	..	..	..	..	Wolstanton.
..	..	7	3	5	2	3	3	3	2	4	4	1	2	1	33	Tunstall.
1	..	70	3	3	1	2	3	4	5	3	6	2	..	2	33	Burslem.
..	..	20	..	..	..	..	..	..	..	1	2	1	..	..	4	Hanley.
..	..	44	..	1	..	3	1	2	..	1	3	4	..	1	20	Shelton.
..	..	29	1	..	2	3	2	2	2	..	3	..	..	..	15	Stoke - upon - Trent.
..	..	1	1	1	..	1	1	..	..	..	..	..	..	..	4	Fenton.
..	..	1	3	2	1	1	2	1	3	2	4	1	..	..	20	Longton.
..	..	2	..	..	..	..	2	1	..	1	..	..	..	3	Norton.
..	..	2	1	1	2	..	2	1	..	1	..	1	..	7	Leek.
..	..	..	..	..	..	..	..	..	..	..	..	..	..	..	Leek Frith.
..	..	..	..	..	..	..	..	..	..	..	..	..	..	..	Longnor.
..	..	1	..	..	..	..	..	..	..	1	..	..	..	1	Alton.
..	..	..	..	..	..	..	..	..	..	..	..	..	..	Ipstones.
..	..	3	..	..	..	1	3	..	3	..	..	1	..	8	Cheadle.
..	..	1	..	..	..	..	..	..	..	..	..	..	..	Uttoxeter.
..	..	..	..	..	..	..	..	..	..	..	..	..	..	Abbot's Bromley
..	..	..	..	..	..	..	..	..	..	..	..	..	1	1	Sudbury.
..	..	1	..	..	..	..	..	..	..	..	..	2	..	2	Tutbury.
..	..	..	..	..	..	..	..	..	..	..	..	..	..	Repton.
..	..	..	..	..	..	..	..	..	..	..	..	..	..	Gresley.
..	..	5	..	1	..	3	..	..	1	1	2	1	1	1	11	Burton - upon - Trent.
..	..	1	..	..	..	1	..	1	..	..	..	1	1	1	3	Tamworth.
..	..	..	..	..	..	..	..	..	..	..	..	..	..	2	Faneley.
..	..	2	1	2	1	1	..	1	..	..	1	..	..	3	9	Lichfield.
..	..	..	..	..	..	..	..	..	..	..	..	..	..	Yoxall.
..	..	3	1	..	1	1	1	..	1	..	..	..	..	5	Rugeley.
..	..	4	1	1	..	..	..	1	..	1	..	..	..	2	Penkridge.
..	..	3	1	1	..	..	..	..	1	1	1	..	..	5	Brewood.
..	..	4	..	..	..	..	..	1	2	1	..	..	2	Cannock.
..	..	4	..	..	..	..	..	1	2	..	1	3	Tettenhall.
..	..	4	..	..	..	1	..	..	1	..	..	..	3	Wombourn.
..	..	..	..	..	..	..	..	..	..	..	..	..	2	Kinfare.
6	..	132	5	4	2	1	4	3	6	34	38	12	7	1	134	Wolverhampton
1	..	201	2	2	..	1	2	1	1	4	14	4	..	..	37	Willenhall.
4	..	470	2	2	4	2	1	1	1	6	27	16	..	..	68	Bilston.
..	..	44	..	..	..	..	..	..	1	1	2	6	..	..	16	Darlaston.
..	..	1	..	..	..	..	..	..	..	..	..	..	..	1	Bloxwich.
6	..	127	..	1	1	..	..	1	2	6	13	1	..	..	27	Walsall.
..	..	3	..	..	..	..	..	1	3	1	..	..	10	Aldridge.
..	..	1	..	..	..	..	..	..	..	..	..	..	4	Handsworth.
2	..	16	1	2	..	2	2	2	..	2	6	5	1	..	21	Oldbury.
2	..	21	..	..	1	..	2	..	2	3	6	13	..	2	32	W. Bromwich (3)
4	..	212	1	2	1	1	3	..	1	1	24	13	2	2	60	Wednesbury.
2	..	14	1	2	1	3	3	1	2	2	2	14	6	7	40	Rowley Regis.
2	1	113	1	2	2	5	5	4	4	4	2	14	6	5	65	Tipton.
14	..	383	1	3	7	5	5	4	4	1	16	10	6	2	80	Sedgley.
14	2	54	5	5	4	3	1	4	4	1	9	13	10	10	96	Dudley.
68	9	..	42	40	36	30	44	40	42	94	253	173	51	39		
8	2															

TABLE IX.

WORCESTERSHIRE.

Districts.	Sub-Districts.	CHOLERA.											
		1848.			1849.								
		Oct.	Nov.	Dec.	Jan.	Feb.	March	April	May.	June.	July.	August.	Sept.
Stourbridge	Hales Owen	.	.	.	.	.	.	.	.	.	1	3	2
	Stourbridge	.	.	.	.	.	.	.	.	.	1	2	15
	Kingswinford	2	.	.	.	.	.	.	.	.	.	4	131
Kidderminster	Chaddesley Corbett	.	.	.	.	.	.	.	.	.	.	.	2
	Wolverley	.	.	.	.	.	.	.	.	.	.	.	1
	Kidderminster	1	.	.	.	.	.	.	.	.	.	.	3
	Lower Milton	.	.	.	.	.	.	.	.	.	.	.	.
	Bewdley	.	.	.	.	.	.	.	.	.	.	.	.
Tenbury	Tenbury	.	.	.	.	.	.	.	.	.	.	.	.
	Bockleton	.	.	.	.	.	.	.	.	.	.	.	.
Martley	Martley	.	.	.	.	.	.	.	.	.	.	.	.
	Witley	.	.	.	.	.	.	.	.	.	.	.	.
	Holt	.	.	.	.	.	.	.	.	.	.	.	.
	Leigh	.	.	.	.	.	.	.	.	.	.	.	.
Worcester	West	.	.	.	.	.	.	.	.	.	.	.	6
	North	.	.	.	.	.	.	.	.	.	7	.	14
	South	.	.	.	.	.	.	.	.	.	7	4	2
Upton-on-Severn	Hanley Castle	.	.	.	.	.	.	.	.	.	.	.	.
	Upton-on-Severn	.	.	.	.	.	.	.	.	1	.	3	2
	Kempsey	.	.	.	.	.	.	.	.	.	.	.	.
Evesham	Evesham	.	.	.	.	.	.	.	.	.	.	.	.
	Broadway	.	.	.	.	.	.	.	.	.	.	.	.
Pershore	Eckington	.	.	.	.	.	.	.	.	.	.	.	.
	Pershore	.	.	.	.	.	.	.	.	.	.	.	.
	Upton Snodsbury	.	.	.	.	.	.	.	.	.	.	.	.
Droitwich	Claines	.	.	.	.	.	.	.	.	.	.	.	3
	Ombersley	.	.	.	.	.	.	.	.	.	.	.	.
	Droitwich	.	.	.	.	.	.	.	.	.	.	4	5
Bromsgrove	Bromsgrove	1	.	.	.	.	.	.	.	.	1	4	10
	Belbroughton	.	.	.	.	.	.	.	.	.	.	.	.
	Tardebigg	.	.	.	.	.	.	.	.	.	.	.	.
King's Norton	King's Norton	.	.	.	.	1	.	.	.	.	.	1	.
	Edgbaston	.	.	.	.	.	.	.	.	.	.	.	4
	Harborne	.	.	.	.	.	.	.	.	.	.	.	.
Number of deaths from Cholera and from Diarrhœa respectively in each month		5	.	.	.	1	.	.	.	1	17	24	200
Number of places in which deaths from Cholera occurred during each month		4	.	.	.	1	.	.	.	1	5	8	14
Number of places in which deaths occurred, whether from Cholera or from Diarrhœa, in each month		.	.	.	9	5	6	9	3	7	11		

—*continued.*

Cholera 1849				Diarrhoea 1849													Sub Districts.
Oct.	Nov.	Dec.	12 months.	Jan.	Feb.	March.	April.	May.	June.	July.	August.	Sept.	Oct.	Nov.	Dec.	12 months.	
.	1	.	7	3	1	.	2	.	.	1	.	.	.	.	1	8	Hales Owen.
22	50	15	95	2	1	1	3	2	1	.	6	11	3	4	3	37	Stourbridge.
73	3	2	215	1	1	.	.	1	3	2	1	8	3	5	2	27	Kingswinford.
.	.	.	2	.	.	.	.	.	.	.	.	.	.	1	.	1	Chaddesley Corbett.
.	.	.	1	.	.	.	.	.	.	1	1	.	.	.	.	2	Wolverley.
7	.	.	11	1	2	3	2	.	1	1	5	3	4	1	1	24	Kidderminster.
.	.	.	.	.	.	.	.	.	.	.	.	1	.	.	.	1	Lower Milton.
.	.	.	.	1	.	.	.	.	1	.	1	3	.	.	.	6	Bewdley.
.	.	.	.	.	.	.	.	.	.	.	.	2	.	.	.	2	Tenbury.
.	.	.	.	1	.	.	.	.	.	.	.	.	.	.	.	1	Bockleton.
.	.	.	.	.	.	.	.	.	.	.	.	.	.	.	.	.	Martley.
.	.	.	.	.	.	.	.	.	.	.	.	.	.	.	.	.	Witley.
.	.	.	.	.	.	.	1	.	.	.	.	.	.	.	.	1	Holt.
1	.	.	1	.	.	.	.	.	.	1	.	1	.	.	.	2	Leigh.
.	.	.	6	.	.	.	.	.	.	2	1	2	2	2	.	9	Worcester—West.
1	.	.	22	1	.	1	1	.	.	.	1	4	2	2	.	12	North.
1	.	.	14	1	.	1	.	.	.	.	.	2	2	.	.	6	South.
.	.	.	3	.	.	.	.	.	1	.	1	1	.	.	.	3	Hanley Castle.
1	6	.	13	.	.	.	.	.	.	.	.	.	.	.	.	.	Upton-on-Severn.
.	.	.	.	.	.	.	.	.	.	.	.	.	.	.	.	.	Kempsey.
.	.	.	.	.	.	.	.	.	.	.	2	2	2	1	1	8	Evesham.
.	.	.	.	.	.	.	.	.	.	.	.	.	.	.	.	.	Broadway.
.	.	.	.	.	.	.	1	.	.	.	.	.	.	.	.	1	Eckington.
.	.	.	.	.	.	.	1	.	.	.	.	2	1	.	.	4	Pershore.
.	.	.	.	.	.	.	.	.	.	1	.	2	.	.	.	3	Upton Snodsbury.
.	.	.	3	.	.	1	.	.	.	.	.	1	.	1	.	3	Claines.
.	.	.	.	.	.	.	.	.	.	.	.	2	.	.	1	3	Ombersley.
9	1	.	19	.	.	.	.	.	1	.	.	1	.	1	1	4	Droitwich.
4	.	.	20	1	.	2	3	1	.	1	2	5	1	.	1	17	Bromsgrove.
.	.	.	.	.	.	.	.	.	.	.	.	3	.	.	1	4	Belbroughton.
.	.	.	.	.	.	.	.	.	.	.	.	.	.	.	.	.	Tardebigg.
.	.	.	2	.	.	.	.	.	.	.	.	5	.	.	.	5	King's Norton.
1	.	.	6	.	.	.	1	.	.	.	1	.	3	.	1	6	Edgbaston.
.	.	.	.	.	.	.	.	.	.	.	.	3	3	1	1	8	Harborne.
121	50	17	.	12	5	9	15	4	8	12	23	64	23	19	14		
10	5	2	.	9	4	6	9	3	6	9	11	21	10	10	11		

WORCESTERSHIRE.

TABLE X.—Showing the Distribution of Cholera and Diarrhœa over during which the Deaths

| | | CHOLERA. | | | | | | | | | |
| | | 1848. | | | 1849. | | | | | | |
Districts.	Sub-Districts.	Oct.	Nov.	Dec.	Jan.	Feb.	March.	April.	May.	June.	July.
Darlington	Darlington										
	Aycliffe										
Stockton	Yarm (with Middlesborough)	2	1	1							4
	Stockton										1
	Hartlepool	1		1							3
	Sedgefield										
Auckland	Bishop Auckland						1				
	Hamsterley										
Teesdale	Staindrop										
	Barnard Castle										
	Middleton										
Weardale	St. John										
	Stanhope										2
	Wolsingham								1		
Durham	Tanfield										
	Lanchester										
	St. Oswald		1		1				2	35	16
	St. Nicholas						3	2	13	39	16
Easington	Easington						1	2			
Houghton le Spring	Houghton le Spring										
	Houghton le Hole					10					
Chester le Street	Chester le Street										
	Harraton				2	10					
Sunderland	North Bishopswearmouth	2	1	1	1		6	1		1	1
	South Bishopswearmouth						1	1			
	East Sunderland						72	1			
	West Sunderland			1	1		52	5			
	Monk Wearmouth	5	12	13	1			3			8
South Shields	Westoe	1	1	1	3		3			2	12
	South Shields			2		4	7		1	4	2
Gateshead	Heworth					2					1
	Gateshead			1	39	22	1		3		
	Whickham				5	14					1
	Winlaton					3					
Number of deaths from Cholera and from Diarrhœa respectively in each month		11	16	21	44	65	147	15	21	81	68
Number of places in which deaths from Cholera occurred during each month		5	5	8	8	7	10	7	6	5	13
Number of places in which deaths occurred, whether from Cholera or from Diarrhœa, in each month					14	11	15	12	11	10	16

the NORTHUMBERLAND and DURHAM "Cholera Field," and the months occurred in each Sub-district.

DURHAM.																		
CHOLERA.							DIARRHŒA.											
1849.							1849.											
Aug.	Sept.	Oct.	Nov.	Dec.	12 months.		Jan.	Feb.	March.	April.	May.	June.	July.	Aug.	Sept.	Oct.	Nov.	Dec.	12 months.
1	.	2	.	.	3		.	.	1	.	.	1	.	12	21	9	.	.	44
.	.	.	.	.	.		.	.	.	.	.	.	1	.	.	.	.	.	1
21	40	21	3	.	93		.	.	.	1	.	1	1	6	2	3	1	.	14
5	11	2	.	2	21		.	.	.	1	.	.	.	3	7	1	2	.	14
9	60	45	.	.	119		.	.	.	.	.	.	2	2	6	11	1	.	22
1	.	1	.	.	2		.	.	.	.	.	1	.	.	1	.	.	1	3
1	.	.	.	3	5		2	.	.	.	.	2	3	.	4	.	2	1	14
.	2	.	.	1	3		.	.	.	.	.	.	.	.	.	.	.	.	.
11	106	18	1	.	128		.	.	.	.	1	.	.	1	3	.	.	.	5
.	.	.	.	.	.		.	.	.	.	.	.	.	.	.	.	.	.	.
.	1	.	.	.	.		1	.	1	.	.	.	.	.	1	.	1	.	4
.	1	.	.	.	3		.	.	.	.	.	.	.	.	.	.	.	.	.
.	.	.	.	.	1		.	.	.	.	.	.	.	.	.	.	.	.	.
.	1	.	.	.	1		2	1	2	3	.	.	.	.	2	.	1	4	15
1	1	1	.	.	69		.	.	1	.	.	2	1	1	2	3	.	1	11
7	4	11	18	9	122		.	.	1	.	.	1	2	4	1	.	2	2	13
6	19	43	.	.	71		1	.	.	.	.	.	.	.	2	2	.	.	5
6	6	.	.	.	12		.	1	1	3	1	.	.	.	.	1	.	.	7
.	.	.	.	.	10		.	.	.	.	.	.	.	1	1	.	.	.	2
10	46	11	.	.	57		.	.	.	.	.	.	.	.	6	1	.	.	7
4	46	7	.	.	66		.	.	.	.	.	.	.	.	.	.	.	.	.
10	22	10	.	.	56		.	.	2	2	1	.	.	2	4	3	.	1	15
6	7	.	.	.	15		.	.	.	.	.	.	.	8	3	2	.	.	13
21	27	14	.	.	135		2	1	.	1	.	.	1	2	4	2	1	.	13
4	30	8	.	.	96		1	2	2	.	2	.	1	1	2	1	.	.	12
14	23	5	1	.	85		.	.	1	1	1	.	.	2	.	5	.	1	11
12	37	50	3	.	125		2	.	7	1	2	1	5	8	10	1	2	.	39
6	19	27	6	1	79		.	.	.	.	.	1	.	2	6	4	.	.	13
2	16	3	.	.	24		1	1	.	.	.	.	.	1	2	.	.	.	5
9	81	8	.	.	168		3	.	.	.	1	1	.	1	9	4	3	2	24
11	9	5	.	.	35		.	.	.	.	.	.	.	.	.	1	.	.	1
2	17	2	.	.	24		.	.	1	.	.	.	.	.	2	.	.	.	3
178	671	289	32	16			15	6	17	13	8	11	16	57	131	56	16	12	
24	24	21	6	5															
25	29	23	13	11															

TABLE X.

NORTHUMBERLAND.

Districts.	Sub-Districts.	CHOLERA.									
		1848.			1849.						
		Oct.	Nov.	Dec.	Jan.	Feb.	March.	April.	May.	June.	July.
Newcastle-on-Tyne	Westgate	.	.	.	3	.	.	2	.	.	
	St. Andrew	.	.	.	.	1	.	.	.	.	
	St. Nicholas	.	.	3	3	3	4	2	.	.	
	All Saints	1	.	3	14	13	17	4	.	.	2
	Byker	.	.	.	20	6	9	2	1	.	1
Tynemouth	Wallsend	1	.	.	.	.	.	.	.	.	
	North Shields	1	.	.	.	.	3	1	.	.	4
	Tynemouth	.	.	.	.	.	.	.	.	.	6
	Longbenton	1	.	.	.	.	.	.	.	.	.
	Earsdon	.	.	.	.	.	.	.	.	.	
	Blyth	1	14	12	5	.	.	1	.	.	1
Castle Ward	Ponteland	.	1	.	.	.	.	.	.	.	
	Stamfordham	.	.	.	.	.	.	.	1	.	
Hexham	Bywell	.	.	.	.	.	.	.	.	.	
	Hexham	.	.	.	.	5	1	.	.	.	
	Allendale	.	.	.	.	.	.	.	.	.	
	Chollerton	.	.	.	.	.	.	.	.	.	
Haltwhistle	Haltwhistle	.	.	.	.	.	.	.	.	.	
Bellingham	Bellingham	.	.	.	.	.	.	.	.	.	
	Kirkwhelpington	.	.	.	.	.	.	.	.	.	
Morpeth	Morpeth	.	.	.	.	.	1	.	.	.	
	Bedlington	.	3	6	.	.	1	.	.	.	
Alnwick	Warkworth	.	.	.	.	.	.	.	.	.	
	Alnwick	.	.	.	.	.	.	.	.	.	
	Embleton	.	.	.	.	.	.	.	.	.	
Belford	Belford	.	.	.	.	.	.	.	.	.	
Berwick	Islandshire	.	.	.	.	.	.	.	.	.	
	Berwick-upon-Tweed	.	.	3	11	2	.	2	.	.	
	Norhamshire	.	.	14	4	1	1	2	1	.	
Glendale	Ford	.	1	3	1	1	1	.	2	.	
	Wooler	.	.	.	.	.	.	1	.	.	
Rothbury	Rothbury	.	.	.	.	.	.	.	.	.	
	Elsdon	.	.	.	.	.	.	.	.	.	
Number of deaths from Cholera and from Diarrhœa respectively in each month		5	19	44	62	31	38	17	5	.	14
Number of places in which deaths from Cholera occurred during each month		5	4	7	9	7	9	9	4	.	
Number of places in which deaths occurred, whether from Cholera or from Diarrhœa, in each month					14	12	13	14	9	6	12

—*continued.*

NORTHUMBERLAND.

CHOLERA.						DIARRHŒA.												
1849.						1849.												
August.	Sept.	Oct.	Nov.	Dec.	12 months.	Jan.	Feb.	March.	April.	May.	June.	July.	August.	Sept.	Oct.	Nov.	Dec.	12 months.
8	17	.	.	.	30	2	.	1	.	.	1	3	5	2	5	2	.	20
1	2	1	.	.	5	1	.	2	1	.	1	.	2	11	7	2	3	28
5	10	4	.	.	34	2	2	1	.	1	.	1	2	3	6	3	4	25
4	52	13	1	.	124	3	.	.	4	1	1	1	2	7	5	6	2	32
7	46	12	2	.	106	.	.	.	1	1	1	.	1	5	1	2	.	12
.	30	5	.	.	36	.	.	.	.	.	.	.	1	1	.	.	.	2
37	147	39	.	.	232	2	.	1	1	.	.	1	4	15	3	1	1	29
38	44	19	4	4	115	1	.	.	.	1	.	1	2	5	10	4	4	28
25	34	16	.	.	76	.	.	1	.	.	.	.	1	1	3	.	2	8
19	97	61	6	.	183	.	.	.	.	.	.	.	1	1	8	8	.	17
.	69	39	8	.	144	.	.	.	.	.	2	.	.	1	2	.	.	4
.	4	.	1	.	6	.	.	.	.	.	.	.	.	1	1	1	.	4
1	8	.	1	.	11	1	.	.	.	.	.	.	.	1	1	.	.	2
1	2	.	.	.	3	1	.	.	.	.	.	.	.	1	.	1	.	2
1	1	2	.	.	10	.	.	.	2	.	2	.	2	2	.	1	1	8
.	.	.	.	.	1	.	.	.	.	1	.	.	.	1	.	.	.	2
.	1	1	.	.	2	.	.	1	1	.	.	.	.	1	.	.	.	2
.	.	.	.	.	.	.	.	.	.	.	.	.	.	.	.	.	.	.
.	4	2	.	.	7	1	.	.	.	.	.	.	.	.	.	3	.	4
1	.	1	26	.	88	.	1	.	1	.	1	.	1	1	.	1	.	5
.	5	.	.	.	5	.	.	1	1	.	.	1	1	.	1	.	.	5
6	63	61	.	.	123	.	1	.	.	1	.	.	1	2	.	.	.	6
6	3	.	.	.	9	.	.	.	.	.	.	.	1	.	.	.	.	1
.	.	3	.	.	3	.	.	1	1	.	.	.	.	2	.	.	.	4
.	2	1	.	.	3	.	.	.	.	.	.	.	.	.	.	.	.	.
.	8	11	8	1	46	.	.	.	.	.	.	.	1	2	1	.	.	4
2	6	6	2	.	41	.	.	1	.	.	.	.	.	1	1	1	.	2
.	3	2	.	.	14	.	.	.	.	.	.	.	5	1	1	1	1	8
.	.	.	.	.	1	.	1	.	.	.	.	.	.	.	.	.	.	1
.	.	.	.	.	.	.	.	.	.	.	.	.	.	.	.	.	.	.
.	.	.	.	.	.	.	.	.	.	.	.	.	.	.	.	.	.	.
206	653	283	58	21		14	7	7	13	6	7	17	43	81	41	28	5	
15	24	19	10	3														
17	25	20	18	6														

TABLE XI.—A List of Places in which the Mortality from [Cholera], during the Year [1]849, amounted to 5 deaths or upwards per 1),000 Inhabitants; the places in each county being arranged according to the months in [which] the first [ ] death occurred during the summer, and the ratio of [mortality] of each [being] distinguished.

NOTE. The following are the [ ] o [ ] Mortality distinguished by the several signs:

5 to 20	[deaths] per 10,000 inhabitants . . . a
20 to 40	" " . . . b
40 to 80	" " . . . c
80 to 120	" " . . . d
120, and upwards,	" " . . . e

The places whose [names] have no signs [ ] suffered the same ratio of [mortality] as the place next above [it], which has a [sign].

Places attacked in the Summer of [1849], in the [month] of

	May.	June.	July.	August.	September.	October.
Northumberland	· · ·	c Norham. b Newcastle - upon- [Tyne].	e North Shields. d B[ ] [ ]. c Tynemouth.	c [Eal.] d Longbenton. a Newburn. Boulmer. Hexham.	e Alnwick. c Wallsend. b Berwick. a Ponteland. Morpeth. Warkworth. Ford.	b Bedlington.
Durham	c Durham.	c Coxhoe. South Shields. Westoe. b Sunderland.	c Yarm. Middlesburgh. Hartlepool. a Stockton. Stanhope.	e Barnard Castle. c Chester le Street. Harraton. Gateshead. Seth [ ]an. Seaham Harbour. b Houghton - le - Spring. a Heworth.	c Dunston. b Blagdon.	

NORTHUMBERLAND and DURHAM Cholera Field.

Yorkshire, East Riding.					
e Hull	.	e Sutton. c Market Weighton. Howden. b York. Hessel. a Naburn. Dunnington.	a Newport. Beverley. Bridlington.	e Hedon. a Pocklington. Bainton. b Ferriby. Cottingham.	
North Riding a Whitby.	a Sutton.	.	a Malton. Thirsk. Marske.		
Wes Riding e Leeds. a Sheffield. Hebden Bridge.	e Stanley. d Thorne. c Gomersal. b Bradford. a Meltham.	d Barnsley. Selby. a Shipley. Pudsey.	e Morley. d Swinfleet. c Batley. Wakefield. Knottingley. Doncaster. Goole. Appleton - Roebuck. b Brightside. Wathe. a Delphe. Strathwaite. Huddersfield. Clackheaton. Bowling. Oulston. Kippax. Cawthorne. Nether Hallam. Ecclesfield Bierlow.	c Pontefract. Worsborough. Attercliffe. b Campbell. a North Bierly. Idle. Dewsbury. Horbury. Ackworth. Kimberworth. Bpworth. Crowle. Snaith. Golcar.	c Knaresborough. Ardsley. Mexborough. Aberford.

TABLE XI.—*continued.*

Countes and Parts of Counties.	May.	June.	Jy.	Jy.	September.	October.
Lancashire	d Liverpool. a Chorley.	c St. Southport. b Prescot. Warrington. Manchester. a Burscough. Bolton. Ramsbottom. Pilkington. Pudham. Biton.	d Wigan. Hindley. c Pemberton. Lancaster. b Ormskirk. a Wh Wootton. Walsall. Standish. Britinwood. Bury. Worsley. Bly.	b H. a Birtle. Ashton - dar - Lg. Clitheroe. Buxton. Croxton.	. . .	a Charnock Heath.
Cheshire	b Northwich.	e Nantwich. b Chester. Poulton. Liscard. a W	b a Stockport. Appleton. Or. Stapeley.	a Bibbington. Su ton.		

LANCASHIRE and CHESHIRE Cholera Field.

Shropshire	.	.	.	d Bridgnorth. c Shrewsbury. b Market Drayton.	b Madeley. Broxley. Condover. a Worfield. Wombridge.	c Much Wenlock. a Yardington. (Whitchurch.)
Staffordshire	.	.	.	e Newcastle-under-Lyne. Bilston. b Burslem.	e Willenhall. Wednesbury. d Wolverhampton. c Darlaston. Tipton. Sedgeley. b Hanley. Shelton. Stoke-upon-Trent. a Wolstanton. Penkridge. Brewood. Seisdon Trysull. West Bromwich.	c Walsall. b Dudley. a Trentham. Meer Button. Tettenhall. Bushall. Oldbury.
Worcestershire	.	.	a Worcester. Upton-on-Severn.	b Bromsgrove. Hales Owen.	Stourbridge. c Kingswinford. b Droitwich.	c Kidderminster. a Chaddesley Corbett.

a Rowley Regis.

WORCESTERSHIRE, STAFFORDSHIRE, and SHROPSHIRE Cholera Field.

TABLE XI.—*continued.*

Places attacked by Cholera in the [ ] Smer of 19, in the Month of

Counties and Parts of Counties.	May.	June.	July.	August.	September.	October.
Monmouthshire .	d Tredegar. v [ ]t. b [ ]in.	e t[ ]th. d Pontypool. c Monmouth. b St. Woolos.	a [ ]ll.	b Llanwrechva. a Abergavenny.		
South Wales .	e M [ ]byr Tydvil.	e Margam.	c Bridgend.			
Glamorganshire .	Cardiff. Gloxton. d Llangafilach.	Neath. Y [ ]alsy. [ ]all. b Caerpelly. Gelligaer. a Llandrisin'	fin. fin.			
Caermarthenshire .	b Llanel y.	c Caermarthen. a Llandillo.	b Llangadock. I dilhfawr.	b Llangende im. a St. Clears.	b Kidwelly. Llandingat. Llangathen.	
Pembrokeshire .		.			a Pembroke. Haverfordwest.	a Slebech. Begelly. Tenby.
Cardiganshire.		.			Lampeter.	

MONMOUTHSHIRE, and SOUTH WALES Cholera Field.

Buckinghamshire	·	·	·	·	·	·
Gloucestershire	·	e Clifton. Gloucester. a Huntley. Boddington.	d Bristol. e Frampton. e Stroud. Rodburgh.	e Weston-under-Edge. b Stonehouse. e Rodwick.	e Llanelly. a Southwick. Cribbbwell.	e Wenvogh. Llanguidoe.	a Upper and Lower Cam.
Somersetshire	·	e Keynsham.	Oldland.	e St. George. a Bath. Yatton.	c Tewkesbury.	c Midsomer ten. Twiverton. a Wells. Glastonbury. Godney Mere. Wrington.	b Midsomer Nor-ten. / d Chatton. Poulten.

BUCKINGHAMSHIRE, GLOUCESTERSHIRE.

Devonshire	e Moss Mayo. d Newton Ferrers.	e Plymouth. c Plympton. Egg Buckland. b Barnstaple.	e East Stonehouse. Devonport. Stoke Damerel. b South Brent.	a Pilton. d Beer Alston. c Tavistock. b Medbury. a Wolborough. Hewitree. Keaton. Kingstenton. Becket. Exeter.	b Ilfracombe. d Brixham. c Torquay. b Totnes. a St. Thomas. Okehampton.
Cornwall		b Falmouth. St. Ives.	e Maker. Moregissey. c Saltash. Truro. Philluck. a Liskeard. Scilly Islands.	c Callington. b Looe. Constantine. a St. Agnes. Gwennap. St. Germans.	c Penryn. b Redruth. Illogan. a Kea. Myler. Wendron.

CORNWALL and DEVON Cholera Field.

TABLE XI.—continued.

Places attacked by Cholera in the Summer of 1849, in the Months of

Counties and Parts of Counties.	May.	June.	July.	August.	September.	October.
Dorsetshire	.	b Poole.	.	c Weymouth. a Dorchester.	a Piddleton. Bridport.	
Wiltshire	.	a Longbridge Deverill.	e Salisbury. a Downton. Ditchampton.	c Potterne. Devizes. b Cliffe. Pypard. a Wilton.	a Lavington. Bradford.	
Hampshire	a South Stoneham. Kingsclere.	d Kingston. c Gosport. Southampton.	e Portsmouth. c Portsea. Landport. Newport. Itchen. b Ryde. Cowes. Romsey. Winchester. a Fareham. Eling. Milbrook. Otterbourn. Alton.	a Compton. Andover. Chalton.		
Sussex		b Pyecombe. Brighton. Shoreham. a Arundel.	a Chichester. b Hastings.	a Rye. Wadhurst.	b Hurstmonceaux. a Pulborough. Ore. Frant.	

Dorsetshire, Wiltshire, Hampshire, and Sussex Cholera Field.

London Cholera Field.

Middlesex .	.	c I , a. / a Isleworth.	d Brentford.	c Staines. Stanwell. Chiswick. b Hillingdon. Twickenham. Finchley. Enfield. a Hornsey.	c Edmonton. b Common Ruislip. Barnet. Cheshunt. a Feltham. Uxbridge. Acton. 1 (eltham. Waltham Abbey.	a South Mimms.
Surrey	.	c London.	b Mitcham. a Guildford.	c Mortlake. b ...gn. Richmond. a Carshalton. Epsom. ...ding. Reigate. Bletchingley. Wimbledon. Kingston.	c Chertsey. Abbey Green.	a Farnham.
Kent .	.	c London. Hm.	e Gravesend. c Crayford. Erith. Strood. b ...tld. a Chislehurst. Doddington.	d Margate. c Ramsgate. Dartford. Milton. Sheerness. ...id. b Farningham. Hoo. Rochester. Canterbury. Northfleet. Herne. Dover.	d East Farleigh. b Linton. a East Peckham. Tunbridge. Chart ...ea. Westwell.	a Yalding.

TABLE XI.—continued.

Counties and Parts of Counties.	Places attacked by Cholera in the Summer of 1849, in the Months of					
	May.	June.	July.	August.	September.	October.
Kent—continued .	.	.	a Aylesford. Mottram. Maidstone. Westgate. St. Stephens. Faversham.			
Essex .	b Leyton.	e Harwich. Ilford. c Stratford. West Ham. Barking.	d Southend. c Dagenham. b Ornett. Mucking. Maldon.	e Great Wakering. d Prittlewell. Leigh. Romford. Rochford. b Grays. Tillingham. a Walthamstow. Longton. Great Warly. Rainham. Upminster. Great Burstead. Bayleigh.	b Wanstead. Steeple. a Epping. Garnon Thoydon. Harlow. White Roothing.	
Berkshire .		a Reading.	c Windsor. b Abingdon. a Egham.	a Thatcham. Greenham. Newbury. Speen. Cumnor.	a Maidenhead.	

County					
London Cholera Field.					
Oxfordshire	·			b Oxford. a Handborough.	c [ ]. Pulbrook.
Buckinghamshire	·	·	d Gt. Marlow. b Gibraltar Gl-dington.	c High Wybe. b Ar. Langley Marsh. a Amersham. Beaconsfield. Ton. Eton.	c Newland. b [ ].
Counties not included in the chief Cholera Fields.					
Cumberland	·	a Keswick.	b St. Bees.	e [ ] tgn. c Maryport. b Whitehaven. a Harrington.	c Cockermouth. a Egremont.
Flintshire	·	·	b Holywell.	c Flint.	
Caernarvonshire	·	a Caernarvon.	b Holyhead.		
Anglesey	·	·	b Holyhead.		b Amlwch, with Port-Amlwch.
Montgomeryshire	·	·	a Llansaintfraid.	b Welshpool. a [ ]n.	
Derbyshire	·	·	a Castle-Donnington.	a Derby.	a Basford. Bulwell. Ratcliff-on-Trent, with Hi ling. a Ilkeston ia.
Nottinghamshire	·	b Newark.	·	a Clarborough. East Betford. Carlton. Lenton.	

TABLE XI.—*continued.*

Places attacked by Cholera in the Summer of 1849, in the Months of

Counties and Parts of Counties.	May.	June.	July.	August.	Sept.	October.
Lincolnshire	.	.	a Barton.	e Gainsborough. b Bra... a Great Grimsby. Winterton. b Owston, with Wet Bu tet-wick and Wet Ferry. M... the, Wet, g ... ish and Wi-keringham. a W lingm.	a ..., ith Miningsby. Caistor. Market Ban.	a Thrapston, with Titchmarsh.
Leicestershire	.	.	a Loughborough.			
Rutlandshire	.	.	.	a Oakham.		
Warwickshire	.	.	a Foleshill. c Coventry.		a Warwick.	
Northamptonshire	.	.		c Hardingstone, with Pidding-ton. b Peterborough.	a Northampton. Stilton.	
Huntingdonshire	b Warboys.	.			.	b Sawtrey.

Counties not included in the chief Cholera Fields—*continued.*

Counties not included in the chief Cholera Fields.					
Bedfordshire			*a* Biggleswade. Potton with Girtford, Sandy.		
Cambridgeshire		*a* Bottisham, with Swaffham Prior.	*c* Leverington. *d* Wisbech. *a* Walpole St. Peter with West Walton. *c* Walsoken. *a* Whittlesey.	*b* Caxton, with Gamlingay. *d* March. *c* Elm.	*b* Chatteris, with Welches Dam. *a* Upwell.
Norfolk			*b* Yarmouth. Norwich.	*b* Buxton.	*b* Coltishall. Sprowston, with Wrexham. *a* Costessey, with Bawburgh.
Suffolk	*b* Lowestoff.	*a* Ipswich.	*a* Beccles.	*a* Gorleston.	

TABLE XIL—Abstracts of Communications received by the Cholera Committee relative to the Sanitary Condition and general Characters of the particular Localities in which Cholera first appeared, in various Towns, Villages, parts of Towns, or Public Establishments.

Place and Reporter.	Local Circumstances.	Number of Cases immediately in same locality.
St. Giles' Parish . (Official Report.)	Church St.: drainage bad; supply of water bad; population dense; ventilation bad; cleanliness very defective.	
Hackney . . (Mr. Appleton.)	Moderately high; drainage good; population of district not dense; ventilation imperfect; cleanliness tolerable; too many persons in the house.	A man and the woman who nursed him.
Upper Clapton . (Mr. Hovell.)	High-Hill Ferry, where Cholera first appeared, is on the banks of the river Lea: the drainage very deficient; miasmata of various kinds. Drains from Warwick Road, &c., pass beneath several of the small tenements, some shut, and others emptying themselves into the Lea.	A woman and three children died within two days.
Shoreditch, Haggerstone District. (Mr. Hooper.)	Houses small, old, and dilapidated; no drainage; slops, heaps of fish, and vegetables allowed to collect in street; ground floors damp; bedrooms ill-ventilated and over-crowded.	Two days after death of first patient, two of his children were seized; then a man who nursed the first patient; and other cases in the neighbourhood followed.
Notting Hill . (Mr. Frost.)	The Potteries: a low and badly-drained district; houses of a wretched class; a large number of pigs kept.	First two cases simultaneous; third case 12 days later; four others within the next week in the same locality, though not in the same house.
Hammersmith . (Mr. Burrows to Dr. Farre.)	Bad drainage and ventilation; a stagnant ditch in the rear of the house, receiving the refuse from a number of pigsties.	
Hammersmith, Willow Place. (Mr. Horton).	A yard without ventilation; water scanty; and bad drain in centre. Privies filthy; stench from the drain very offensive.	Seven cases and three deaths in one family in nine days; afterwards no inhabited house in the yard escaped.
Penge . . (Mr. Ray.)	Situation unobjectionable, except a small drain near and trees around; inhabitants sober and cleanly.	A solitary case of Cholera; two attendants had severe diarrhœa.

TABLE XII.—*continued*.

Place and Reporter.	Local Circumstances.	Number of Cases immediately in same locality.
Walham Green (Messrs. Rouse and Rowland.)	Low badly-drained houses, crowded and badly ventilated; inhabitants not cleanly.	A single case at that time.
Dulwich . . (Mr. Ray.)	Site low; drainage bad; rooms over-crowded, badly ventilated, and dirty.	
Tooting—Drouet's School. (Mr. Kite.)	Want of space and ventilation; 1400 children; a dense fog causing children, on two days preceding outbreak, to be kept in schoolroom during play-hours, with closed doors and windows; all first cases on ground floor.	
Brixton, Surrey . (Mr. Ray.)	Open ditches at front and back of the house; privies and drains in a most offensive state; cottages over-crowded and ill ventilated.	
Maidstone . . (Dr. Plomley.)	Site elevated, and distant from river, but very bad as to sanitary condition; no water; no drainage; badly-constructed and open cesspools, contents of one soaking through wall of house of first case. The lodging-house in Bristow's Yard, site of renewed outbreak, contained three small rooms and a landing-place without ventilation of any kind, in which 17 persons slept; there is no back door, and the cellar, used as a wash-house, is the receptacle of refuse.	First case a woman, and second case a man who assisted to carry her to the grave, and therefore had, doubtless, been in the house; both died. First case in Bristow's Yard was a vagrant; the mistress of the lodging-house, and five other persons in the same yard.
Canterbury . . (Dr. Lochée.)	As regards elevation, drainage, supply of water, density of population, and cleanliness, very bad indeed.	The first case a travelling tailor—died; 36 hours later, two children were attacked, not in the same house, but within 100 yards of it.
Brighton . . (Dr. Ormerod.)	First case in close, ill-drained, and dirty neighbourhood; cesspools often annoying.	
Hertford County Gaol. (Dr. Davies.)	Nothing in locality to account for outbreak. Prison generally healthy; no open cesspool or drain near prison.	Twelve cases in first four days in the same part of the gaol.
St. Albans . . (Mr. Lipscombe.)	Situation healthy; favourable in every respect.	First a single case; only single cases occurred.

TABLE XII.—continued.

Place and Reporter.	Local Circumstances.	Number of Cases immediately in same locality.
Ware . . . (Mr. Butcher.)	Cottages detached from each other, and adjoining a lime-kiln.	
Hemel Hempstead (Mr. Merry.)	A cluster of cottages most healthily situated on Box Moor; no drains or offensive matter near.	
Reading . . . (Mr. Vines to Dr. Bradshaw.)	Locality low, damp, and badly drained; no densely-populated houses; dirty in the extreme, and ill ventilated.	
Downton . . (Dr. Welch.)	Ill-ventilated, thickly-tenanted, and dirty houses.	Four cases immediately following each other: first on 23rd August; second a woman in next house, then her husband, and on following day her mother-in-law.
Oxford . . (Dr. Kidd and Dr. Ogle.)	Spot low, ill drained, and dirty; an offensive open drain in the neighbourhood.	No second case in the same locality immediately.
County Gaol . (Mr. Allen.)	In unhealthy neighbourhood, but itself well drained and ventilated; well supplied with water and very clean.	First case fatal on Aug. 18th; second case Aug. 20th; third case Aug. 31st; and eight other cases within the nine following days.
Exeter . . (Dr. Shapter.)	Situation low, and circumstances generally insalubrious.	No case followed immediately on the first case.
Plymouth . . (Dr. Yonge.)	Average as regards density of population, drainage, and ventilation.	
Stonehouse, Market Lane. (Mr. Perry.)	Drainage very defective; houses densely crowded; situation flat; water-supply bad; houses ill ventilated; filth proverbial.	Two boys, a woman who nursed them, and one other person who came to the house; afterwards, not a house exempt in the locality.
Torquay . . (Dr. G. Black.)	Elevation not bad; no drainage; water-supply bad; population dense; ventilation very bad; cleanliness very defective.	
Gloucester . . (Mr. Hicks.)	Situation badly ventilated; damp; and water very impure.	

TABLE XII.—continued.

Place and Reporter.	Local Circumstances.	Number of Cases immediately in same locality.
Shrewsbury House of Industry. (Dr. H. Johnson.)	Situation very healthy; apartments airy and lofty; house clean and well-ventilated.	Almost simultaneously 11 or 12 cases in different parts of the asylum.
County Prison . .	Air in courts confined by the high double walls; otherwise, ventilation good.	
Bridgnorth . . (Dr. Strange.)	In houses of early cases, no ventilation; no drainage; filthiness extreme; of first case, site not low; of the next, level with the river.	No case immediately followed the first in the same locality.
Dowlais . . (Mr. White.)	Not in a populous district, but not very cleanly; damp and ill ventilated; within six yards of a heap of horse-dung, into which an overflowing privy was constantly draining.	The second was the child of the first patient in the same house; two other cases within 48 hours, but at some distance.
Holyhead . . (Mr. Walthew.)	Locality airy and salubrious.	
Birmingham Workhouse. (Dr. Bell Fletcher.)	Neighbourhood dirty and crowded; drainage imperfect; cesspools sometimes offensive; supply of water abundant; all cases but one in the insane ward.	
Walsall . . (Dr. Burton.)	A wide open street.	A lady; no case followed in the house nor in the town for ten days.
Stockport . . (Mr. J. Rayner.)	About lowest level of town, within 100 yards of river; drainage and water very good; population not dense; ventilation and cleanliness above the average; ventilation of street good; house and persons cleanly.	The first patient died; the second patient, her husband, recovered; a servant had diarrhœa.
Manchester . . (Dr. Pincoff.)	Tolerably well drained, but as bad as possible as regards water, density of population, ventilation, and cleanliness.	Not stated.
Bolton . . (Dr. Black.)	Residences confined, close, and densely populated; ventilation and cleanliness imperfect.	No case after the first for 20 days; then several occurred simultaneously; always more than one in the same house.

U

TABLE XII.—continued.

Place and Reporter.	Local Circumstances.	Number of Cases immediately in same locality.
Preston (Dr. Fearnside.)	Situation filthy in the extreme; no supply of water; drainage and ventilation bad; inhabitants low Irish; the cases occurred in cellars below level of street.	Second case two doors off first case, after six days' interval.
Lancaster (Mr. Harrison.)	Elevation and sanitary condition average.	
Hull (Dr. Sandwith.)	At first limited to ill-drained localities.	
Hedon (Dr. Sandwith.)	Several open sewers in neighbourhood of first cases recently cleaned out and very offensive; other cases about same time in healthy localities.	The person from Hull died, and the woman who nursed her.
Leeds (Mr. Bearpark.)	Low, damp, and ill ventilated, badly drained, densely populated, and dirty.	The first four cases occurred all within 150 yards during eight days.
Titchmarsh (Mr. Williams to Dr. Burrows.)	Drainage fair; water unexceptionable; but an offensive smell from offal in a tub in yard of first patient (Edgson).	First patient and his mother died; wife and two daughters were attacked with diarrhœa, and the nurse died.
Pocklington (Dr. T. Wilson.)	Rather close, but not so much so as many other localities in the town; an open yard, with pigs, privies, and drains common to the cottages.	A travelling man, the keeper of the lodging-house, and four other persons living in the same range of houses.
Wakefield Lunatic Asylum. (Dr. Wright.)	Ward clean and well ventilated; one of most healthy in institution, but site of building unfavourable as to drainage and ventilation; damp; dysentery prevalent.	Five cases and four deaths in first ward.
Wakefield (Dr. Wright.)	On elevated ground; supply of water good; ventilation and cleanliness not defective.	A single case in that neighbourhood; the second case occurred three days later in different parts of the town.
Wakefield (Mr. Statten.)	First case in proximity of some privies, but they are still unremoved, and no other case has occurred within their influence; some much more offensive depôts of privy soil, &c., lower down same street, and there no cases occurred. In the ground floor of the Corn Exchange, the man in comfortable circumstances.	

TABLE XII.—*continued.*

Place and Reporter.	Local Circumstances.	Number of Cases immediately in same locality.
Sunderland—Monkwearmouth. (Dr. Brown.)	First case on shore: the reputed sources of the disease were wanting; an isolated farm-house. Second case: population of colliery dense, but sanitary condition by no means unusually bad; in various parts of the town of Sunderland, there was just as much filth.	A single case only in this house; there had been previous cases amongst the shipping. After a case on the 6th Nov., no other case till the 17th; on the 24th or 26th the disease became general in the colliery.
Seaham Harbour . (Dr. Brown.)	Houses in a court, ill constructed, and without thorough ventilation; a dirty ash-pit very near it.	The first patient died, and a man who lived with him was attacked and recovered.
Broom Hill, near Dalkeith. (Dr. Moir to Dr. McWilliam.)	Private house on elevated ground in a considerable inclosure a mile from any town.	The first patient, a gentleman, and his daughter, and a woman who had visited the house, died.
South Brent . (Dr. Yonge.)	A lodging-house for vagrants.	A vagrant, the mistress of the house, and a lodger.
Tewkesbury . (Dr. Viner Beadle.)	An alley containing a slaughter-house, pigsties, and bone deposit.	For more than a month it lingered there, spreading thence over the town.

Table XIII.—*Statistics of the Lunatic Asylums in England*

Names of Asylums.	Classes of Patients.	Number of Patients.	Number of outbreaks.
Peckham House.....	Men	199 {	1st men 2nd men
	Women	285 {	1st women 2nd women
Grove Hall, Bow	Men	144	1st men
	Women	263 {	1st women 2nd women
London House, Hackney	Men	15	...
	Women	13	
Althorpe House, Battersea	Men	16	...
	Women	28	...
Bethnal House, Bethnal Green	Men	264	
	Women	348 {	1st women 2nd women
Camberwell House........................	Men	133 {	1st men 2nd men
	Women	195	...
St. Marylebone Infirmary................	Men	26	...
	Women	47	...
St. Luke's	Men	92	...
	Women	123	...
Cowper House, Old Brompton.........	Men	33	...
Hoxton House	Men	160	...
	Women	279	...
Kingsland Asylum	Men	51	...
	Women	41	...
Vernon House, Briton Ferry............	Men	78	...
	Women	73	...
Hull Borough Asylum	Men	38	...
	Women	35	...
Bristol Asylum	Men	30	...
	Women	49	...
Wreckenton Asylum...	Men	21	...
	Women	16	...
West Riding Asylum	Men	296	...
	Women	324	...

attacked by Cholera during the Epidemic of 1848-49.

Date of first case or death.	Date of last case or death.	Number of days in each outbreak.	Number of cases.	Number of deaths.	Number of wards attacked.
22nd October	15th Nov.	25	90	3	2
25th June	4th Sept.	72	20	13	3
17th October	15th Nov.	30	33	16	7
12th July	17th Aug.	35	16	11	6
10th Feb. 1849	19th Feb. 1849	10	4	3	1
13th Nov. 1848	29th Nov. 1848	17	21	7	4
18th Oct. 1849	...	...	1	1	1
5th Feb. 1849	...	...	1	1	1
22nd Nov. 1848	...	...	1	1	1
10th Jan. 1849	19th Jan.	10	3	3	?
12th Jan.	2nd Feb.	22	5	3	?
31st Aug.	13th Sept.	14	20	18	18
14th Feb.	6th March	21	28	25	11
11th Sept.	27th Sept.	17	13	13	10
1st July	6th Aug.	37	9	8	3 ?
7th Sept.	...	...	1	1	1
16th July	26th Aug.	42	13	9	2 ?
21st July	30th Aug.	41	4	4	2
11th Aug.	6th Sept.	27	4	3	2
23rd July	8th Sept.	46	6	1	2
20th Aug.	23rd Aug.	4	4	3	1
12th Sept.	28th Oct.	47	7	3	2
10th Sept.	11th Oct.	32	32	18	7
25th July	16th Aug.	23	11	9	4 ?
25th July	...	...	2	2	?
29th July	1st Aug.	4	4	4	1
29th July	18th Aug.	21	5	4	3
9th Sept.	16th Sept.	8	3	1	2 ?
27th Aug.	5th Sept.	10	6	3	3 ?
24th Sept.	7th Oct.	14	6	3	2
1st Sept.	24th Sept.	24	6	2	3
12th Sept.	20th Sept.	9	14	11 }	several
12th Sept.	20th Sept.	9	10	7	
15th Oct.	15th Nov.	32	70	53	13
22nd Sept.	27th Nov.	67	63	45	12

TABLE XIV.

SHOWING THE ORDER IN WHICH THE EPIDEMIC BEGAN AND CEASED IN THE SEVERAL WARDS OF FIVE LUNATIC ASYLUMS, WHICH SUFFERED SEVERELY FROM CHOLERA.

Name of the asylum.	Whether the first or second outbreak, and whether among men or women.	Designations of the wards.	Date of the first case in each ward.	Date of the last case in each ward.	Duration of the epidemic in each ward (in days).	Number of cases of Cholera in each ward.	Remarks.
Peckham House.	1st outbreak, women.	Laundry.	17 Oct. 1848	...	...	1	
		No. 1	19 „	4 Nov. 1848	17	11	
		11	20 „	5 „	17	8	
		12	21 „	... „	16	4	
		9	22 „	15 „	25	8	
		13	...	8 „	13	2	
		10	1 Nov.	5 „	6	6	
	1st outbreak, men.	2	22 Oct.	31 Oct.	10	2	
		3	23 „	15 Nov.	23	11	
	2nd outbreak, women.	9	13 July, 1849	13 July, 1849	1	3	
		12	...	...	...	1	
		8	...	15 July,	3	2	
		10	16 „	25 „	10	3	
		Mansion House. 19	„	...	...	1	
		No. 1	20 „	17 Aug.	29	4	
	2nd outbreak, men.	No. 2	25 June	16 Aug.	52	11	
		4	28 „	27 July	30	6	
		3	20 Aug.	4 Sept.	16	3	
Grove Hall, Bow.	1st outbreak, women.	No. 5	13 Nov. 1848	29 Nov. 1848	17	10	
		1	16 „	19 „	4	5	
		4	17 „	25 „	9	3	
		7	18 „	20 „	3	3	
	2nd outbreak, men.	No. 2	10 Feb. 1849	19 Feb. 1849	10	4	
	3rd outbreak, men.	No. 5	18 Oct.	...	...	1	
Horton House.	Women.	Pitt's	10 Sept.	29 Sept.	20	7	
		Batchelor's	...	2 Oct.	23	5	
		Weston's	19 „	26 Sept.	8	9	
		Edgecombe's	24 „	...	...	1	
		Wright's	26 „	3 Oct.	7	3	
		Smee's	27 „	11 „	14	5	
		Keeley's	29 „	...	...	1	
	Men.	Pitt's	12 Sept.	28 Oct.	47	4	
		Infirmary	18 „	23 Sept.	6	2	
		Lane's	2 Oct.	...	...	1	

TABLE XIV.—*continued.*

Whether the first or second outbreak, and whether among men or women.	Designation of the wards.		Remarks.
1st women.	No. 12	14 Feb.49	
	18		
	17	...	
	6	17 „	
	13		
	19	...	
	15	19 „	
	11	24 „	
	10		
2nd men.	No. 6	1 Aug.49	
	Infirmary	2 Sept.	
	No. 5	...	
	1	3 „	
	8		
	3		
	7	...	
	2	4 „	
	4		
	10	10 „	
Women.	No. 1	11 Sept.4	
	5	13 „	
	7		
	17		
	11	16 „	
	18	19 „	
	14	...	
	6	23 „	
	12	25 „	
Women.	New Building, 3	22 Sept.4	1 case subsequently on the 1st Nov.
	„ 1	16 Oct.	
	Old Building, 12		
	„ 16	18 „	
	„ 18		
	New Building, 2		
	Old Building, 11		
	New Building, 10	21 „	
	„ 4		
	Old Building, 15		
	„ 14		
	„ 13		
	„ 18	30 „	
Men.	Old Building, 4		
	„ 3		
	„ 7		
	New Building, 5	...	
	Old Building, 6	19 „	
	„ 2		
	New Building, 6	...	
	Old Building, 9	20 „	
	New Building, 7		
	Old Building, 1		
	New Building, 8		

TABLE XV.

ABSTRACTS of the ACCOUNTS received by the Cholera Committee of the appearance of Cholera subsequently to the probable introduction of infection in Seventy-three Towns, Villages, and Public Establishments.

Place and Reporter.	First Cases of Cholera.
1. Spitalfields Workhouse. (Mr. Byles.)	On four several occasions cases of Cholera were admitted into the Workhouse, the inmates being previously healthy, and on each occasion one or two cases of malignant Cholera followed. [No details are given.]
2. South Hackney ...... (Mr. Appleton.)	*First Case* in this district of Hackney, a jobbing bricklayer had been to Old Street Road, where Cholera prevailed on the 11th August; at 3 A.M., on the 14th August, was attacked, and died at half-past 4 P.M. *Second Case.* Mother-in-law of first patient nursed him, but did not sleep at his house, was attacked on August 16th, and died in 14 hours. *Third Case.* A young man, who was much in the houses of former two patients, at death of latter, and assisted in wringing sheets they had used. Attacked on morning of 17th, and died on 19th. *Fourth Case.* Son of second patient had also been with his mother while she was dying, was attacked on morning of 18th, fell into collapse, but recovered. *Fifth Case.* Another son of second patient similarly exposed to infection by her was attacked at the end of a week, recovered. *Sixth Case.* A woman who had visited the first and second patients attacked 10 days after death of second patient; removed to Union, and there died.
3. Royal Free Hospital and Holborn Union House. (Dr. Peacock.)	155 children were received from Tooting on the 5th January, and on the 6th, 7th, and 8th, there were sent in from the Holborn Union House to take charge of them about 14 nurses and 4 male attendants, all of whom slept in the wards, and none of whom had visited Tooting except the matron, who had been there one night before the removal of the children. During the first two or three days, three or four of the nurses were sent back to the Union, and others came in their stead, and there were also several men who were much with the children during the day, but slept in the Union at night. So that, in all probability, about 20 to 25 persons had free intercourse with the children during the first fortnight, while 9 of the children suffered from Cholera, 30 from severe vomiting and diarrhœa, and 45 from simple diarrhœa.

Place and Reporter.	First Cases of Cholera.
	On the 13th January, 1845, the eighth day from the reception of the children from Tooting, two of the attendants in the Hospital were taken ill with Diarrhœa, and one who had come to the Hospital on the 7th and slept in the Boys' Ward till the 11th, and since that date in the Union, presented symptoms of Cholera on the 13th, and died in the Union house. Between 13th and 21st, ten cases of serious diarrhœa, three becoming Cholera, and one proving fatal, occurred among the attendants at the Hospital. At the same time there were from 50 to 60 persons in another part of the building, situated not many yards from the children's wards, but having little intercourse with them, none of whom laboured under any similar form of affection. From the first the freest intercourse existed between the Union and the Hospital. And on the same day that the attendant above referred to as having slept in the Boys' Ward till the 11th was taken ill, namely, on the 13th, another man in the Union, who occupied the opposite bed to him, was seized, and shortly after died; and from this time the disease manifested itself among the inmates. [According to the weekly returns in the Registrar-General's Report, no fatal cases had occurred previously in the Holborn district. But three deaths are recorded as occurring in the week ending January 20th, and thirteen in the next week. All in the Union Workhouse.]
4. Sydenham .... (Mr. Ray.)	*First Case*, 11th July. A gentleman who came from Bath to attend the funeral of a friend who had died of Cholera in Bridge Street, Blackfriars, London. *Second, Third, and Fourth Cases* were sons of the woman who washed the linen and clothes of the first patient. They were washed in a yard to which the second and third patients (children of eight and ten years) had access. And the fourth patient, a young man of 25 years, had carried them washed and unwashed from one house to the other. These cases, all fatal, occurred a few days after the first case. Only one other fatal case occurred in Sydenham about the beginning of September.
5. Southend .... (Mr. W. R. Warwick to Dr. Fincham.)	The first case, on the 28th June, and eleven others (namely, Cases 2, 6, 7, 8, 9, 10, 12, 20, 21, 32, and 34), out of a total of 35 cases, were all from infected districts. *Case 2.* A man had been at Greenwich two or three days before, died at Southend on the 5th July; had neglected diarrhœa. Cholera attacked him on his way home. *Case 3.* Came on July 5th to nurse Case 2; returned home on July 7th, was seized the same night with Cholera, and died next day. *Case 4.* Brother of Case 2; came home on evening

Place and Reporter.	First Cases of Cholera.
	of July 5th, had diarrhœa on 6th, Cholera at noon on July 8th, and died on 11th. Case 5. Mother of Cases 3 and 4; nursed them; attacked early on morning of July 10th, died same day. The father and two daughters were subsequently affected with Diarrhœa. At this time no other case existed in the place, nor did other cases occur in other parts of the Union for a month after these, except imported cases, Nos. 6, 7, 8, 9, 10, and 12, between July 15th and August 17th. Cases 11 (August 5th) to 18 (August 30th), are attributed by Mr. Warwick to atmospheric influence. But between Cases 13, 14, 15, 16, and 17 there seems to have been indirect communication. Between Cases 22, 23, 24, 25, 26, 27, and 28 there was communication. Case 22 had nursed a lodger ill with rice-water. Diarrhœa, September 4th, died September 5th. Cases 23 and 24, her children, seized September 6th; Case 23 died September 10th. Case 25, of same family, seized September 9th. Case 26 lived two miles off, had been to and fro the houses of previous patients, and her mother had nursed Case 22; was seized September 9th. Cases 27 and 28, brother and sister of 26, attacked September 12th and 15th.
6. Gravesend, Officers of Customs. (Dr. McWilliam.)	A tidewaiter, placed on board a French vessel (from Dunkirk, where Cholera prevailed, and with a case of Cholera on board), on the 19th March, returned to Gravesend on 23rd with Diarrhœa, on 25th had Cholera, and died in 12 hours. The man in whose house he lodged had Cholera 13 days afterwards, but recovered. There were no other cases of Cholera for many weeks before or after at Gravesend.
7. Margate Infirmary ... (Mr. Field.)	*First Case* on 25th August. A man had visited friends in the town where Cholera existed, was brought back in a state of collapse, and died 9 hours after. *The Second Case* occurred in the same ward in which the first case lay. There are twenty-one wards in the hospital, and eleven on the male side. Soon the disease broke out on the female side; all the patients were removed from the ward in which the first woman was attacked. The second was a child who lay close to the door communicating with this ward. The two next cases were nurses who waited constantly and exclusively on Cholera patients.
8. Hertford County Gaol and House of Correction. (Dr. Davies.)	*First Outbreak. First patient* attacked 30th December, 1848, committed to the House of Correction four days previously, then in good health; had resided in a locality where two or three cases of Cholera existed at the time. He died. *The Second Case* occurred on December 31st, in a

Place and Reporter.	First Cases of Cholera.
	man in the same yard of the prison. On January 1st three more cases occurred. On January 2nd, seven new cases, and then the disease spread rapidly. The debtors, who have no communication with the prisoners in the Gaol and House of Correction entirely escaped. *Second Outbreak.* J. B., a man attacked October 9th, 1849, had been in prison since the 15th June, had had Diarrhœa since October 6th. The prison had not been free from Diarrhœa of a specific character since the previous outbreak of Cholera. The disease had disappeared from the town for some weeks previously. "There is no reason to suspect the introduction of fresh contagion." *Second Case.* A female prisoner, attacked October 23rd, having had Diarrhœa since the 18th; was in a ward at a distance from that in which the first case occurred. *The 3rd and 4th Cases* occurred on the 24th October, one a male the other a female prisoner, both had Diarrhœa the previous day. Another case occurred on the 27th, and four on the 28th, when the disease became general.
9. Lower Whitby, near Oxford, consists of one farm-house and a double cottage with two families. (Mr. T. Allen and Mr. Rusher.)	*First Case.* A boy, farm servant at the farm-house, visited his mother, ill of Cholera, at Abingdon on August 12th, returned the same day to Whitby, attacked with Cholera on the 14th, and died on 15th. *Second Case.* Wife of cottager, nursed first patient, a week after had Diarrhœa, on 31st August had developed Cholera. Recovered. *Third Case.* Husband of second patient, had a mild attack on September 2nd. Recovered. *Fourth and Fifth Cases.* The other cottager and his wife, father and mother of third patient, both attacked on September 2nd. Both died. Some of the farmer's family had Diarrhœa, but recovered.
10. Long Handborough. (Mr. T. Allen, Mr. Shurlock, and Mr. Palmer.)	*First Case.* A woman from Shoe Lane, London, which she left on 13th August, in the morning reached Long Handborough at 8½ P.M., felt ill before arrival, immediately afterwards seized with vomiting and purging. Died in sixteen hours. *Second and Third Cases* on the 16th August. One lived in the house in which the first patient died, the other lived in a house fifty yards off, but had nursed the first patient. Recovered. *Fourth Case.* The child of a neighbour, who had been frequently in house of first and third patients, on the 21st August. Died. *Fifth Case.* On the 26th August, the father of this child. Died.

Place and Reporter.	First Cases of Cholera.
	Sixth Case. On the 28th August, the mother of the child. Died.
	Seventh Case. On September 1st, another neighbour, who had communicated through medium of his daughter. Died.
	Eighth Case. Also on September 1st, a boy who lived with this daughter of the seventh patient.
	Ninth Case. The child of third patient and niece of first, on September 4. Diarrhœa existed before. Died.
	Tenth Case. Another child of the third patient, on Sept. 6th. [The names and all particulars are given.]
11. Tichmarsh, near Thrapston. (Mr. H. Williams.)	1st. A butcher had been to Peterborough and visited a house there infected with Cholera on the 3rd October. His bowels became very loose on the morning of the 6th; he soon became collapsed, and died the same night. "His bowels had been out of order for a month previous, and any excitement invariably set them going." 2nd. His mother was attacked on the 18th and lingered to the 24th. His wife, two daughters, and son, were also ill with severe Diarrhœa. 3rd. The woman, who nursed the first case, was attacked in his house on the 13th, moved to her own 400 or 500 yards off on 14th. Recovered. 4th. This woman's daughter was attacked on the 17th; mother removed her to her house half a mile off. Recovered. 5th. The husband of the last patient was attacked on the 22nd. Nine cases (six fatal) occurred within a few doors of last patient, between the 21st October and 15th November. The sister of "Case 5," who nursed both Cases 4 and 5, was attacked on the 4th November, and died in twelve hours. Two men living next door to first case were attacked on the 9th and 14th November. Both died. A woman, who nursed them, was attacked on the 17th, and died in twelve hours.
12. Bedford .... (Dr. G. F. D. Evans.)	*Lucy Flemming* had just returned from Northampton where Cholera prevailed, she was seized with Diarrhœa on the 15th September and died on the 19th. *Ann Lichfield* had been in frequent communication with Lucy Flemming, was attacked on the 21st, and died in twelve hours. This patient was attended by Mrs. Barker and Mrs. Alva, her next door neighbours, they were taken ill on the 22nd, and died, one the 25th the other on the 27th. After this Diarrhœa and Cholera spread rapidly. [In the Registrar-General's Report the death of Lucy Flemming is not recorded as due to Cholera.]

Place and Reporter.	First Cases of Cholera.
(Dr. Dick and Mr. Gates.)	" The disease appeared suddenly, and many persons were taken ill at the same time." " We could not discover that the first cases had any contact with patients in the disease far or near."
13. South Brent, Dartmoor. (Dr. Davie and Dr. Lang.)	*First Case*, on 23rd July, an Irishman just arrived from Plymouth. He died. *Second Case*, soon after, a woman in same house. *Third Case*, the mistress of the house. Both died. Then the disease spread until a dozen persons died, and every case could be clearly traced back to the Irishman. [The facts do not appear to have been personally investigated either by Dr. Davie, or by Dr. Lang, and no dates are given after that of the first case, but each separately gives the facts with confidence in their accuracy.] (The Registrar-General records a fatal case as occurring at South Brent on July 17th.)
14. Swansea, and 15. Swansea Gaol. (Dr. G. G. Bird and Mr. W. H. Michael.)	A few cases from infected districts about the beginning of July.—Mr. Michael. [Dr. Bird does not mention the occurrence of cases in the town before those in the gaol; nor does the Registrar-General's Report record any fatal cases before the 6th July. But it is there recorded that one fatal case occurred at Llangafaast, a subdistrict of Swansea district, on the 31st May, two in June, and three in July.] On 6th July, a prisoner in the gaol, who had come on previous day from Neath, where Cholera existed, was attacked with Cholera, and died. In the next fortnight four other prisoners, who had likewise come from Neath on the 5th July, and one who had not been there, were attacked fatally. In all, 14 cases occurred, 8 in prisoners who had not been at Neath or Cardiff; and 2 prisoners who had not been at those places being discharged were attacked immediately afterwards and died. They had had diarrhœa previously. [Cholera had prevailed in May and June at Neath and Cardiff, but became more prevalent in July.] On the 20th July, a girl who had nursed a patient with Cholera in the gaol on the 19th, was seized with Cholera immediately after her discharge. On the 23rd July, one of the policemen who had cleansed the house the last patient died in, was attacked and died. On the 25th July two cases occurred not far from the house of the policeman, without any intercourse traced between them. On the 27th two other cases, and after this time the cases became numerous.
16. Walsall Union Workhouse. (Dr. Burton.)	*First Case.* A man came two days previously from Wolverhampton, moribund when admitted on 31st August. *Second Case*, on 10th September, had come to Wal-

Place and Reporter.	First Cases of Cholera.
	all two or three days previously from Portobello, where she had been exposed to contagion. Died of effects of Cholera on 26th. *Third Case.* A man who had come from Bilston to Walsall two days previously, attacked and admitted on 13th September, died on the 14th. *Fourth Case.* A man from a house where people from Cholera locality lodged, 14th September. *Fifth Case.* The most active attendant on the third patient was attacked on the 17th, and died on the 18th. *Sixth Case,* on 18th September, also imported. Of 8 female attendants on this woman, one had Cholera, and two rice-water purging, followed by consecutive fever; dates of their attacks not mentioned. *Seventh and Eighth Cases.* Two female inmates not exposed to contagion were attacked on the 19th September with rice-water purging, followed by fever. *Ninth Case.* The most constant attendant on the fifth patient, who had attended also on the fourth and sixth patients, was attacked on the 22nd. *Tenth Case.* A man exposed by attendance on third patient and others; attacked on 23rd September. There were in all 51 cases (28 fatal) of Cholera or rice-water purging; of these 18 were brought in already infected, 14 were inmates exposed to infection or contagion, 18 not exposed to infection or contagion.
17. Wolverhampton...... (Dr. Topham.)	A man from Liverpool (a street there in which Cholera existed), first night in Wolverhampton, slept in lodgings in a court, next day went into another house in a neighbouring street, there had Cholera, August 4th, and died. *The Second Case* occurred in the lodging-house where first patient slept on night previous to attack. *The Third* in house in which first patient died. *The Fourth Case* in next house but one to this. *The Fifth Case* in the house in which second patient died. *The Sixth Case* in the house of fourth patient. *The Seventh and Eighth Cases* about fifty yards from some of former cases. *The Ninth* on 13th August, a mile distant. The next cases without known communication.
18. Barton on Humber.. (Mr. Morley, Mr. W. H. Eddie.)	A vagrant from Hull, where she had had premonitory symptoms, was attacked with Cholera on August 21st and died in Tindall's lodging-house. [Previous to this case, namely, on July 4th, one fatal case is recorded by the Registrar-General, possibly a case of English Cholera.] 2nd. The child of the woman who nursed first case, was attacked on the 24th and died on 27th. The woman herself was attacked on 26th, and recovered. Two other women living in same lodging-house were at-

Place and Reporter.	First Cases of Cholera.
	tacked on the 27th, one died in eight hours, the other on September 6th, of consecutive fever. *6th Case.* A woman took the clothes of the patient who died on the 27th to Tomlinson's lodging-house on the 28th, but did not remain there. A vagrant from Grimsby, where Cholera was not prevalent, was attacked on night of August 28th, in Tomlinson's lodging-house. Tomlinson's daughter was attacked and died on September 1st. An old woman living under the same roof was attacked and died on September 5th. Thirty-seven cases in all reported by Mr. Morley and Mr. Eddie; twenty-seven fatal. *Five* occurred in Tindall's lodging-house; *Four* in Tomlinson's (including a vagrant attacked on 16th); *Nine* occurred in houses near Tomlinson's; *Six* others were cases imported from Hull (not including the first case); *Thirteen* occurred at Fleetwood and Newport, not traced. So that twenty-four out of thirty-seven might be ascribed to contagion or infection more or less direct. Mr. Eddie makes the proportion of probably infected cases larger.
19. Hedon in Holderness. (Dr. Sandwith.)	An Irishman, from Mill Street, Hull, where Cholera raged, attacked with Diarrhœa on the road, fell into Cholera at Hedon next morning, on 26th August, 1849. No other case at this time. A Mrs. Harpur came from Yarmouth to Hull, there dined in a house in which there had recently been cases of Cholera, on following day went to Hedon, on next day, September 14th, was attacked with Cholera, and died on the day following. Nurse Brown, who was in attendance, was speedily attacked, and died on second day. Another family under the same roof were also attacked, and one died. A case had occurred at village of Preston, one mile from Hedon, on September 12th, fatal in a few hours; the case was an isolated one, i. e. not traceable to contagion, and other cases occurred in neighbouring houses in Preston. A day or two after the death of Mrs. Harpur, a woman with two children came through Hull (where Cholera prevailed) to Hedon, to visit a grandmother. Within a day or two one of the children fell into Cholera and died in a few hours. The mother and grandmother, both living in same house, were next attacked, and, in the course of a fortnight, seven more individuals residing in the same square or alley of eight or ten houses died of Cholera.
20. Kilnsea .... (Dr. Sandwith.)	A man and woman from Kilnsea visited a daughter dying of Cholera at Hedon, twenty-one miles distant. On their return home, two days afterwards, both fell into Cholera and one died. The grandmother, who had not left Kilnsea, but dwelt in the same house, took

Place and Reporter.	First Cases of Cholera.
	the disease and quickly died. [These deaths are not recorded by the Registrar-General. There were four deaths in males at Partington subdistrict, a few miles from Kilnsea.]
21. Howden Union Workhouse. (Dr. Sandwith?)	A child of a vagrant, just arrived, died in about two hours without being seen by a medical man. Another child (an inmate) which was in same room was seized on following day with Cholera, and died in twenty-four hours. The mothers of both children were attacked on the next day and both died. A healthy woman, who nursed them, was the next victim. Another employed in like manner also died of the disease. The Cholera then spread through the Union-house and carried off eleven persons. [These deaths occurred (Registrar-General's Report) between January 5th and February 11th. Deaths from Cholera occurred at Clifton Workhouse, on January 3rd, at Walingate (York), late in January, South Cave, Beverly, on January 3rd; all in the East Riding. The vagrant may have come from one of those places.]
22. Pocklington, Yorkshire. (Dr. T. Wilson?)	A travelling man arrived from York on September 2nd and died in a few hours in a lodging-house. The keeper of the lodging-house was attacked on the 7th September and died on the 11th. A man living in same range of houses was attacked on the 11th and died in a few hours. Three other cases occurred in same range of buildings on the 16th, 17th, and 22nd. Two cases, not traceable to same source, occurred on the 12th September. No others of any severity occurred in the town.
23. Church Stretton ... (Mr. Wilding to Dr. Wallich.)	*First Patient.* The driver of the mail cart from Shrewsbury to Church Stretton died August 11th, after three or four days' illness. *Second Patient.* A married sister of the first patient, who had nursed him, and at whose house he died, had diarrhœa three or four days, and died August 19th. *Third Patient.* An old woman, residing at a distance, who assisted in nursing the second patient, died on 21st August. There was no diarrhœa prevalent in the town at the time. The first patient was taken ill while in Shrewsbury, where he was staying for a few days, and his worst symptoms came on during his journey to Church Stretton on August 11th. The town of Church Stretton lies high and dry on a deep stratum of gravel, with excellent natural drainage, and pretty constant currents of wind. The house was clean and well ventilated. The nearest places at which Cholera prevailed were Shrewsbury and Bridgnorth, about 11 and 18 miles distant.

Place and Reporter.	First Cases of Cholera.
34. Stonehouse .... (Dr. Yonge.)	On the 20th July, when the Cholera was raging in Stonehouse Lane, Plymouth, a boy left his home, wandered about the streets, and was taken into a house in Market Lane, Stonehouse. On the 21st he was attacked and died at 2 P.M. On same day, at 7 P.M., a boy who slept with him the previous night was attacked and died in three hours and a half. The woman in whose room these boys died, after attending some other cases, also died. And one other person who came to the house from Devonport was attacked. There was no case in this locality before the boy came from Plymouth. Afterwards it spread.
35. Wakefield Lunatic Asylum. (Dr. Wright's Official Report.)	*First Patient.* Eliza Fenton, admitted on 17th September, 1849, from Gomersal workhouse, where two persons had died of Cholera the previous night. At 9 P.M., on same day, was found to be suffering from Diarrhœa; on night of 25th September Cholera supervened. She recovered. *Second Patient.* Mary Morley, in room opposite to Eliza Fenton's, in same gallery, attacked in the night of 22nd September, and died the following day. *Third Case.* Sarah Atkinson, ten days after, 2nd October, slept in a room occupied for four hours by Mary Morley (second case) during her attack, and died. *Fourth Case.* In same ward as the other three, on 6th October. *Fifth Case.* Also in a room in same ward, on 8th. On October 9th, all patients transferred from this ward to another range of rooms, before uninhabited, and no further cases occurred amongst them. On October 15th, a male patient in another part of the building attacked, and nearly at same time, on 17th, a woman in different part. On the following day others, and at length not a single ward escaped. N.B.—Previous to the appearance of Cholera in the Asylum it was gradually spreading its ravages over the surrounding district. But in 1832, when the same thing occurred, the Asylum escaped.
36. Seaham Harbour ... (Dr. J. Brown.)	Between 21st July and 28th August ten seamen from London were landed; eight treated in the infirmary, of whom two died, and two, both of whom died, out of the infirmary. First indigenous case occurred on 15th August, fatal on the 16th, not traced to direct communication with sick sailors. House in a court very near the harbour. Next Case, brother-in-law of former and living with him, occurred on 16th. This patient was removed to his mother's house. The mother-in-law sickened on the 21st, her grandson, living with her, on the 28th. Their next door neighbour on the 1st September. Mr. Smith, surgeon to the infirmary, who had likewise attended all the cases in the town, was attacked

Place and Reporter.	First Cases of Cholera.

on the 24th of August, and died on the 28th. The matron and sole nurse of the infirmary was attacked on the 25th of August, but recovered.

Two other cases not traced to contagion, and not fatal, occurred on the 16th August, and others subsequently to the 21st, and prior to the 28th.

Crews of ships in the harbour had suffered from Cholera.

First. A trimmer employed in these ships sickened on 3rd October, and died in 14 hours.

Second. A woman who nursed him and washed his clothes, sickened and died on 5th October.

Third and Fourth. A married daughter of the former and her husband, who had visited and attended upon him in his illness, sickened and died on the 5th. The two last lived in a distant part of the town from that of former cases.

Fifth Case. A next door neighbour of last two, sickened and died also on the 5th.

Sixth. A child in part of same house as third and fourth cases sickened on 6th, and died some days later in Fever.

Seventh. Mother of No. 5, sickened on 7th, but recovered.

Eighth. A young neighbour of third and fourth cases, much in their house during their illness, sickened on the 8th or 9th, but recovered.

27. Gateshead Low Fell (Dr. J. Brown.)

A woman, who had nursed her husband with Cholera at Wrekenton, at his decease came to Gateshead Low Fell, and shortly afterwards she sickened and died.

A week after, her brother, with whom she stayed, sickened and died. An old woman at Gateshead Low Fell received the clothes of the man who died of Cholera at Wrekenton to wash, took Cholera, and her husband, who nursed her, also took it. Both died. These were the only cases at Gateshead Low Fell.

28. North Shields, Tynemouth. (Dr. J. Brown.)

A man, who had been to Durham, where Cholera prevailed, and there buried his wife and daughter, dead of the disease, on his return fell ill of Cholera, and died. A woman from a different street nursed him till his death, then returned to her home, sickened, and died. Then Cholera spread in the street where she lived, and became generally diffused. [Dates not given.]

29. South Shields ...... (Dr. J. Brown.)

After an equivocal case, the first was a woman coming from a vagrant lodging-house in Sunderland to a similar house in South Shields, suffering from Diarrhœa. On arrival, attacked with Cholera. Died same day, 16th March, 1849. A young, strong woman in same lodging-house attacked on 18th, died on 21st. Another inmate attacked on 19th, died on 21st. The mother of former, also in the house, attacked on 25th.

Place and Reporter.	First Cases of Cholera.
	Died. [One case fatal had occurred at Yarrow, two or three miles distant, on February 13th. See Registrar-General's Report.]
30. Broomhill, between Dalkeith and Lasswade (distant a mile from either). (Mr. Moir, of Musselburgh.)	First Case. (Slight.) Mrs. A., 21st December; had been exposed to infection at Dalkeith and Lasswade. Second Case. Col. A., husband of first, on 24th December. Fatal. He had not been out of his own grounds for some weeks previously. Third Case. Daughter of first and second, on 26th December. Fatal. Fourth Case. A woman who laid out body of second, on 27th. Fatal on 28th.
31. Musselburgh .... (Mr. Moir.)	A series of importations; the last was as follows:— a woman from Queensferry, found on the road, taken to a lodging-house. Recovered. Three women who had been with her in the house were attacked and died. Thence it spread to others in same street. Twenty-two died. No other locality in the parish was attacked, in a population of 9000. [Dates and other details wanting.]
32. Tooting (Drouet's School.) (Mr. W. J. Kite.)	The child first attacked, January 1st, had not been in an infected place, but had been living and sleeping in the same rooms with children from Wandsworth Union Workhouse, where cases of Cholera had occurred, and also with other children from different metropolitan parishes. [Cases of Cholera had occurred in the Wandsworth Union Workhouse in November and December, 1848.] The child attacked was removed to the sick ward on the first complaint of illness, and remained there surrounded by other patients until the symptoms began to indicate Cholera. No case occurred in the sick ward for some days. The next cases after the first came from the same ward as the first, and from an adjoining one (both on the ground floor).
33. Maidstone .... (Dr. Plomley.)	First Case. July 2nd, 1849. An intemperate woman, whose husband had returned home from the Borough, London, on the 30th June (two days previously). The wife had Diarrhœa on the 1st July. Fatal. Second Case. July 5th. Had assisted in carrying the person of the first case to the grave. Fatal. No other cases till the 15th July : between that date and 3rd August, Ten Cases, none traced to communication with patients in disease. One was a vagrant. Another had been to Tunbridge Wells on the previous day. Thirteenth Case. Attacked August 8th. No. 14 and 15 on the 11th and 13th of August, not traced to communication. No. 16, a vagrant attacked on August 13th, in a lodging-house in Bristow's Yard.

Place and Reporter.	First Cases of Cholera.
	Nos. 17, 18, 22, 24, 25, and 26 all occurred in Bristow's Yard, on the 13th, 14th, 16th, 17th, 18th, and 21st August. The 21st Case had nursed the 13th Case, was attacked August 15th. Of thirty residents attacked fatally, twelve were either certainly or probably exposed to contagion or infection. Many cases were those of vagrants.
34. Ashford Union Work-house. (Mr. H. Whitfell.)	A labourer, who had been in search of work, was attacked with Cholera, and being removed to the Work-house, died there in a few hours. His fellow-labourer, who attended him during the night, was attacked just previous to their going to the Union-house, and also died in twenty-four hours. Immediately after the introduction of these patients several cases occurred in this Union, some of which were fatal. [It is not clearly stated that the cases following the two imported ones were the first indigenous cases, nor are the intervals between the cases given.]
35. St. George's Parish, Canterbury. (Dr. Lochée.)	On September 24th a woman died of Cholera near the river: her niece, Mrs. Cheeseman, who nursed her, removed certain articles of clothing to her own home, in St. George's Parish, at least a quarter of a mile distant. On October 2nd Mrs. Cheeseman's husband and one of her sons were attacked with Cholera, and both died. Four persons in the adjoining cottage were seized about the same time (October 2nd) and two died. On October 3rd the woman Cheeseman herself was seized with Cholera and died in twenty-four hours. On the same day three more of the children of this woman were attacked. They recovered. On the 7th October the husband's father, who had visited the family during their illness, was seized and died. He had suffered from slight Diarrhœa about a week previously. Four persons who had nursed the patients in the two cottages took Cholera, and two of them died; and two labourers sent to purify the cottage on October 10th were attacked and one died. There were no other cases than these.
36. Birmingham Union Workhouse. (Dr. B. Fletcher.)	The disease broke out in the Male Insane Ward, the keeper of which had gone to Walsall (where Cholera prevailed), and on his return had slept three nights in the Insane Ward. The only case in the Workhouse, out of the Insane Ward, was that of an old man who assisted at the Post Mortems of the insane who died of Cholera. [Several imported cases of Cholera seem to have occurred in Birmingham without the disease spreading.]

Place and Reporter.	First Cases of Cholera.
37. Swanland (a village six miles west of Hull). (Dr. Sandwith.)	Margaret Peart, aged 62, had slight Diarrhœa, when a daughter arrived from Hull, had malignant Cholera in the night and died in eight or ten hours. The daughter, who attended on Margaret Peart, was taken ill with Cholera two days afterwards and died in about eight hours. The son, who attended the funeral of the mother on the 8th September, went to his house three miles from Swanland, had Cholera and died at midnight on 9th. Two or three brothers who remained in the street and did not enter the house remained well.
38. Noss, Devon .... The first attacked of the group of villages in eighth district of Plympton St. Mary's. (Mr. M'Laren.)	French vessels passed to and fro Noss and Dieppe, an infected place from end of April. *The First Patient* had several times been on board these vessels as late as 11th May. On the 10th he had purging. On 11th, after being on board the vessel, became worse, fell into collapse, and died in consecutive fever on 17th. *The Second Patient* was his partner, boatman, who had been to sea with him on 10th May, and on board the French vessel on the 11th. On the 15th he was attacked with Diarrhœa. He recovered. *Third Patient.* A child of second patient, had Cholera severely; recovered. *Fourth Patient.* A niece of first patient, and in same house, attacked, while first patient lay dead, and died in twenty-four hours. *Fifth Patient.* Another child of second patient, attacked on 24th, and died in twenty-four hours. *6th, 7th, 8th, and 9th Patients,* on June 3rd. One of these had had dealings with the Frenchmen, another was his wife, the other two were a labourer and a labourer's child. *Tenth Case and Eleventh,* on June 4th or 5th. *Twelfth Case.* Mother and nurse of one of the cases on June 3rd, was attacked on June 7th. *Thirteenth Case.* Her daughter on the 8th. *Fourteenth Case.* The partner-boatman of one of cases on 3rd, attacked and died on 9th June. [The disease was now epidemic in Noss, but existed in no other part of the south-western counties.]
39. Cairnbulg .... (Mr. Grieve.)	A boat had been at Montrose where the crew with that of Inveralochy boat went through the town. One of the crew died with symptoms of Cholera on way home on 22nd September. Others of crew had serous Diarrhœa. On the 29th and 30th September two persons, first and second cases, who had been employed in removing the cargo at Cairnbulg, were attacked with Cholera. No other cases occurred until the 3rd October. There were two cases which could not be traced to communication with the sick, but one of them had

Place and Reporter.	First Cases of Cholera.
	attended a funeral, when he was brought into contact with those who had attended the sick.
40. Inverlochy .... (Mr. Robb and Dr. Jamieson.)	A boat from Inverlochy had been at Montrose, where Cholera prevailed. The crew saunterd through the town, and on their way home several had severe Diarrhœa, of which they had not recovered on reaching Inverlochy. On 28th September, three or four days after the arrival of the boat, the father of one of the crew who had been engaged in removing the cargo was attacked with Cholera. *The Second Case* was in the wife of the first patient. *The Third Case.* A daughter living with her parents. *The Fourth.* Another daughter living in a different house, but who had nursed her father and mother. *The Fifth.* The husband of the fourth patient. *The Sixth.* The mother of the fifth patient. Three cases occurred which were not known to have communicated with the preceding, but in two of these the houses were near a stream, where the clothes from the suspected boat were washed.
41. Manchester .... (Dr. Pincoff.)	*First Case*, on 11th June, in a prize-fighter from Liverpool. *The Second and Third Cases* in two different parts of Ancoats, without communication with first patient. The second also said to have come from Liverpool. The disease spread from these different points. [A similar account is given in the History of Cholera in Manchester by Messrs. Leigh and Gardner, and a fortnight elapsed between first and second cases.]
42. Boston .... (Mr. Clegg.)	A sailor, of brig "Orr," died of Cholera at sea: a week afterwards the vessel entered the Port of Boston: next day, 29th July, a second sailor was attacked on board the vessel and died in a few hours. On 30th July, an old man, previously healthy, was attacked with Cholera in Boston Union-house and died same day. Other cases occurred in the Workhouse, and the town was not entirely free from the disease from the above date until September 25th. [There had been a fatal case of Cholera at Holbeach, Gidney-hill, on 11th May, at Lincoln on 9th May, and one in Boston Union-house 30th May (July?), (Registrar-General); at Deeping 11th July; at Morton (Bourn) 29th June; at Grantham 29th July.]
43. Sunderland, Monkwearmouth, and Bishopwearmouth. (Dr. J. Brown.)	Cases in ships in harbour, October 1st, from Hamburgh; October 3rd, from Hamburgh; October 13th, from London. Two others in harbour in ships not from infected places. October 10th, from Nantes. October 17th, from Lynn. Quarantine ceased on 14th. *First Case* on shore. A lady, in isolated house, quarter of a mile from the river, nearly a mile from the

Place and Reporter.	First Cases of Cholera.
	ships; Diarrhœa on 16th October, vomiting on 25th, collapse and death on 26th. *Second Case.* In a house fifty yards from ship, in which an imported case died on 14th October, sickened on 5th, and died on 6th November. No evidence of direct communication with ships, though it is possible. *Third Case.* Man who worked in same coalpit with second Case, attacked twelve days afterwards, his house much more remote from river, and 200 yards from house of second case, probably communicated with second case while the latter had Diarrhœa. Third case died on 18th November. On 26th November four new cases, three fatal. On 27th, eleven cases, five fatal in colliery. The disease then became epidemic in colliery.
44. Sunderland Parish... March 5 to April 6. (Dr. J. Brown.)	Prior to the *Second Outbreak*, sick had been landed from ships come from infected places. Direct communication not traced.
45. Bishopwearmouth ... (from 28th June.) (Dr. J. Brown.)	*Third Outbreak.* A sailor had Cholera on passage from London, landed with consecutive Fever, on 28th June, and died on July 2nd. Sailor's mother attacked on July 4th, died on July 6th. Other cases occurred speedily in other parts of Sunderland not traceable to this sailor, but perhaps due to infection from other seafaring persons who arrived ill of Cholera. Previous to landing of the sick sailor, there had been no Cholera in the town for three months.
46. Bolton .... (Dr. Black.)	A cattle-dealer, three days previously from Liverpool, where Cholera prevailed, 11th June. The next cases occurred after an interval of twenty days without communication with first. Several cases immediately after occurred simultaneously. In several instances there was evidence of communication with preceding cases.
47. Buddam, Peterhead. (Dr. Jamieson and Mr. Robb.)	Boats from Peterhead had been at infected ports. Crews returned in perfect health ten days before. *First Case,* which occurred in woman who had been in no infected locality, nor in any way exposed to infectious influence.—Dr. Jamieson. It is said one of the fishermen had Diarrhœa when he returned, and that his mother-in-law washed his clothes, and was attacked with Cholera in a few days after and died.—Mr. Robb. *Second Case.* Son of first patient, whom he attended in her illness. The disease now spread rapidly, and the attacks were confined to blood relatives of the first case. The disease, in its progress, attacked those who were more immediately in contact with the patients who previously suffered.—Mr. Robb.

Place and Reporter.	First Cases of Cholera.
48. Plymouth .... (Dr. Yonge and Mr. J. H. Eccles.)	The first fatal case, on the 25th June, a butcher, without communication, direct or indirect, with infected persons or localities. The next case, a baker's wife; her shop was frequented by persons coming from Noss Mayo, where Cholera was most intense. No definite evidence of communication between the first patients and those next attacked.—Dr. Yonge. [The Registrar-General records the death of a labourer from Cholera on the 9th June, in Stonehouse Lane, Plymouth, and this death is the second mentioned by Dr. Roe in his interesting "Account of Cholera in Plymouth," *Medical Times*, vol. i. new series, pp. 196 and 453. The first case, according to Dr. Roe, was that of a man just come from Noss, where Cholera was raging, who died in a few hours at the South Devon Hospital. The second case was that of an Irish emigrant landed from a Cork steamer, and conveyed to a public-house in Stonehouse Lane on June 8th, where he died on June 9th. The third patient (the baker's wife), was attacked on the 13th, and died on the 14th. The next cases had intercourse with persons belonging to Noss, and lived in Stonehouse Lane. It appears, too, from the reports made to the Director-General of the Navy, that a convict ship with Cholera on board anchored in the Sound in the month of April, but remained in Quarantine till she continued her voyage. That on the 5th June an emigrant vessel, the " American Eagle," on board which Cholera had broken out, arrived in the Sound, and that the people on board were allowed to land and mix with the inhabitants of Plymouth.]
49. Wells, Somersetshire (Mr. H. W. Livett.)	*The First Case.* A vagrant from Bristol where Cholera prevailed, on 10th August. *Second Case* on 2nd September, not traced to communication with first case, or with other infected persons. *Third Case*, September 5th, also not traced to infection. *Fourth and Fifth Cases*, on September 5th and 6th, in a different quarter of the town, but in a house where the linen of the second patient was washed. *Sixth Case.* Mother of second patient, whom she nursed, attacked September 6th. *Seventh Case.* In house where the linen of second patient was ironed by this seventh patient, attacked September 6th. Of nine succeeding cases, four might be referred to communication, direct or indirect, with previous cases, and one other was an imported case from Shepton Mallet, where the disease prevailed.
50. Downton .... (Dr. E. A. K. Welch.)	*First Patient* had been to Salisbury, where Cholera raged, on the 17th July, was attacked on 20th, and died in ten hours.

Place and Reporter.	First Cases of Cholera.
	Second Patient. A gleaner, attacked in the field, on 23rd August.

Second Patient. A gleaner, attacked in the field, on 23rd August.

Third Patient lived in next house to second patient, and nursed her, seized on the 25th August.

Fourth Patient. Husband of last, attended her, seized and died on 28th August.

Fifth. Mother-in-law of second patient, helped to nurse her, fell ill on 24th August, and removed to further end of village, and there seized with Cholera. Died.

Sixth. Daughter of fifth, whom she visited during her illness, was in a very short period attacked.

Seventh, Eighth, and *Ninth.* Children of a woman who attended on the second and third patients, attacked on 29th August, 4th and 5th September.

Tenth. Nursed the ninth patient, fell ill on September 6th, and in a very short time was attacked and died.

Eleventh. A child living next door to seventh, eighth, and ninth patients. There was likewise a fatal case in the village, a mile and a half off, not traceable to communication with the previous cases.

51. Monmouth ....
(Dr. Price to Prov.
Med. and Surg.
Association.)

In the first week of June the disease first attacked a person from the Forest of Dean, and three persons of an Irish family just landed at Newport. It commenced in the Workhouse, and all the cases happened in the Workhouse, except three in a house in the immediate neighbourhood, the windows of which looked directly on the windows of the hospital. [Exact dates and details not given.]

52. Hastings ....
(Dr. Mackness.)

First Patient. A lady who had arrived in the morning from London.

Several other cases occurred simultaneously about ten days or a fortnight after the first case without probability of communication.

53. Chelmsford ....
(Dr. Badeley.)

The person first attacked was an itinerant Jew, that day arrived from a most infected part of London; the only other case happened a fortnight after without evidence or probability of near approach.

54. St. Albans ....
(Mr. Lipscombe.)

First patient attacked 20th July, had returned home only a few hours from Lambeth, where Cholera prevailed. The *Third, Fourth,* and *Fifth Cases* appear also to have been imported cases. [Interval fourteen days after first imported case. Of seven cases, four or five were imported.]

The *Second Case* occurred on the 3rd September, the *Third* on the 4th September, *Fourth* and *Fifth* on the 5th, *Sixth* on the 8th, *Seventh* on the 12th, and *Eighth* on the 25th October.

There was no communication between the first and the subsequent cases.

Place and Reporter.	First Cases of Cholera.
55. Offchurch, near Leamington. (Dr. Turner.)	*First Cases* in three persons who arrived in a boat from London by the canal, all ill of Cholera, and all died. The disease immediately spread through the village, and carried off upwards of twenty persons. [Facts not investigated by Dr. Turner himself. There were only three deaths from Cholera, and at most one from Diarrhœa at Offchurch, in 1849, according to Registrar-General.]
56. Wakefield Old Prison. (Messrs. Dunn and Milner.)	During December, 1848, a few cases at a village eight miles distant; but prisoners then healthy. No unusual amount of Diarrhœa. On 19th December, a batch of convicts from Millbank, where Cholera had been fatal, slept in cells of Old Prison. On 22nd December, a prisoner committed on 24th November who had occupied a cell which a convict from Millbank had slept in was seized with symptoms of Cholera, and died on 29th December. This was recorded as severe Bilious Cholera. No farther case till 8th January, when a case of Asiatic Cholera, fatal in fourteen hours, occurred, and was speedily followed by other cases, of which there were in all sixteen in January, besides the one in December. [Three cases occurred in the Wakefield district after second case in the prison, namely, on January 11th and January 16th, but no others until August. Registrar-General's Report.]
57. Chorlton-upon-Medlock. (Dr. Pincoff.)	*First Case*, 28th June. A child had died on 23rd, of Diarrhœa, in same house, soon after coming from Liverpool. Two daughters of first patient died in the same house on the 2nd July. No more cases in this neighbourhood. In a different street a woman and a man died on the 30th July.
58. Stockport (Dr. Rayner and Mr. J. Rayner.)	*First Patient* returned on 17th July from Southport (where deaths had occurred from Cholera in the vicinity of her lodging), had Diarrhœa there, on the 18th was attacked with Cholera, but recovered. *Second Case*. Husband of first patient, had been to Southport for his wife on the 17th July, attacked and died on the 23rd. *Third Case* (profuse Diarrhœa, recovered from), on 23rd July. This patient had nursed the first patient, was her domestic servant. *Fourth Case* in another street on 29th July. *Fifth*, in different street, at beginning of August. On 16th August several cases. [Two cases of Cholera had occurred previously in May, in Stockport, and one at Cheadle in February.—Registrar General.]
59. Exeter (Dr. Shapter and Dr. Lang.)	*First Case*, on 19th July. A German musician from Plymouth, where some of his companions had died, came ill of the disease, but recovered.

Place and Reporter.	First Cases of Cholera.
	Second Case, on 9th August. An officer of 82nd Regiment, which had come from Plymouth on previous day, several deaths having occurred among the men at Plymouth. Recovered. [A child died in the barracks the same night, and four other cases occurred among the men, two fatal, on the 13th, 14th, and 15th; there were none later.] Of forty-three fatal cases, thirteen were in strangers direct from infected places. The next cases after the second (and the child) were on the 10th August, in the west quarter of the city. These persons had had Diarrhœa for some days, and had had no contact with the persons from Plymouth. In no one instance did it spread in the eastern and higher part of the city.
60. Sampford Peverell, near Cheltenham ? (Dr. Merson.)	First and only case had been in contact with a person coming from an infected locality.
61. Halton, near Lancaster. (Mr. W. Hall to Prov. Med. and Surg. Association.)	First patient, a woman, who had left an infected district of Liverpool two days previously, died in twenty-four hours. The following day her mother, and a woman who assisted in nursing her, were both seized and died in a few hours. No other case occurred in the village before or since. The village healthily situated on the side of a hill; the house a new one, detached, and with no unhealthy influences about it. [No dates or names given.]
62. Stoke Prior, near Bromsgrove. (Mr. Horton to Prov. Med. and Surg. Association.)	First patient, a boat-boy on Birmingham and Worcester Canal, attacked on his way from London, reached Stoke 21st August, died the same evening at his father's house. The bedding and clothes of the boy were removed to a house a quarter of a mile distant, and washed there; in a few days two persons died of Cholera in that house, and four persons in all in the same row, besides the first patient.
63. Stourbridge .... (Dr. Norris to Prov. Med. and Surg. Association.)	First patient, a man who had been sleeping a few nights at Wolverhampton, where Cholera was raging, died the latter part of August. His father, mother, and child took the disease and all died. Others in the house (a lodging-house crowded with inmates in an unhealthy situation) also suffered. Next, a case occurred in a filthy locality about a hundred yards distant, and after this others in various parts of the town. [The Registrar-General records two cases of Diarrhœa in the early part of the year, and one case of Cholera on 22nd July.]
64. Dudley .... (Mr. Farnday to Prov. Med. and Surg. Association.)	First patient, about the middle of September, a man from the neighbourhood of Tipton, was brought into the Dudley Poor-house and died next day. Shortly

Place and Reporter.	First Cases of Cholera.
	after several of the cases occurred in the Poor-house, most of which were fatal. Other cases soon after appeared in different parts of the town and neighbourhood. [No dates or other details given.]
65. Dorchester .... (Dr. Cowdell to Prov. Med. and Surg. Association.)	First Case, about 10th of August, that of a poor man employed in chopping rags, collected without care to exclude those of Cholera districts. Second Case, eight days after, that of a man who had been staying in London with a connection who was carried off by Cholera during his visit; he himself a fortnight later. A few hours after his death, one of his children was seized and died.
66. Northampton ...... (Mr. Bryan to Prov. Med. and Surg. Association.)	First Patient. A boatman just arrived from Paddington (London), was seized while still in his boat, and died in a few hours. The next case occurred in a court about 400 yards from where the boatman was. Also fatal. Several deaths took place in the same spot within two or three days. Mr. Bryan believes there had been some communication between the second and first patient.
67. Kingsthorpe, one mile from Northampton. (Mr. Bryan.)	A man who whitewashed a house where deaths had occurred in Northampton fell ill with symptoms of Cholera, but recovered. His wife, however, was attacked and died of the complaint, which did not spread further in Kingsthorpe. [It is not stated whether the wife had been in Northampton recently.]
68. Ramsgate .... (Mr. H. Curling, through Mr. Reid, to Prov. Med. and Surg. Association.)	First case, July 14th, that of a boy who had come four days previously from London, where his father resided; fatal. Second case that of a Licensed Victualler from London, who had Diarrhœa before he left London, died July 19th. Fourth case, July 24th, a young woman who had been only a few days in Ramsgate, from London. (Third, fourth, and fifth cases on July 21st, 25th, and 27th, not described.) Seventy deaths registered as from Cholera; sixteen visitors, the rest residents, all of lower class.
69. Margate .... (Mr. G. H. Hoffmann, through Mr. Reid, to Prov. Med. and Surg. Association.)	First Outbreak. About 6th or 7th January, thirty children were brought from Drouet's School at Tooting to a similar establishment at Margate, situated on the side of a chalk hill, surrounded by extensive grounds and with lofty, spacious, well-ventilated rooms, and free from bad smells from privies or drains. Placed for the most part in a very large room with invalid children already there. On the 7th January several of the children brought from Tooting were attacked with Cholera. One died on the 8th. Of the previous inmates of the house several were attacked and three died, two on the 11th, and one on the 29th January (28rd, Registrar-General). This last noted as nurse.

Place and Reporter.	First Cases of Cholera.
	The disease disappeared in three weeks, and did not extend beyond the establishment. *Second Outbreak.* A sailor from Blackwall was landed at Margate in a state of collapse on 19th July, and died in a few hours. Second case was that of a young sailor, who lived near the house of first patient, and was said to have assisted at his funeral; he died, and then his mother. Then the disease appeared in other parts of the town and became epidemic. In this second outbreak it did not invade the Pauper School, which moreover was not visited in 1832.
70. Newport, Isle of Wight. (Mr. Bloxam to the Prov. Med. and Surg. Association.)	The *first* case occurred on July 9th (with the exception of two or three seamen put on shore at Cowes, this was the first case in the island). It was the case of a man come from Portsmouth, where the disease was prevalent. He began to suffer from it on the journey. Ten hours after his arrival in Newport, he was removed to an isolated building, where he died fourteen hours after his arrival. The *second* case, July 13th, was that of a child three years old, who lived in a court in the same street, 180 paces from the site of the first case. The *third* and *fourth* cases, in children of two or three years, occurred in the same court on July 14th. On July 21st eight cases had occurred in the same court, seven fatal, and ten cases in other parts of the town; three of them in the same street with first case. Mr. Bloxam has not heard that there was any direct communication between the parties of the first and other cases.
71. Carisbrook (one mile distant from Newport). (Mr. Bloxam to the Prov. Med. and Surg. Association.)	Seven fatal cases occurred within one week. All the seven persons were attacked and died within forty-eight hours after eating of some stale cowheels which had been brought from Newport from the house of a man who died of Cholera on August 20th. (Two women who laid out the body of this man, and a third who washed his clothes, also died of Cholera, and "it is supposed that they had eaten of the cowheels, though the fact is not known for certain.") No other cases of Cholera occurred in Carisbrook. [From further information obtained by Dr. Snow from Mr. Bloxam, it appears that eleven persons in all partook of this food, that eight of them were attacked with Cholera, and that seven died. Who conveyed the cowheels to Carisbrook?]
72. Catterick, Yorkshire (Dr. Blagbrough.)	" A tramp from Barnard Castle, where the disease had been very frequent and fatal, entered a low lodging-house in Richmond at 10 P.M. on the 6th September, was seized with all the symptoms of Cholera, at 2 A.M. of the 7th, and died at 2 A.M. on the 8th." . . . . " His widow came here on the 8th, continued her tramp to Catterick, five miles distant, was there

Place and Reporter.	First Cases of Cholera.
	seized with Cholera, and died also in 24 hours. The lodging-house keeper at Catterick, who had no fear of infection, carried the corpse down stairs to the coffin, took the disease, and died in about 24 hours also. No other cases occurred either here, Richmond, or at Catterick."
73. Tavistock .... (Dr. Lang.)	The first case in a vagrant who imported the disease. [No details given.]

TABLE XVI.

ABSTRACTS of the ACCOUNTS received by the Cholera Committee of the appearance of Cholera independently of any known introduction of Infection in Forty-six Towns, Villages, and Public Establishments.

Place and Reporter.	Order of Cases.
1. Holloway .... (Dr. Wilkinson.)	The first three cases were isolated, not traced to infection, occurred between 20th August and 11th September. [Details not given.] The disease was not communicated by either of first three patients to other persons. On 11th September the disease became epidemic in Holloway.
2. Upper Clapton ...... (Mr. R. R. Welsh.)	First four cases simultaneous on 26th January. A woman and four children; the mother and two children died. Fifth case, a child for some time in same room with the first four cases, on 27th January, died the following day of Cholera.
3. St. Luke's Hospital... (Dr. J. A. Sutherland.)	First Case. A female patient admitted into the Hospital on 24th December, 1847, attacked 9th October, 1848. No infection could be traced. The Second Case occurred in August, 1849. No infection traced. The Third Case, a day or two after second case, in the room adjoining that of the second patient, but there was no evidence of direct communication.
4. Haggerstone, West District, Shoreditch. (Mr. E. R. Hooper.)	First Patient, attacked 10th July, 1849, died in about twelve hours. Two days after two of his children were seized and died; then a man, two doors off, who, with his wife, assisted in nursing the first patient. Then the wife of this man; she was taken for one night to sleep on the bed of an opposite neighbour. The next day this neighbour was seized and died. A woman, who nursed the man and his wife above-mentioned, took the disease and was removed to her home a stone's throw off and died, but did not communicate the disease to any one. Two other women, who

Place and Reporter.	Order of Cases.
	came in contact with one or more of the former cases, also a child living two doors from the first patient, died of the disease, making ten victims in seven days. [The Registrar-General records one death from Cholera in January, and one in July before the 10th.]
5. Notting Hill .... (Mr. Chas. M. Frost.)	*Two Cases* occurred early in the morning of August 8th in the Potteries; they had not been in an infected place, nor received into their houses clothes which could have conveyed infection, nor been in contact with persons coming from an infected locality. There was no communication between the first patients and those next attacked. [Deaths occurred in the subdistrict of Kensington Town in January and February, and a death from Cholera is recorded as occurring in the Potteries on July 8th.]
6. Walham Green, Fulham. (Mr. Rouse and Mr. Rowland.)	*First Case.* A man attacked while at work cleansing some foul ditches, no infection to be traced. *Second Case.* A child had been in the neighbourhood of the same ditches, had no communication with first patient; attacked a week afterwards. *Third Case.* Attacked fifteen days later; had also *not* communicated with first patient. Several were attacked thirteen days after third case, and the disease became general.
7. Deptford and Dockyard (Dr. Bruce.)	The first cases could not be traced to any medium of infection. [Details not given.]
8. Brighton .... (Dr. Ormerod.)	*First Case.* A scavenger not known to have been exposed to contagion. Two children died in same house about the same time, it was said of Smallpox that would not come out, and one with vomiting, not purging. Medical attendant and wife not affected. Two young women had vomiting, not purging or cramp. His clothes were burnt. None of his connections or friends took the disease. "The man himself had little or no communication with an infected place (beyond the cesspools) as far as could be ascertained." *Second Case.* A gentleman whose symptoms commenced in London. Was attended by his reputed wife, with the assistance of a woman who laid him out. "His reputed wife shortly left the place; the woman who laid him out had no Cholera. The three medical men who saw him were not attacked. His clothes were carried by two children to their mother to wash. Neither the mother nor the children had any Diarrhœa or illness subsequently. There were no cases of Cholera in the neighbourhood at the time."
9. Hertford, First Outbreak. (Dr. Davies.)	*First Case* occurred on December 13th, 1848; there was another suspicious case in the same locality. [Six

Place and Reporter.	Order of Cases.
	fatal cases are recorded as occurring in January, besides those in the prison.] *Second Outbreak. First Case.* A woman living in a dirty court, attacked August 19th, died on seventh day. A woman living at some distance from first was attacked on August 20th, and died on August 23rd. The first and second cases became two separate centres of Choleraic influence during the whole epidemic.
10. Ilford .... (Dr. T. K. Chambers.)	*First Case,* July 17th. A mile and a half from Ilford, not traced to any source. *Second Case.* Probably imported. *Third Case,* July 28th. A short distance from Ilford, not traced to any source. *Fourth Case,* August 16th. Probably imported. *Fifth Case,* same day, but not in immediate vicinity. *Sixth Case,* not traced, August 11th. *Seventh, Eighth,* and *Ninth Cases* in communication with sixth case. *Tenth Case.* Son of a woman who had been to London to see a sister who died of Cholera; some of deceased's sister's clothes and bedding had been sent to Ilford. *Eleventh Case.* A brother of tenth, five days later, and *Twelfth.* A child fourteen months old, three days later, in same house. *Thirteenth Case.* A woman who had had constant communication with the family of tenth, eleventh, and twelfth cases. Communication was clearly traced in several subsequent cases.
11. Canterbury .... (Dr. Leebée.)	A travelling tailor came on July 15th, direct from Chatham (where Cholera did not then prevail), and apparently in good health; was seized in the evening, and died in eighteen hours. Nothing could be learned of his previous habits and doings. *The Second* and *Third Cases* occurred nearly simultaneously, thirty-six hours after the first, in children aged six and three years; there was no communication between them and the first patient, though they lived within a hundred yards of the house where he lodged. [The first case of Cholera at Chatham occurred on July 30th, but the disease was rife at Milton, which lies near the road from Chatham to Canterbury, from July 7th.]
12. Faversham .... (Mr. W. P. Hoare, through Mr. Reid to Prov. Med. and Surg. Assoc.)	*The First Case* was that of a woman travelling from Canterbury on 14th July. *The Second Case,* on July 16th, was that of a labourer in a neighbouring village, the first symptoms having appeared while he was at work near Milton, an infected place.

Place and Reporter.	Order of Cases.
	The Third Case. A gun-stock maker, seized on arriving, July 27th, from Sittingbourne, near Milton. *Fourth, Fifth,* and *Sixth Cases* were those of a man and two children in the house where the subject of third case lodged (31st July). No other case till October 7th, then one. All seven cases fatal. [The first case of Cholera at Canterbury occurred on 15th July in a man who, in coming from Chatham, would pass through the neighbourhood, first of Milton, and afterwards of Faversham. There were deaths from Cholera at Milton from July 7th to September 20th, seventeen in the workhouse at Milton in July, and four in August, and two deaths at Sittingbourne on 3rd and 5th of July.]
13. Dowlais, Merthyr Tydvil. (Mr. White.)	Merthyr, Pen-y-darran, and Dowlais are continuous, Merthyr resembling the body of a bird, Pen-y-darran a long neck, Dowlais the head. A ravine not more than fifty yards broad separates the two latter. Cholera raged with the greatest intensity in Pen-y-darran before the first case appeared at Dowlais. This was in a poor woman who lived from 200 to 300 yards from nearest point to Pen-y-darran, and had not left her house for several days, if not weeks. Nor was it discovered that any clothing from an infected district had come to her house, or that she or any of her family had been in contact with persons from an infected district. *The First Case* occurred on the Sunday morning. *The Second,* in the child of the first patient in the same house, on Sunday evening. *The Third, Fourth,* and *Fifth Cases* occurred on the following Tuesday; only one other case during the next fortnight. The third and fourth cases occurred at some distance from, and had had no communication with, the first two, though they had both been in contact with Cholera elsewhere. [Details fully given, except the dates.]
14. Oxford .... (Dr. Kidd, Dr. Ogle, and Mr. T. Allen.)	*First Patient.* A male prisoner in County Gaol since April 3rd, attacked on August 12th; no communication suspected. Died on 13th. *Second Patient.* A prostitute, at a fair at Nuneham, a few miles off, on 12th August; attacked on 13th, and died same day in Orpwoods Row. *The Third Case* occurred on the 18th August. *The Fourth* and *Fifth* on the 20th, without communication with first and second case. *Sixth Case.* A turnkey in the gaol was attacked on the 21st August, who had had communication with first patient during his illness; he recovered. *Seventh Case.* A woman in Orpwoods Row, where second patient lived, on 21st August. *Eighth Case.* A man employed in digging a drain,

Place and Reporter.	Order of Cases.
	close to a drain and locality of third case. No communication traced. *Ninth Case.* A woman in whose house second patient had lodged, and who had nursed her during her illness, and had washed her clothes after death, attacked on 22nd. Died. *Tenth to Fifteenth Cases* in different localities in Oxford not traced to communication. Succeeding cases down to 22nd September in different parishes, not traced to communication. In the gaol a third case occurred on September 13th, and within next nine days eight cases occurred to male prisoners. On the female side the disease showed itself on 22nd September in women recently admitted. On 22nd August a girl, living in same house with second and ninth patients, whom she had nursed, sickened with Cholera and died.
15. Southampton .... **(Dr. Oke.)**	*First Patient.* Wife of a beershop-keeper, no evidence leading to supposition of the attack being caused by infection. *Second Case.* On 30th June, thirteen days after the first case, about 100 yards distant; there had been no communication between the families. Shortly after this cases occurred in a higher and quite distinct part of the town.
16. Gloucester .... **(Mr. Hinton.)**	*First Patient.* An old woman had Cholera and died in a court on the island. *Second Patient.* Niece of first patient, and her attendant during her illness. Others who held communication with the first patient were attacked, and from her the disease apparently spread by communication to another part of the city, about half a mile distant. But, at the same time, a child living in a neighbouring court had a fatal attack, without intercourse between the families having taken place. [Dates and names are not given.]
17. Barrow, five miles from Tewkesbury, and four from Cheltenham. **(Dr. Bartle.)**	The patient had had no personal communication with an infected district, though Cholera was raging at Gloucester, five miles off. The sister of first patient came to nurse her, and washed the linen, returned home a mile and a half distant, and in three days was attacked with malignant Cholera. The disease then passed through the village. [No names or dates are given.]
18. Bridgnorth .... **(Dr. Strange.)**	On 24th July, an old woman, who had not left the neighbourhood, nor had any communication with infected districts. *Second* and *Third*, on 8th August, had had no communication with first patient.

Place and Reporter.	Order of Cases.
	Fourth. In a different part of town. *Fifth Patient,* son of fourth, had returned from Birmingham on night after his father's funeral; attacked next day. Subsequent cases spread in two different directions from site of first case. No local causes.
19. Shrewsbury House of Industry. (Dr. H. Johnson.)	*First Case.* An inmate of House of Industry, not off premises for some time previously. Attacked on 25th July. [An isolated case before, at Wyle Copes, St. Julian, in February.]
County Prison	*First Case.* A man, in prison since April 13th, attacked 27th July. Almost simultaneously ten or eleven other cases occurred, not in the same ward with this man, but here and there over the house.
20. Chapel-en-le-Frith, Derbyshire. (Mr. Goodman.)	*First Case.* A girl thirteen years of age, who had never been from home. There was no infected locality within several miles. She recovered. *Second Case.* Husband of a woman who had been with first patient, was attacked at night after coming home to his wife, and died on third day. Of two women and a man who laid him out, two had forthwith severe purging, the third had purging for a few days and then fatal collapse. [No dates.]
21. Holyhead .... (Rev. C. Williams.) (Mr. W. Walthew.)	In December, 1848, two men were attacked almost simultaneously. End of July, 1849. A case, as far as is known, isolated. Middle of August. A man died of Cholera who had been three or four days before at Kingstown, where Cholera prevailed. Soon after, a seaman belonging to mail-packet from Kingstown came home with symptoms of Cholera, but recovered, having consecutive fever. His wife took Cholera, and died in nine hours. His mother, who washed their clothes, also took the disease, and died. A child also was ill, but recovered. [More details were desirable.] A man had Choleraic symptoms, but recovered. His mother nursed him and washed his clothes, took Cholera, and died. A next-door neighbour who visited these patients also took the disease and died. September 19th. A woman, whose mother had nursed those who died about the 10th, was attacked, and died five days later. She was a washerwoman. Ten days later another house had two fatal cases, and one not fatal. On the 29th a case occurred, and after beginning of October, cases were very numerous. [Mr. Walthew gives no dates. It is probable that he does not mention the first case.]

Place and Reporter.	Order of Cases.
22. Lancaster .... (Mr. J. L. Harrison.)	A child aged 2½ years, *First* fatal case. *Second Case.* Not in communication with first, lived in a different street, 800 yards distant. *Third, Fourth,* and *Fifth Cases.* In communication with second case. Of 87 cases, 21 were exposed to direct communication with other cases, 27 to indirect communication, and 22 not exposed. [The negative fact is not stated, but is implied. The exposure to possible infection was direct in 21 cases, and indirect in 27 cases out of 87.]
Lancaster .... (Mr. W. Hall to the Prov. Med. and Surg. Association.)	During the first week five or six cases occurred within a few yards of each other, on the Quay. In the second week only a single case, not fatal. In the third week it broke out in Henry Street, at the opposite extremity of the town, most violently. After a few days it again ceased, and then, after almost a week's absence, it appeared in a new and opposite side of the town, raged several days, and was very fatal. After this there was a cessation for almost ten days, and then it again broke out in Henry Street more virulently than before. After ten days it left the town entirely and crossed the river to Skerton, a straggling suburb. Thus there were four distinct outbreaks of the disease, each preceded and accompanied by warm foggy weather.
23. A district of Leeds . (Mr. G. H. Bearpark.)	The person first attacked in Mr. Bearpark's district had not recently been in an infected district; a friend who visited her had not come from a place in which Cholera was known to exist. No clothes or other articles likely to convey infection had been received into the house. The first four cases occurred successively, all within 150 yards; three days elapsed between the first and second cases, one day between the second and third, and four days between the third and fourth. The first and second were not at all together, the second and third were, the third and fourth were not.
24. Wakefield (Town)... (Dr. Wright and Mr. Statter.)	A porter at the Exchange, where he may have mingled with strangers from an infected locality (Leeds), attacked August 20th. Recovered. *The Second Case,* on 23rd August. *Third* and *Fourth Cases* on the 25th and 26th, and several on 29th, 30th, and 31st. No communication whatever can be discovered between the first patient and those next attacked.—Dr. Wright. *Second Case* seen by Mr. Statter, no communication with first case. [This is properly a renewed outbreak of the epidemic, since cases had occurred in the prison, and three cases in other parts of Wakefield in January. It ought not, perhaps, to be reckoned among the cases showing the mode of *origin* of the disease.]

Place and Reporter.	Order of Cases.
25. Bristol Lunatic Asylum. (Mr. Stansbury to the Commissioners in Lunacy.)	Cause of outbreak unknown. The disease did not not prevail in the immediate neighbourhood. Twelve cases, five fatal, occurred between the 1st September and 7th October. Six female patients were attacked between September 1st and September 24th. On the latter day, the first case occurred in the male wing. The five other male patients were attacked during the first week of October. The first patient had been seven or eight years in the asylum; the others, periods varying from one year five months to eleven years. [The disease prevailed in Bristol from June to November.]
26. Kingsland Asylum, near Shrewsbury. (Mr. Heathcote to the Commissioners in Lunacy.)	Cause of outbreak unknown. The disease did not prevail in the district, nor in Shrewsbury, till the 25th July, when four cases occurred in the asylum, all fatal. Nine other cases followed, the last on the 16th August; all but two fatal. The disease appeared indiscriminately throughout the asylum. The four patients first attacked had been in the asylum for periods varying from eleven months to four years. [The asylum forms part of the same building with the House of Industry. Cholera appeared on the same day in this building and in the gaol. See under head of Shrewsbury.]
27. Wrekenton Asylum, near Gateshead. (Mr. R. Davies to the Commissioners in Lunacy.)	Cholera prevailed to a fearful extent in the neighbourhood at the time; there were numerous cases in houses closely adjoining the asylum. It appeared in the asylum three or four days after it had thus prevailed in the village. The first three cases occurred on September 12th; twenty other cases followed, the last on the 20th September; fifteen were fatal. The disease, when it broke out, seized several patients in different wards, both in the male and in the female wings. Of the three first attacked, one had been four months, another six months, and the third six years in the asylum.
28. Bethnal Green Asylum.	Cause of outbreak unknown. The disease was prevalent in the district. Two fatal cases occurred in the asylum on the 14th February, 1849; twenty-six other cases followed before the 7th March: only four patients recovered in this early outbreak. The disease, in this outbreak, was confined entirely to pauper females. Of the two patients first seized, one had been four and a half years, the others three years and ten months in the asylum. [With the exception of the twenty-two deaths in the asylum, very few occurred in this district at this early period of the year.] The second outbreak occurred on August 31st, and continued to September 27th. There were thirty-four cases, all but two fatal. This outbreak began with pauper males, and ended with pauper females. [In other parts of the district the second outbreak began in July.]

Place and Reporter.	Order of Cases.
29. Camberwell House Asylum. (Mr. J. H. Paul to the Commissioners in Lunacy.)	Outbreak attributed to "atmospheric causes." The disease was prevalent in the district. On July 1st, the first case (fatal) occurred in the male infirmary. On that day week it spread to the male refractory wards, and eight days subsequently to the female refractory wards, thence it extended to the male and female convalescent wards. There were twenty-three cases, eighteen fatal, besides four fatal cases of Diarrhœa. Eleven fatal cases occurred between the 8th and 24th of July; the last fatal case on the 7th September, one not fatal on the 12th. The three patients first attacked had been respectively two years and seven months, three years and two months, and five months and one week in the asylum.
30. Peckham House Asylum.	*First Outbreak* on October 17th, 1848, attributed to atmospheric influence and the emanations from drains which were not quite covered in. The disease was not prevalent in the district (though cases had occurred in the south districts nearer to the river). The first case was that of a laundry-maid; she recovered. Two days afterwards (19th October), four cases, three fatal, occurred in the female epileptic ward, situated near the laundry. It prevailed principally in this ward, in the wards near the chapel, and in those in connexion with the principal female airing yard, and latterly in the male epileptic ward. Eighteen women and three men died. The first death amongst the men occurred on the 4th November; five cases, not fatal, had occurred between 22nd and 31st October; the first, fourth, and fifth of which were not patients, but a farm-servant, an attendant, and a carman, residing in London. The first four cases occurred in female patients who had been respectively one and a half year, four years, four years, and two and a half years in the asylum. [The last case of Cholera in this outbreak was on the 15th November, the last fatal case on the 13th. Number of lunatics, males, 214; females, 288.] *The Second Outbreak* occurred on 25th June, was fatal to twelve men and eight women. Six men had been attacked, and four had died before the disease appeared amongst the women on the 13th July. The last case among the women occurred on the 17th August, the last amongst the men on the 15th September; both fatal cases. At the time of this outbreak the disease was prevalent in the neighbourhood. The first patient was a lunatic who had been four years in the asylum. No attendant was attacked. [Number of lunatics, males, 184; females, 282.]
31. Grove Hall, Bow ...	Cause of *First Outbreak* unknown. Date 13th November, 1848. One fatal case had occurred a few days previously in the immediate neighbourhood. [Only this one fatal case occurred in the Bow subdistrict

Place and Reporter.	Order of Cases.
	before those in the asylum, and only one had occurred in the subdistrict Poplar, one in the Limehouse subdistrict, two in Ratcliffe, three in Shadwell, and two in the Mile End Old Town upper and lower subdistricts.] The first four cases, two fatal, occurred in the same woman's ward on the 13th and 14th November, and five other cases, one fatal (including the last in this outbreak, on November 29th), occurred subsequently in the same ward. From this ward it passed to an adjoining laundry, thence to a detached wing at the other extremity of the building, and subsequently a few cases occurred in the body of the house, and an adjoining wing, but *all* in wards appropriated to females. Total number of deaths, seven. [Number of lunatics, males, 144; females, 263.] The first four patients had been respectively 224 days, 13 days, 748 days, and 15 days in the asylum. *The Second Outbreak* occurred on the 10th February. No females were attacked, but four male lunatics in the same ward between the 10th and 19th of the month; three died. The first attacked had been fifty-six days in the asylum. A single death occurred on the 18th October, 1849, in the same female ward in which the disease first appeared. [But during 1849, twenty-seven persons died of Dysentery, and twenty-one of Diarrhœa.]
32. St. Marylebone Infirmary Asylum. (Dr. Allen to the Commissioners in Lunacy.)	Date of outbreak, 21st July, 1849. Cause unknown. Cholera had prevailed in the district from July 7th. The first patient was attacked while in the airing yard; what ward he had previously been in is not stated. The only three subsequent cases (all fatal) occurred in No. 1 Male Ward, on August 3rd, 22nd, and 30th. No female patients were attacked. The first patient had been three years in the asylum. [Number of lunatics, males, 26; females, 47.]
33. Hoxton House ...... (Mr. E. L. Bryan to the Commissioners in Lunacy.)	Date of outbreak, 10th September, 1849. Cause unknown. Was, and had been for some time previously, very prevalent in the immediate neighbourhood. On the 10th September, three cases occurred simultaneously in three different wards. One of the first three patients was a laundry-maid; she recovered. The first male patient was attacked on September 12th. The disease prevailed in eleven different wards until the 28th October, proving fatal in twenty-one cases; eighteen women and three men died. The two lunatics first attacked had been, one three years, the other two years four months in the asylum. [Number of lunatics, males, 160; females, 279.]
34. Althorpe House, Battersea. (Dr. Wing to the Com-	Date of outbreak, 10th January, 1849. No cause known. A few cases occurred at this period in various parts of the parish. [In the subdistrict Battersea only

Place and Reporter.	Order of Cases.
missioners in Lunacy.)	seven deaths from Cholera occurred previous to the 10th January (three of them were in the union workhouse), one in October, one in November, four in December, and one in January.—Registrar-General.] Three male lunatics were attacked on the 10th, 12th, and 19th of January, and five females on the 12th, 13th, 16th, and 22nd of January and the 2nd of February. After the first case, others appeared indiscriminately on the male and on the female side of the house. The first patient had been two years and three months in the asylum. [Number of lunatics, males, 16; females, 28.]
35. Cowper House Asylum, Old Brompton. (Mr. W. V. Pettigrew to the Commissioners in Lunacy.)	Date of outbreak, August 20th, 1849. Attributed to eating unripe mulberries, and imperfect drainage. A few cases in the district at the time. The cases all occurred in the western ward, in the outhouse. No cases occurred in the large house. The patient first attacked had been nine years in the asylum. The last case occurred on August 23rd. [Number of lunatics, all males, 38.]
36. Vernon House, Briton Ferry. (Mr. Player to the Commissioners in Lunacy.)	Date of outbreak, July 29th, 1849. Cause unknown. Cholera prevailed in the district, which is a rural one and not densely populated. Eight cases occurred, seven fatal; the first three on the same day: one of them was a woman, the two others males. They had been, the woman four years, the men each one year, in the asylum. The last case occurred on the 11th August. On the 28th August a woman was brought in while sick of Cholera, and died at the end of ten days. Of the patients attacked in the house four were men and four women. Number of lunatics, males, 78; females, 73. The disease appeared only in four wards.
37. Hull Boro' Asylum. (Mr. Casson to the Commissioners in Lunacy.)	Date of outbreak, 27th August, 1849. Cause unknown. Cholera prevailed in the district. There were nine cases and four deaths. Six women were attacked and three died. Three men were attacked and only one died. From the 27th August to the 5th September, the disease was confined to the women's ward, in which it broke out, attacking there five women. On 9th September it appeared in the men's wards, affecting two men on that day and one on the 16th September. The sixth woman was seized on the 10th September, but suffered slightly. Number of lunatics, men, 38; women, 35.
38. London House, Hackney. (Mr. Ayre to the Commissioners in Lunacy.)	Date of outbreak, 23rd November, 1848. Cause unknown. A few cases of the disease occurred in the neighbourhood at the same time. Only two cases occurred. The first a lady, who had been fourteen years in the asylum. The second on February 5th, 1849, a gentleman who had been between thirteen and

Place and Reporter.	Order of Cases.
	fourteen years in the asylum. Both occupied private rooms. [Very few fatal cases had occurred in the Hackney district at this period.]
39. Romsey .... (Mr. Buckle to the Prov. Med. and Surg. Association.)	First patients attacked, July 2nd, were two children in an ill-ventilated, poor person's home. The next victim was an old woman who lived near, and nursed and laid them out. The parents and brothers and sister escaped. All the cases (fourteen fatal) occurred within twenty yards of the first cases, in an insalubrious locality.
40. Farnham .... (Mr. Slowman to the Prov. Med. and Surg. Association.)	Four cases occurred, all in one family residing in a row of houses a quarter of a mile from the town, in a low damp spot, surrounded by a nuisance. The husband had suffered from severe Diarrhœa for several days before his wife was attacked with Cholera, of which she died in fourteen hours. The son was attacked the same evening, and died in thirty-six hours. The rest of the family, five in number, were removed to a house kept as a receptacle for cases of infectious disease, and two children died there.
41. Preston .... (Dr. Fearnside.)	*First Case*, on 24th July. Fatal in nine hours, not in any infected place, nor received goods from such place, nor communicated with strangers. *Second Case.* In cellar two doors from first (had not communicated with first patient, but his wife had been in cellar of first patient during his illness), on 30th July. Fatal in ten hours. *Third Case*, on July 31st. Quarter of a mile distant, had not communicated, directly or indirectly, with first two patients. Recovered. *Fourth Case.* In part of town remote from former cases, on August 6th. Rapidly fatal. *Fifth Case.* At opposite extremity of town, August 9th, had not communicated with any person in the disease. Fatal in twelve hours. *** Out of eleven subsequent cases, five had had communication, more or less direct, with patients in the disease.
42. Torquay .... (Dr. Nankiwell to the Prov. Med. and Surg. Association.)	The disease broke out in the first week in September, and first attacked one person in an unhealthy locality in a house built against the shady side of a hill, ill ventilated, undrained, and ill supplied with water. In this locality, in houses similarly circumstanced, the epidemic chiefly prevailed at its commencement. It afterwards extended chiefly along the defective sewers. The houses of the richer inhabitants, with one exception, situated near the open mouth of the main sewer, escaped.

Place and Reporter.	Order of Cases.
42. Torquay .... (Dr. G. Black.)	*The Two First Cases* occurred simultaneously without communication, direct or indirect, with infected persons or localities. [No details given.]
43. Herne Bay .... (Mr. Godfrey to the Prov. Med. and Surg. Association.)	The few cases of Cholera were confined to one row of houses, away from the main part of the bay, and occupied by the extremely poor; all the patients were females, and all of one family. "I must also add one case that was brought on shore here, in a dying state, from the Margate steamer." [No dates given.]
44. Millbank Prison ... (Dr. Baly.)	The prisoner first attacked on October 15th, 1848, had been more than five months in the prison. No communication with any person, clothes, or stores, which could have conveyed infection, was traced at the time. It has since been ascertained that the officer of his ward had a day or two previously been at Woolwich. But he had not been near the Convict Hulks in which alone at that time Cholera prevailed. The succeeding cases occurred in different parts of the prison, two or three in each ward visited; there being, in most instances, intervals of several days between the outbreaks in the several wards.
45. Woolwich Hulks ... (Dr. Parkes.)	The convict first attacked on the 2nd of October, was seized in the "Justitia" Hulk. The convicts are allowed no intercourse with other persons, and are watched by an armed guard. No merchant-vessel anchors, except on account of the tide, at this part of the river. There was no Cholera in Woolwich at the time.
46. "Dreadnought" Hospital Ship. (Dr. Parkes.)	A man was attacked on the 5th October. The "Dreadnought" lies three or four miles distant from "Justitia" Hulk, with which it holds no communication. The man had been on board for another complaint a month before his seizure. No sailor arriving from any infected place had been admitted for some considerable time. The "Dreadnought" lies in a clear part of the river, several miles below the Pool, where the merchant-vessels lie.

TABLE XVII.

Instances of supposed infection by clothes, linen, and bedding, with facts of an opposite character.

Place and Reporter.	Circumstances related.
1. Tewkesbury .... (W. Viner Beadle, M.D.)	Some bedclothes were removed from a poor lodging-house where a man and two children had died of Cholera; some of the bedclothes were removed to the house of relatives, a man and his wife, both very aged. They were suddenly seized, and died in a few hours. The bed on which they slept was taken to another house, and there two boys, who slept on it, were seized and died. [No dates are given, but Dr. Beadle vouches for the accuracy of the facts.]
2. Loanhead, N. B. .... (Dr. Smith, of Lasswade, in a letter to Dr. McWilliam.)	A shepherd from the hill country, after being a short time in a house where a man had died of Cholera two days previously, went to the house of his nephew, a mile distant; the next morning was in collapse from Cholera, and died the same day. The same evening the nephew was attacked, and next day died. On the evening of that day the nephew's wife was attacked, and in 24 hours died. The bedding of these persons was sent to a woman living a mile off; she washed the clothes, took the disease the following day, and died. [All details except dates given.]
3. Hammersmith .... (Philip Burrows, Esq., to Dr. Farre.)	A washerwoman carried on her business at some distance from her home, in a locality where there had been many fatal cases of Cholera. She had also, on the day before her attack, washed and laid out the body of a woman reported to have died of the disease. She and her two children, living in the same room, were attacked and recovered. A child living in the room below was attacked and died.
4. Wandsworth .... (J. Howell, Esq.)	Mrs. S., living in Garratt Lane, died of Cholera. Mrs. B., her daughter, nursed her, and after her funeral returned home to Ann Street, York Road, Battersea, taking some clothing of the deceased Mrs. S.; the next day was seized with Cholera, and died. The woman who nursed her, and the one who took her infant, were also attacked, but recovered.

Place and Reporters.	Circumstances related.
5. Boston............................ (Walter Clegg, Esq.)	On the 2nd December, 1848, a woman and two children died of Cholera in Snow Fields, Southwark. The clothes of the children were sent to Boston for the use of a third child, living at its grandmother's. The old lady and the child unpacked the parcel, and both were attacked with Cholera, and were with difficulty saved. No other cases in Boston until eight months afterwards.
6. Sunderland .... (Dr. J. Brown, a note.)	The instances "are innumerable." Two examples are given.
7. Sydenham .... (W. Ray, Esq.)	No. 4 in Table XV.
8. Gateshead, Low Fell ... (Dr. J. Brown.)	No. 27 „ „
9. St. George's Parish, Canterbury. (Dr. Lochée.)	No. 35 „ „
10. Peckham Lunatic Asylum. (Dr. Turner.)	A man not resident in the house was employed to remove a quantity of straw, on which several Cholera patients had lain; he observed that the smell was peculiarly offensive, and next day he was attacked with Cholera, but recovered.
11. Wells, Somerset ...... (W. H. Livett, Esq.)	No. 49 in Table XV.
12. Stoke Prior, near Bromsgrove. (Mr. W. Horton.)	No. 62 „ „
13. Ilford.................... (Dr. T. K. Chambers.)	No. 10 in Table XVI.
14. Preston................... (H. Fearnside, M.B.)	The linen of a woman who had died of Cholera was washed by a woman living in an adjacent street. On the following day she was attacked by diarrhœa, and three or four days afterwards had a slight attack of Cholera.
15. Notting Hill .... (Mr. C. M. Frost.)	No case of Cholera was seen or heard of at a large laundry establishment in the neighbourhood. And no case of the kind was seen in private families. In two reputed instances investigated by Mr. Frost, the evidence was not satisfactory. Cholera was prevalent in the immediate neighbourhood of both cases.
16. St. John's Wood ...... (Mr. J. H. Roberts.)	A gentleman died of Cholera. His coachman's wife, living "at the stable at the bottom of the

Place and Reporter.	Circumstances related.
	garden," washed his linen, and two days after died of Cholera. But she had had diarrhœa before she washed the clothes.
17. Holyhead .... (Mr. W. Walthew, Rev. C. Williams.)	No. 22, in Table XVI.
18. Boddam................... (Dr. Jameson and — Robb, Esq.)	No. 47, in Table XV.
19. Wakefield Prison ...... (Messrs. Dunn and Milner.)	Of the 27 prisoners attacked in January, 1849, 7 were employed in washing clothes. They had washed the clothes of Cholera patients. About 25 men were generally employed in the washhouse, so that they were attacked in the proportion of 1 in 3·5, while the proportion of attacks among the whole number of prisoners (137) was 1 in 4·7.
20. Wandsworth and Clapham Union Workhouse. (Mr. H. Knapp, Master of the Workhouse.)	Two laundresses died in August, 1849, and three who were attacked recovered. [Names, dates, and ages are given.] Afterwards, all the clothes and bedding used by Cholera patients were burnt, and no further case occurred amongst the laundresses. [Number of laundresses not mentioned.]
21. St. Luke's Hospital ... (Dr. J. O. Sutherland.)	Three laundry-maids had severe diarrhœa. [The cases occurred in the summer season.]
22. Exeter .... (Dr. Shapter.)	Two other cases of the kind have occurred. [Particulars of one case given. The woman had been a day and night in the house of the person who died of Cholera, and whose clothes she washed.]
23. Woolwich Hulks ...... (Mr. Dabbs, R.N.)	The second patient had washed the clothes of the first, who died, and attributed his disease to their smell.
24. Stockport .... (Dr. Rayner.)	Two cases. Of one of the cases no dates are given ; in the other the woman washed the clothes at the house where three persons had died of Cholera. A nurse who had attended on a Cholera patient, who died, took the foul linen home, and buried them in the dust-bin in the backyard. She was attacked in 48 hours, and died.
25. Manchester .... (Dr. Ogden.)	A man, removing the bed on which a Cholera patient had died, took hold of it with his teeth. Three days afterwards he was attacked with Cholera, and died.
26. Drouet's Pauper School, Tooting. (Mr. W. J. Kite.)	" Those who were employed in washing the bed-clothes, and other articles of the Cholera patients, did not suffer from diarrhœa or Cholera. The pro-

Place and Reporter.	Circumstances related.
	cess of washing occupied several weeks after the disappearance of Cholera from the establishment. The sheets, blankets, bedding, and clothes of the Cholera patients accumulated to such a degree, that they remained unwashed for weeks; but not a single person of all who came in contact with them suffered from one symptom of Cholera." "Chloride of lime in solution was employed at first to the clothes to be washed, but not a tenth part were in any manner wetted with the solution."
27. Leeds...................... (Mr. G. R. Bearpark.)	"A great number of women were employed by the Sanitary Committee to wash the linen of Cholera patients generally; none were affected."
28. Oxford .... (Mr. T. Allen.)	"At least 50 bundles, containing blankets, coverlets, &c., were sent [from the Cholera Hospital] to be washed at the hospital washhouse. Two women and a man were employed for several weeks in washing these things and others from the hospital, all saturated with evacuations. Not one of these persons had developed Cholera: all had diarrhœa, and took medicine." But 16 city policemen, who never came near the hospital, suffered equally.
29. Brighton .... (Dr. Ormerod.)	No. 8, in Table XVI.
30. Bedford.................... (Dr. Dick.)	No washerwoman who washed the clothes sent from the hospital was affected with the disease, but several of them suffered from small pox, of which there were cases at the same time.
31. St. Giles and Bloomsbury Poor House. (Dr. Reid.)	No washerwoman was attacked.
32. Haslar Hospital......... (Dr. Wilson.)	None of the women who washed the foul linen were attacked.
33. Royal Hospital, Plymouth. (Dr. Rae.)	The washerwomen who washed the clothes and bedding in which the patients lay, which are commonly saturated with the rice-water discharge, did not suffer even from diarrhœa.
34. University College Hospital. (Dr. Parkes.)	Four women washed the clothes; none were attacked.
35. Millbank Prison ...... (Dr. Baly.)	Thirty women were employed in the laundry; one who did not wash the dirty linen, but ironed those which had been washed, was attacked, and died. Eight other women died who had not been in the laundry. The whole number of women was 130.

TABLE XVIII.

Instances of supposed communication of the disease by the sick to nurses and others in contact with them.

Place and Reporter.	Circumstances related.
1. Boston.. .... (Mr. Clegg.)	A traveller passing through Boston (4th August) was seized with Cholera, and was taken to a lodging in Warmgate. A nurse residing in the house took charge of him. On the 6th of August this woman died of Cholera; the man recovered. These were the only cases in this populous street.
2. Stockport .... (Dr. Rayner and Mr. J. Rayner.)	Sarah Dixon went to Liverpool, September 1st, to bury her sister, who had died of Cholera there; returned to Stockport on September 3rd, was attacked with Cholera on the 4th, was taken home by her mother to her mother's house, a quarter of a mile distant, was in collapse, but recovered. Her mother was attacked on the 11th, and died. The brother, James Dixon, came from High Water to see his mother, and was attacked on the 14th.
3. Bolton..................... (Mr. G. Mallet.)	A man employed on the railway between Bolton and Wigan (Cholera raging at the latter place, scarcely commencing at the former) was attacked with Cholera, and died at his house at Bolton. His wife and daughter, who nursed him, were both attacked, and the daughter died. The mother's seizure occurred two days after the man's death; the daughter's three days later. The disease did not spread, although the locality was unhealthy and crowded.
4. Hackney.................. (Mr. De Berdt Hovell.)	A gardener at Upper Clapton went to Wandsworth to attend the funeral of a relative who had died there of Cholera, returned home, was attacked with Cholera, and died. His wife, who nursed him, was also attacked, and died.
5. Liverpool................. (Mr. Henry Taylor.)	A nurse attended a patient in Great Howard Street (at the lower part of the town), and on her return home, near Everton (the higher part of the town), was seized, and died. The nurse who attended her was also seized, and died. No other case had occurred previously in that neighbourhood, and none followed for about a fortnight.
6. Hedon .... (Dr. Sandwith.)	Mrs. N. went from Paul, a village close to the

Place and Reporter.	Circumstances related.
	Humber, to Hedon, two miles off, to nurse her brother in Cholera; the next day, after his death, went to nurse Mrs. B., also at Hedon; within two days was attacked herself, was removed to a lodging-house; the son of the lodging-house keeper was attacked the next day, and died. Mrs. N.'s son removed her back to Paul, was himself attacked two days afterwards, and died.
7. Wakefield Prison ...... (Messrs. Dunn and Milner.)	Two of the persons attacked were nurses in the hospital, and one had been in the infirmary under treatment for itch, and had been in communication, not with the Cholera patients, but with the nurses who were in attendance on them. All three recovered.
8. Wandsworth and Clapham Union Workhouse. (Mr. H. Knapp to Dr. Paris.)	"Three Cholera nurses died of Cholera. Four others were attacked, and recovered." "In the earlier visitation (December, 1848, and January, 1849), the patients were kept in wards exclusively appropriated to Cholera, and there almost every nurse was attacked. During the later visitation, the patients were separated, and no nurse was attacked."
9. Woolwich Hulks .... (Mr. Dabbs.)	Of 47 convicts attacked in 1849, nine (of whom eight died) "had attended on the sick." Two were hired nurses (of whom one died). Two guards, not in attendance on the sick, also died of Cholera.
10. St. Luke's Hospital ... (Dr. J. A. Sutherland.)	One man had severe diarrhœa. "The apothecary had Cholera. The effluvia from the evacuations of the first patient had a decided effect on him."
11. Shrewsbury House of Industry. (Dr. H. Johnson.)	"A very healthy woman, employed as nurse, and attending on the Cholera patients, had the disease, and died."
12. Shrewsbury County Gaol.	"Two of the attendants, who resided out of the precincts of the prison, had the disease."
13. Lewisham Workhouse (Mr. J. J. Haycraft.)	Nine cases of well-marked Cholera were admitted. Seven occurred in inmates of the house, of whom four were nurses. One of the nurses died; another narrowly escaped. The one who died had just attended some severe and fatal cases of choleraic diarrhœa. All the nurses were affected with Cholera or diarrhœa. Mr. Haycraft and his brother, who assisted him, suffered from diarrhœa.
14. Drouet's School, Tooting. (Mr. W. J. Kite.)	"Three adults of the establishment died of Cholera. Two of these were nurses, the third a housemaid. Some of the other nurses suffered from a choleraic disposition."

Place and Reporter.	Circumstances related.
15. Millbank Prison ...... (Dr. Baly.)	One male attendant on the sick was the close of the epidemic, and died. T wife, who had no intercourse with the and had been absent from the prison height of the epidemic, was attacked after her return, and died. [The numl soners and officers are given at pp. 177 the Report.]
16. Hemel Hempstead ... (Mr. R. Newry.)	"The two nurses I employed to atter lera patients removed to the Union H seized most violently, and one died in a i
17. Seaham Harbour ...... (Dr. J. Brown.)	"The only constant attendants on the infirmary," namely, the surgeon and t both took the disease, and the former di of the general population of the place th amounted to only one in about 500.
18. St. Giles's Workhouse (Dr. Reid and the Sanitary Committee's Report.)	No "Cholera nurse" was attacked. employed about the sick, and in removi bodies, was attacked, and died. With thi the medical officers and nurses have a No large number of patients was collect ward. They were distributed amongst t wards. In 1832 there was a Cholera H ten of the attendants died.
19. St. Bartholomew's Hospital. (Dr. Burrows.)	[The principal facts are given at pagu 183 of the Report.] The following mus here :—" The resident medical officer of I lomews' Hospital, who was in constant upon the Cholera patients there, had se attacks of severe diarrhœa, that he was to relinquish those duties, and absent hi the Hospital. During the same period, resident civil officers, who were not in with the Cholera patients, did not su addition to the foregoing facts, several a assiduous clinical clerks, whilst in attend the Cholera patients, had attacks of diarr
(Dr. Roupell.)	"The nurse who died in St. Bartholo pital attributed her seizure to the exhal the bed-linen of a patient whom she had b ing, and who died."
20. Liverpool Cholera Hospital. (Dr. Dickenson and Dr. Burgess.) Liverpool Workhouse ... (Mr. Henry Taylor.)	"Many of the nurses and of the mem carried the Cholera patients from their c to the Cholera Hospital, were seized, and "Out of 30 healthy inmates of the I took the offices of nurses and attending Cholera hospitals, 9 died."

Place and Reporter.	Circumstances related.
	one of these was fatal. Of lawyers in the south of England, I have known of one only being attacked, and he had been exposed to contagion."
25. Plymouth .... (Dr. Yonge.)	" In the Cholera hospital temporarily established here, every nurse was more or less affected with Cholera."
26. Dowlais................. (Mr. J. N. White.)	" At the height of the epidemic, fully half the population were engaged in attending on, or were in the habit of visiting the sick; and it was impossible, therefore, to draw any inference on this subject. They were, doubtless, frequently attacked, but I do not think in a more than ordinary proportion."
27. University College Hospital. (Dr. Parkes.)	" None of the physicians, 3 in number, resident medical officers, 5 in number (viz. 1 apothecary, 2 physicians'-assistants, and 2 house-surgeons), or Cholera nurses (viz. 2 head nurses, and 4, or sometimes 6 assistant nurses), were attacked. The apothecary and physicians' assistants were constantly in contact with the patients; and the house-surgeons, from the interest they took in the subject, were also frequently exposed. In addition to these individuals, some of the students bestowed great attention on the Cholera cases. I am unable to state the number, which varied, indeed, from day to day; but it was not great, as the majority of the students were out of town for the vacation. None of these gentlemen were attacked." "None of the ordinary nurses, porters, or attendants at University College Hospital, were attacked." "One patient took the disease in hospital. This person was a woman, whose case will be found among those already forwarded. She was confined to bed, and lay at the extreme end of a long female ward. At the further end of the ward was the female Cholera ward, and there was a door between the two rooms which was used by the nurses. The patient in question had not been into the Cholera ward, nor had any of the convalescent Cholera patients been brought at this time into the long ward. No other patient, male or female, was attacked, except this person. The male Cholera patients were at this time placed in a room corresponding to the female Cholera ward, and situated at the end of a long men's ward. So that the men of this ward were equally exposed with the women of the corresponding ward."

ACCOUNT OF THE ORIGIN OF CHOLERA IN SUNDERLAND IN THE YEARS 1848 AND 1849.

BY DR. J. BROWN.

" In no town in this neighbourhood where I have had an opportunity of investigating its origin has the epidemic appeared till after the arrival there from an infected district of persons either ill of the disease or sickening there immediately after."

(Dr. Brown gives, on authority of Mr. Mordey, the quarantine surgeon, notices of several cases of Cholera that occurred in the five following ships —October 1, 1848, the *Orb*, from Hamburgh ; October 3, the *Volant*, from Hamburgh ; October 13, the *Roberts*, from London ; October 14, the *Chasse Marée*, from Nantes ; October 17, the *Anne*, from Lynn.)

" These were the first cases imported. All quarantine ceased on the 14th of October ; still many ships arriving with sick crews continued to sail to the upper part of the river." . . . " The first unequivocal case which took place here " (on shore) " occurred in an isolated country house, large, well-ventilated, and perfectly cleanly ; the only supposable objection to it as a residence being, that it stood on clayey and undrained land, and consequently that the adjacent ground was damp in wet weather*. It was situated about a quarter of a mile from the river, on its north bank, and about three miles above our bridge. The ships in quarantine lay in the direction of the house, but no one of them so high up. The subject of the case was a delicate female recovering from her accouchement. She had diarrhœa on the 16th of October, for which medicines were prescribed. She was understood to be better for a period ; but was attacked with vomiting on the 25th, and when her medical attendants were summoned to her on the 26th, they found her in a state of hopeless collapse from Cholera ; and she died about five hours after their arrival." . . . .

" It is true, that the house was situated at some distance, nearly a mile, from where the ships lay, but exactly in the direction in which the prevailing easterly winds would convey any effluvia from the vessels, without interjacent obstacles to its reaching the house."

The ships " had continued to accumulate in the same part of the river, and beyond it, up to the period of her attack."

---

* Dr. Brown subsequently says of this case :—" A lady, certainly under circumstances rendering direct intercourse with any one affected with the disease impossible, and any communication with those who had visited the infected very improbable."

" The next case that occurred, except some on board of ships lying in the river, was likewise on the north bank of the river, a good deal lower down than the situation of the last case, but still above the bridge. It took place in a house belonging to Monkwearmouth Colliery, but not, strictly speaking, within the colliery, situated immediately over the point of the river where the *Chasse Marée* (No. 4 on Mr. Mordey's list of ships infected), on board of which a boy, Francis Monsey, died on the 14th of October, lay at the time of his death, and where she continued to lie for some time after. The subject of the case was a collier, 18 years of age. He sickened on the 5th and died on the 6th of November. The house in which he lived was not above fifty yards from where the *Chasse Marée* lay." . . . .

This case " may have arisen by direct communication with the crew of the infected vessels, for all quarantine ceased on the 14th of October : there is, however, no evidence of such direct communication, and there is no difficulty in conceiving that some emanation from the infected vessels should reach and infect an inhabitant of a cottage very near that point of a narrow river at which the vessels lay, and with no intervening obstacle between the cottage and the river." . . . .

" On the 17th of the same month " (November, 1848), " another pitman named Spence, aged about 50, was brought up from his work in the pit ill of Cholera, and died on the 18th. This person lived in the centre of the colliery, in one of those long rows of cottages which are built by the colliery owners, and let to the workmen as part of their wages. It was certainly at some distance, perhaps two hundred yards, from the residence of the former man ; but this distance has no bearing on the probability of proximity between the former man and the present one during the illness of the first, because persons of the class we are at present speaking of constantly continued at work in spite of the diarrhœa, and did not quit till collapse compelled them, and the men were workmen in the same colliery." . . . .

" The man Spence . . . . might have received the disease from the boy, his fellow-workman, in the close atmosphere of the pit. His house was in the centre of the colliery buildings, much more remote from the river than the residence of the boy, with its front to the north, or away from the river, and many buildings interjacent between it and the river." Twelve days intervened between the attack of the boy and that of Spence, but " the class of persons in question always dated the disease from the stage of collapse, not from the initiatory or diarrhœal stages, which may last for days." . . . .

" On the 24th of November, a fatal case occurred on board of the brig *Welcome*, opposite Ayre's Quay, on the south side of the river, and nearly opposite the colliery, so often mentioned, on the north. She arrived here on the 22nd from London, whence she had sailed on the 15th. The man sickened on the night of the 23rd, and died at 10 A.M." . . . .

" On the 26th of November, the disease became so general in the colliery as to merit the name of epidemic; for on that day four sickened, of whom three died, and on the following day (27th) eleven sickened, of whom five died. From this period it continued to prevail in the colliery, and in its environs, among people connected with it, till the early part of January, when it totally ceased. In the meantime the *town in general* remained exempt from the disease." . . . .

" That Spence had been the *focus* whence these individuals received the infection, is the most reasonable supposition that the subject admits." . . . .

" At intervals (after the epidemic in the colliery), persons ill of the disease continued to arrive from London, or other places where it prevailed, and again we had an outbreak of Cholera, commencing March 5th of the present year. I cannot, however, connect this outbreak with any particular case or cases of importation, although many such had occurred. Its main range was Sunderland parish: that is, the eastern part of our town on the south side of the river, whereas the preceding seizure was in the western part on the north side; so that a mile intervened between the affected localities. It appeared simultaneously in various parts of the parish, and with such severity that, from the 7th to the 11th of March, forty-four persons sickened, of whom twenty died, and on the 12th and 13th twenty-eight persons were attacked, and twelve died. This epidemic . . . . commenced on the 5th of March, and ended on the 6th of April. One hundred and thirty persons perished in Sunderland parish alone." . . . . " Prior to this outbreak there had been the arrival of vessels from infected ports, and the landing of sick from them into the part of the town where this epidemic especially prevailed, that part where seafaring persons and their families principally reside. One such case, and that a fatal one, in the person of a master mariner, landed sick from London, I visited on the 15th of February, or just eighteen days before the outbreak, in this very locality, and other cases occurred seen by other parties. But when *foci* of infection become multiplied in a crowded locality, and the number attacked is considerable, it is impossible to trace the contamination from individual to individual." . .

" From the 6th of April to near the close of June, we enjoyed here a total exemption from Cholera, ... when on Thursday, the 28th of June, a sailor of the name of Maynard was landed from a ship from London. He had suffered from the ordinary symptoms of Cholera on the passage, and was in the febrile stage when he was landed and conveyed to his father's house, which was in Bishopwearmouth, immediately behind my own. He lingered in this stage till Monday, July 2nd, when he died. The family now consisted of only the father and mother. On Wednesday, July 4th, the mother became affected with diarrhœa, and when she was first visited on Friday morning, July 6th, by a respectable surgeon and myself, she was in a state of hopeless collapse, and she died that night. The father did not take the disease, nor did I hear of any case apparently derived from the sailor boy, excepting his mother's. But I speedily heard of cases of Cholera in various parts of the town, especially among pilots and their families—a class of men very likely to be brought into proximity with the disease ; and I found on inquiry that the father of the family first sickened, and then the other members became affected. At the same time it should be remarked that what occurred in the case of the sailor boy Maynard was going on in various parts of the town. Seafaring persons were arriving from London ; some by ships, others, for greater expedition, by railway, ill of the disease, and dying shortly after their arrival. Under these circumstances, it will surprise no one familiar with epidemics and their propagation to learn that Cholera is at this moment (September, 1849) prevailing extensively in Sunderland." . . . .

"The sickening of Mrs. Maynard " (took place) . . "in a clean and comfortable house, on the 4th July, where there had been no Cholera in the town for nearly three months, that is, from the 6th April." . . .
"She attended incessantly on her son from the 28th June, the time when he landed ill of Cholera from London, to the time of his death, July 2nd, there being no other case of the disease existing in the town at the time. I can discern no sources of the disease but the body of her sick son." [Extracts from Dr. Brown's Report, received by the Cholera Committee of the Royal College of Physicians, on the 8th October, 1849.]

[The preceding extracts give the facts. The following contain the more important of Dr. Brown's remarks on the first indigenous case :—]

"The most reasonable explanation that the first of this group of cases admits of appears to me that proposed by Drs. Russell and Barry, with respect to the outbreak of Cholera at Dantzic in 1831." . . . .
"It did not reach Dantzic till after the arrival there of ships, some of them infected, from St. Petersburgh, shortly after which the disease spread through the former place, although no communication had been allowed between the crews of the infected vessels and the town. The best explanation these gentlemen found to offer was, that the emanations from the infected vessels, conveyed by the wind, had spread the disease through the town."

"In the case of the party first attacked" (at Sunderland), "only some such explanation is discoverable." . . . . "That the vessels were infected is beyond a question, for all had lost at least one, some more, of their crews ; and those acquainted with the diffusion of malaria, which, it is well known, is often conveyed at least a league, as in the case of the exhalation from Lake Agnano reaching the Convent of Camaldules, will have no difficulty in understanding how the contaminated atmosphere from these vessels, whether the taint be considered to have proceeded from the bodies of the sick, to have been engendered by the dirt and foulness within the vessel, or from both combined, may be wafted by a favourable wind to the distance of a mile, and there affect a person predisposed by debility to its action. Whatever may be thought of this view, it must be deemed much more reasonable and probable than that of an epidemic atmosphere extending its *influence* over thousands of square miles, and yet affecting only a few square feet in the township of Hylton and parish of Bishopwearmouth, and two points at the opposite extremities of this vast area—London and Dundee."

Note.—At page 38, reference is made to the Appendix for particulars of the visitations of Cholera in Glasgow and Paisley, and for descriptions of those parts of the same towns most severely visited by the Epidemic, which it was intended to quote from Dr. Sutherland's Report to the General Board of Health. But, on further consideration, it has appeared unnecessary to print here matter which is already before the public. It is sufficient to state that the passages referred to will be found at pages 34 and 35, 70 and 71, of Dr. Sutherland's Report; and that some further valuable information relative to the outbreaks in Dumfries and Glasgow, communicated by Dr. Barker and Mr. J. M. Adams, is contained in the ninth volume of the Monthly Journal of Medical Science, at pages 940, 1012, and 1066.

REPORT

ON THE

MORBID ANATOMY, PATHOLOGY, AND TREATMENT,

OF

EPIDEMIC CHOLERA,

BY

WILLIAM W. GULL, M.D.,

ASSISTANT PHYSICIAN TO GUY'S HOSPITAL.

JOHN AYRTON PARIS, M.D., D.C.L., F.R.S.,

PRESIDENT OF THE ROYAL COLLEGE OF PHYSICIANS OF LONDON.

SIR,

   This Report is, from the state of our knowledge, necessarily fragmentary.

The design has been to set down the principal ascertained facts, and to draw such conclusions as were possible from them. It is obviously not intended to be an Essay on the disease.

The section on treatment contains little that is positive; its value, if any, lies in removing the obstructions which prevent a simpler view of the subject; since having learned what is useless, we gain a better ground for future success.

The epidemic of 1849 was already declining when this Report was undertaken; hence no opportunity was afforded for original inquiry.

The thanks of the College are due to those Members of the Profession who favoured the Committee with communications;—some of which were of great value.

The principal writers in this country and on the Continent have been consulted, and their statements, when introduced, generally rendered *verbatim*.

   I have the honour to be, SIR,

      Your faithful servant,

         WILLIAM GULL, M.D.

8, Finsbury Square, December, 1853.

CORRIGENDA.

Page 46, in the Table, *for* Inorganic constituents to 1000 parts of organic, *read* Inorganic constituents to 100 parts of organic.

Page 47, in the upper Table the bracket should include only the two upper lines, thus :

Transuded fluid (vomited and dejected). }
Intercellular fluid.

Page 47, the lower Table gives the analysis of Blood Cells.

CONTENTS.

MORBID ANATOMY.

PATHOLOGY.

TREATMENT.

REPORT

ON THE

MORBID ANATOMY AND PATHOLOGY

OF

CHOLERA.

CONDITION OF THE BODY AFTER DEATH IN THE COLD
STAGE OF CHOLERA.

Rise of Tempera-
ture, &c.
DURING the former epidemic, it was noted by
several observers, that the icy coldness of the body,
which occurs to so marked a degree in the collapse of cholera, passed
away after death, the surface becoming in some cases actually warm.
No precise thermometrical details were given; the evidence resting
upon the vague impressions received by the hand.

The following cases are therefore of more value, since they un-
equivocally prove, by careful measurements, that a rise of temperature on the surface of the body after death did occur. In Case 2,
during life the coldness of the surface was very marked, two hours
and a half after death the thermometer indicated 102·12°. In Case 6,
ten minutes before death, the temperature in the axilla was 103·1°:
five minutes after death it was 104°. In Case 9, twenty-five minutes
after death, the temperature of the uncovered abdomen was 89°;
forty-five minutes after death it was 90°; and fifty minutes after
death it was 91°. Some of the cases are equivocal, as the temperature was noted at so long a period before death, that it might afterwards have risen before death took place:—thus, in Case 5, at a
quarter to five o'clock, P.M., the temperature in the axilla was 99·14°;
death occurred two hours later, and five minutes after death, the

B

temperature in the same place was 101·12°. It is to be observed that signs of reaction had manifested themselves in this case when the first observation was made, and hence it is probable, that in the two hours which elapsed before death, there was a gradual increase of temperature, accounting for the high degree noted in the second observation. The same objections cannot be made in Case 7, for it is stated that the patient remained collapsed until death.

Where an absolute increase of temperature was not observed, the length of time during which the body retained its warmth was in many cases remarkable. In Case 1, five hours before death, the temperature was 95° in the axilla; the patient remained in the same collapsed state, and died half an hour after mid-day; three hours and a half after death the temperature in the axilla was 95·36°, and in the groin, 97·16°, being an increase of nearly half a degree above that noted during life. In Case 2, the temperature was 101·12°, two hours and a half after death. In Case 3, the temperature of the room being 75·2°, the body, two hours and a quarter after death, was 98·24° in the axilla, and 100·4° in the groin. In Case 9, the surface of the abdomen retained its temperature unaltered for forty-five minutes. In Case 10, the heat observed at the moment of death was not only maintained, but an hour afterwards was nearly 2° higher.

Mr. F. W. Barlow, of the Westminster Hospital, recorded the particulars of a remarkable case of slow cooling of the body after death in cholera [*]. It occurred in the practice of Dr. Green, of the Bristol Infirmary. The patient was a gentleman who was attacked with the usual symptoms of the epidemic, and died in collapse rather suddenly, after 15 hours, at 2 A.M., on the 13th of October.

" At 6 A.M.," says Dr. Green, " I saw the body; the skin was warm; limbs not rigid; features not collapsed. I directed that he should not be buried until I had seen him again.

" At 6 P.M. I found he had been screwed down in his coffin: the lid was removed by my direction, the body taken out, and found still warm, and in the same condition as in the morning. The entire body and extremities were then closely packed in sawdust.

" Oct. 14th.—Had remained during the night in the sawdust; the warmth still continued; there was no rigidity; a vein in the arm was opened, but no blood came.

---

[*] Observations on the Condition of the Body after Death from Cholera.—*Med. Gazette,* 1850.

" At 12 at noon, tepid salt and water were injected slowly in a vein of the arm; some frothing of the mouth followed; next powerful galvanic shocks were passed from the back of the neck in the direction of the heart for half an hour: no other means were used.

" The sawdust was then removed, and the body laid out in the usual way.

" 15th.—Heat less.

" 16th.—Body cool.

" 17th.—Body quite cold; limbs rigid; appearances of decomposition over the abdomen."

" As to the long retention of warmth," says Mr. Barlow, " it will doubtless have struck the reader that the packing of the body in sawdust had, in every probability, much to do with the retention of the heat. It would be against reason not to conclude so; and such is the opinion of Dr. Green, Dr. Wallis, and Mr. Kelson; such that of Dr. Alfred Taylor and others to whom I have mentioned the facts of the case. Still, it seems clear that there was something not a little uncommon in the temperature of the body, and that the long-continued heat was far from being altogether owing to the bad non-conductor wherewith it was surrounded: the corpse, as we see by the account, had less heat on the 15th, was called 'cool' on the 16th, and not pronounced quite cold until the 17th, though it was removed from the sawdust about noon on the 14th. Inferring from Dr. Green's narration that the face was left uncovered whilst the rest of the body was completely enveloped in the sawdust, I made inquiry of that gentleman whether the exposed part did not become more quickly cold than the rest of the body. Dr. Green says in a note, ' I took care that the face should be entirely uncovered. The next morning there was not much, if any, difference between the temperature of the face and other parts; but on the morning of the 15th the face was decidedly colder than the rest of the body.' From this we may gather that the sawdust operated in keeping, or helping to keep, the body warm: indeed, it could not have done otherwise; but the corpse appears to have been very slow in cooling even when there seemed nothing to prevent its doing so. I asked Dr. Green to inform me of the circumstances under which the body lay subsequently to its being removed from the sawdust, of the temperature of the atmosphere meanwhile, &c., and I learn from him that it was laid on a board, dressed as the dead are usually, and covered with a sheet. No fire was in the room it lay in. The window was open in the day-time and shut at night. The following was the temperature of the weather at Bristol in four out of the five days wherein the corpse was watched : —

Saturday,   Oct. 13th, 45°, wind East.
Monday,   „   15th, 45°, „   East.
Tuesday,   „   16th, 47°, „   E.S.E.
Wednesday,   „   17th, 60°, „   W.S.W.

" From hence we may conclude that the body was slow in cooling, even when by no means unfavourably situated for losing its warmth quickly, when the temperature was moderately low, the wind being in the east the while, when the window of the room was open at day-time, and the body lightly covered."

Observation	Age	Sex	Time of observation before death.	Temperature.	Time of death.	Time of observation after death.	Temperature.	Remarks.
1	54	Female.	7 h. 30 m. A.M.	In axilla, 95°.	12 h. 30 m. noon. In collapse.	4 h. P.M.	In axilla, 95·36°. In groin, 97·16°.	Body lightly covered after death. Briquet and Mignot.
2	42	Female.	Before death coldness of surface very marked.		8 h. P.M.	10 h. 30 m. P.M.	101·18°.	Cadaveric rigidity well marked. Briquet and Mignot.
3	58	Female.	9 h. A.M.	In axilla, 101·8°.	10 h. 15 m. A.M.	12 h. 30 m. noon.	In axilla, 98·24°. In groin, 100·4°.	Temperature of room 75·2°. Briquet and Mignot.
4	50	Female.	9 h. A.M.	In axilla, 97·52°.	4 h. 45 m. P.M.	5 h. 15 m. P.M. 7 h. 15 m.	In axilla, 100·4°. In axilla, 98·26°.	Body covered after death. Briquet and Mignot.
5	50	Female.	4 h. 45 m. P.M.	In axilla, 99·14°.	6 h. 35 m. P.M.	6 h. 40 m. P.M.	In axilla, 101·18°.	Slight reaction, with cerebral congestion. Briquet and Mignot.
6	18	Female.	4 h. 45 m. P.M.	103·1°.	4 h. 55 m. P.M.	5 h.	104°.	Briquet and Mignot.
7	71	Male.	10 h. A.M.	In axilla, 96·98°.	11 h. 58 m. A.M. In collapse.	2 m. after 12 noon.	In axilla, 98·06°.	Briquet and Mignot.

* Traité du Choléra Morbus, 1850, page 381.

Observations.	Age.	Sex.	Time of observation before death.	Temperature.	Time of death.	Time of observation after death.	Temperature.	Remarks.
8	56	Male.	8 h. A.M.	In axilla, 98·2°.	8 h. 40 m. P.M. In asphyxia.	8 h. 50 m. P.M. 4 h. 50 m.	In axilla, 95°. In axilla, 98·08°.	Brinton and Mignot.
9	30	Male.	Immediately after death.	Mouth, 81·5°. Abdomen, 94°.	8 h. 40 m. P.M.	8 h. 47 m. P.M. 4 h. 4 m. 4 h. 18 m. 4 h. 25 m. 4 h. 55 m.	Mouth, 87°. Abdomen, 92·5°. Mouth, 87°. Abdomen, 98°. Mouth, 86°. Abdomen, 94°. Mouth, 87°. Abdomen, 94°. Mouth, 87°. Abdomen, 90·5°.	Muscular movements in various parts for an hour after death. The skin gradually becoming of a lighter color. Dr. Purkinje.
10	58	Female.			9 h. A.M.	9 h. 25 m. 9 h. 30 m. 9 h. 45 m. 9 h. 50 m. 9 h. 60 m.	Mouth, 84°. Abdomen recovered, 89°. Mouth, 84°. Abdomen, 89°. Mouth, 88°. Abdomen, 90°. Mouth, 88·6°. Abdomen, 91°. Mouth, 86°. Abdomen, 91° (nearly).	Muscular movements after death. After one hour, fingers of right hand contracted. After one hour, extremities rigidity commencing. Dr. Fisher.

The phenomena detailed above are not peculiar to Cholera. Cruveilhier* speaks of a rise of temperature after death from asphyxia; Dr. Dowler † observed the same in cases of yellow fever; and Briquet and Mignot made similar observations in peritonitis, pneumonia, &c.:—

Age.	Sex.	Time of observation before death.	Temperature.	Time of death.	Time of observation after death.	Temperature.	Remarks.
28	Female.	9 h. A.M.	In axilla, 104·86°.	5 m. after noon.	20 m. after noon.	In axilla, 106·16°.	Puerperal peritonitis.
60	Female.	9 h. 20 m. A.M.	In axilla, 104·9°.	10 h. 35 m.	10 h. 45 m.	In axilla, 105·44°.	Pneumonia of right lung.
Aged person.	Male.	9th July.	In axilla, 100·94°.	11 July, 6 h. 30 m. A.M.	8 h. A.M.	In axilla, 101·12°. In groin, 102·56°.	Chronic inflammation of spinal chord.

Anatomie Pathologique, livre 16me, p. 35.

Experimental Researches, &c., New York, 1846.

Muscular
contractions.

Amongst the phenomena presented by the body after death from Cholera, are the well-known contractions of the muscles, which often occur to so great an extent, and last for so long a period, as to excite horror in the ignorant, and add in such minds a further mystery to this disease. The muscles affected were principally those of the extremities, but contractions were likewise occasionally observed in all the other voluntary muscles. These movements varied in extent, from flickering and tremulous undulations in a few fibres, scarcely to be seen or felt, to contractions sufficiently powerful to move the limbs from their position, or even to displace the body itself. By a rare coincidence, in which one or more sets of muscles were simultaneously affected, the results had sometimes a voluntary character ; thus both arms were in one case observed to be flexed, and the hands approximated together as in the attitude of prayer*: in another the eyes opened and moved slowly downwards: and in a third the right arm was brought over the chest and the hand lifted to the throat. We refer these results to *coincidence* of contraction in different muscles, and not to any co-ordinating influence of the nervous centres, not only because such an explanation is more in accordance with the whole phenomena, and is in itself sufficient, but because the manner in which the contractions took place, even when they had such a complex character, was altogether different from the action of voluntary muscles under nervous stimulus, being either slow and creeping, like the movements visible in separate fibres under the microscope, or, when more lively, like the twitchings seen in the muscles of a slaughtered animal.

They began shortly after death, and lasted a variable time, from a few minutes to two hours, as in a case observed by Mr. Kesteven†, in which the lower jaw was moved at intervals for that period. They were rarely so enduring as this. In the case of a female reported to us by Dr. Parkes, they continued for an hour in the flexors of the fingers and fore-arm, cadaveric rigidity at the same time beginning in both knees, and in the elbow of the opposite side, the temperature of the abdomen continuing as high as 91°.

When not occurring spontaneously, they could still be excited by percussion or other mechanical stimulus of the fibres.

* Observations on the Muscular Contractions which occasionally happen after Death from Cholera, by W. F. Barlow, M.R.C.S.—*Med. Gazette*, 1850.

† Supplement to some Observations on the Muscular Contractions, &c., by W. F. Barlow, M.R.C.S.—*Med. Gazette*, 1850.

They were more commonly observed in those who died rapidly of the disease, in the middle period of life, when the muscular system was vigorous and well-developed, which will, perhaps, account for their greater frequency in males than in females.

Post-mortem contractions are not peculiar to Cholera. Mr. Barlow observed such in a case of severe apoplexy, fatal after six hours. In this case they affected the lower extremities principally, but the hands were slightly moved once or twice, and the fingers flexed several times. They lasted for three quarters of an hour, the temperature in the axilla, half an hour after death, being 104°; discernible movements could not be excited by striking or pricking the muscles. Dr. Dowler * readily produced contractions by percussion after death from yellow fever and some other diseases. The muscles of slaughtered animals are well known to exhibit for a long time similar contractions.

" We have often," observe Reinhardt and Leubuscher † " seen contractions of individual muscles after death. In one instance they were remarkable, affecting the muscles of the inner side of the right thigh, the toes of the same side and the fingers of the left hand. They continued very active for more than a quarter of an hour, and then gradually lessened. . . . Irritation of the skin increased them, and pressure upon the ulnar nerve, and the nerves of the axilla, several times produced flexion of the fingers." Briquet and Mignot‡, on the contrary, state that they never saw these movements.

Rigor mortis. Cadaveric rigidity often supervened very quickly; in one case, mentioned above, it began at the end of an hour after death. Briquet and Mignot observed it after forty minutes, and in most cases before two hours had elapsed. Its occurrence was not retarded by the high temperature which the body retained ; in one case being very marked, whilst the temperature in the axilla was as high as 100·58°.

Rigidity occurred not only at an early period, but lasted from 20 to 40 hours.

Putrefactive Changes. Cruveilhier§ says, putrefactive changes were slow, as in all cases where much blood has been lost, and adds, " in the alimentary canal, on the contrary, de-

* Experimental Researches on the Post-Mortem Contractility of the Muscles, &c. New York, 1846.
† Archiv. für Pathologische Anatomie, &c., 2ter, ! and, 1849, p. 442.
‡ Op. Citat., p. 395.　　　　　§ Anatomie Pathologique.

composition was rapid, as commonly occurs where the digestive organs are the seat of considerable sanguineous congestion."

Most observers confirm the former part of this statement, but with respect to the intestinal canal the conditions were variable, and often the contrary of that noted by this great authority. The intestines containing little more than pure water, and being entirely devoid of fœcal and ammoniacal contents, were certainly not prone, in most cases, to undergo rapid decomposition.

MORBID APPEARANCES IN CHOLERA WHEN DEATH OCCURRED DURING COLLAPSE.

THE stomach was pale and generally more or less
Stomach. distended. It contained turbid, mucoid fluid, grey, or
colorless, or tinged of a chocolate, or reddish brown hue, by admixture
with blood. The surface of the mucous membrane was covered with
tenacious mucus, having in some cases a puriform character from the
large admixture of exfoliated epithelium. It was pale in 12 out of
30 cases; in the others, there was hyperæmia, in different degrees,
usually most marked at the greater cul-de-sac and along the greater curvature, either in a continuous arborescent form, from fulness of the
smaller veins, or in irregular patches of punctate redness, occupying
the summits of the rugæ, and often accompanied with spots of ecchymosis.

The membrane was generally rather thickened and opake; the
texture firm and the surface mammillated. In 2 cases out of 30
there was some softening at the left end, probably the result of post-
mortem digestion.

In one instance, death having occurred 36 hours after the onset of the acute symptoms, there were slight traces of granular
fibrinous exudation (diphtherite), extending along the greater curvature towards the pylorus. In 4 cases the solitary glands are
stated to have been enlarged; in 2 they were seen near the cardia
and termination of the œsophagus, and in 2 near the pylorus. At
this part also the membrane was occasionally dotted over with small
pits, probably produced by the bursting of these glands from serous
effusion into their cavities, a result, as will hereafter be seen, frequently observed in the solitary glands of the small intestines.

According to Reinhardt and Leubuscher*, " after death in the cold
stage, the mucous membrane of the stomach commonly presented
patches of hyperæmia more or less extensive, sometimes with ecchymosis. The fundus was their usual seat, but they also frequently
occurred at the pylorus, or were uniformly diffused over the whole
surface. The glands were sometimes unaffected, but not rarely they

* Archiv. für Pathologische Anatomie, &c., 2ter Band, p. 492, 1849.

were swollen. The surface of the membrane was almost constantly covered with a thick layer of tenacious mucus, for the most part of a whitish color, but sometimes reddish brown or blackish brown, from the effusion of blood."

Briquet and Mignot[*] of La Charité write as follows:—

" The state of the stomach is mentioned in 32 cases. In most instances it was much distended, and seemed to have lost its contractile power (?). In 7 cases there was general pulpy softening, and in 10 others the softening was limited to the greater cul-de-sac. In no instance," say they, " did we observe traces of gelatiniform softening (from digestion ?)."

" In 11 cases there was general aborescent venous injection, in 5 this was intense, in 6 slight. In 3 there were numerous patches of a bright punctate redness, giving the membrane the appearance of crimson velvet. The hyperæmia was limited to the greater curvature in 8 cases, and in 2 to the pylorus."

Dr. Leudet, who, as an Interne under Louis, had extensive opportunities, at the Hotel Dieu, of studying the morbid anatomy of cholera, and who favored us with a record of his observations, gives the results of 91 post-mortem examinations. In speaking of the state of the stomach he says:—" In most cases, the stomach was healthy, its color varied from a white to a reddish brown at the greater cul-de-sac. In 9 cases there was general softening of the mucous membrane; when observed in others this change was limited to the cardiac end. Patches of punctate injection were very rare. Enlargement of the gastric glands (solitary ?) seemed to be the exception. The reaction of the mucous membrane was always either neutral or acid."

Pirogoff[†] gives a plate (Tab. xii) of a very remarkable appearance of the stomach, produced by the exudation of large masses of granular amorphous matter on the surface of the highly vascular and ecchymosed mucous membrane. He terms it a rare form of diphtherite, and adds that he observed such a condition but twice. It appears to be an extreme instance of that change which was apt to occur in the mucous membranes, in cholera, wherever the hyperæmia was intense and long continued. According to this observer, " the stomach was affected by the *cholera process* in a much less degree

[*] Traité Pratique et Analytique du Cholera Morbus, p. 399.
[†] Anatomie Pathologique du Cholera Morbus, par N. Pirogoff, *Atlas*.

than the intestines, and less frequently than the lungs and brain (!),
at least so far as regarded morbid alterations of tissue."

Pharynx and The state of the œsophagus and pharynx is not
Œsophagus. generally mentioned in the communications we received. In one case, fatal after 12 hours of acute symptoms, we
observed that the lower part of the œsophagus was deprived of its
epithelium.

The state of these parts is described by Reinhardt and Leubuscher *
thus : " In the first (algide) stage we several times found the mucous
membrane of the pharynx and œsophagus in a state of intense hyperæmia. The lower part of the œsophagus was principally affected :
the hyperæmic and ecchymosed membrane being not unfrequently
denuded of its epithelium, especially along the ridges of the longitudinal folds."

Briquet and Mignot † examined the œsophagus in 11 instances,—
in 4 it presented a general but moderate degree of rose-colored
injection, and in one there was intense congestion throughout the
lower third. In most cases the surface was dry; in one it was
covered by a white pultaceous substance.

According to Leudet, " The pharynx and œsophagus were constantly covered with a soft pulpy detritus (exfoliated epithelium?).
In one instance only was there a development of the follicles.

Peritoneum. The small intestines had generally externally a pink
  or rose tint from hyperæmia of the portal venous
system. In some instances they had a remarkably dark color, the
venous trunks being large and full of pitchy blood. The different
tints soon changed upon exposure to the air.

In most of the reports received, no note is made of the state of
the peritoneal surface : in some it is stated to have been rather drier
than natural, and covered with a slight layer of a tenacious mucoid
secretion.

Briquet and Mignot ‡, in their report, state that " The peritoneum
was carefully examined in 32 cases. In 11 there was universal
and intense injection of the small capillary veins of the sub-
epithelial cellular tissue. In the other cases the same condition
existed, but in a less degree. It was in general most marked on
the depending surface of the intestines, and on the organs contained
in the pelvis, and especially on the genital organs of the female."
They many times noticed along the convexity of the intestinal con-

* Op. Citat., p. 492. † Op. Citat., p. 399. ‡ Ibid., p. 398.

volutions, red stripes and patches in which the injection was greater
than at other parts; this hyperæmia being, according to them,
nothing more than an intense degree of the same venous engorgement which existed elsewhere. " There were no traces of inflammatory action. In 5 cases, a drachm or two of yellow serum was
found in the cavity of the peritoneum; but in no instance fibrinous
exudation. The surface of the membrane was frequently covered by
a thin layer of a semi-solid glutinous matter, which caused the convolutions to adhere slightly together. It was not great on the other
serous membranes, and where it existed had not the importance
some observers have attributed to it."

In one case noted by these authors, in which death occurred after
reaction, with symptoms of inflammation of the brain, the peritoneal
surface of the small intestine was covered with numerous small
crystals, probably of the ammoniaco-magnesian phosphate. The intestine was scarcely at all injected, and contained a greyish rice-water
fluid.

Virchow (" Medicin. Reform," No. 12) says, " The surface of the
peritoneum was constantly found covered with an adhesive fluid of
a yellow colour having a pungent sour smell, and commonly an acid
reaction; by rubbing it between the fingers a lather was formed like
that produced by a concentrated solution of albumen."

According to Leudet, " The digestive tube was covered externally
with a glutinous matter readily adhering to the finger. This exudation was principally observed in persons who died during the cold
stage, and was generally absent where the patients had sunk in the
more advanced periods of the disease."

Small   The coats of the small intestine were thickened and
Intestines.   pulpy from œdema of the mucous membrane and submucous tissue.   The duodenum and ileum were more commonly
affected, and to a greater extent than the jejunum. In some instances the mucous membrane was pale throughout, in others the
lower part of the ileum only, or the duodenum only was hyperæmic.

The vascularity of the mucous membrane presented itself under
two conditions, as uniform arborescent venous injection, affecting
large tracts of the intestine, particularly the lower part of the ileum;
or as patches of variable extent, in which the redness was punctate,
and of a bright color, frequently with spots of ecchymosis and an
exudation of tenacious bloody mucus.

The villi were also swollen and prominent from œdema, especially throughout the jejunum. Their appearance and the condition of the epithelium covering them was minutely described by Böhm * during the last epidemic in 1832–33. According to his observations the villi had sometimes a swollen and rounded appearance, from the presence of fluid enclosed beneath the loosened yet partly-adherent epithelium ; but more frequently they were quite denuded, or with only here and there a solitary cell upon their surface, indicating the previous disposition of the epithelium, and rendering more obvious the change that had taken place.

Upon the surface and into the tissue of the mucous membrane, where the morbid process was most intense, as shown by the vascular injection and ecchymosis, there was sometimes observed an effusion of a yellowish finely-granular fibrinous matter, such as occurs in ordinary diphtherite. The textures thus affected subsequently underwent a gradual process of disintegration, leaving an irregularly-abraded surface, often rendered more distinct by a stain of color from the contents of the intestine. The lower part of the ileum was most commonly thus affected, but occasionally the pharynx, the œsophagus, as well as the stomach and the other parts of the intestinal tract, were the seat of similar changes.

In the majority of cases, the affection of the villous surface did not pass beyond the stage of congestion, ecchymosis, and œdema of tissue, with exfoliation of epithelium, the granular fibrinous or diphtheritic exudation described above, being by no means common or extensive; it is, however, probable that, without careful observation, the minor degrees of it might have been overlooked, from the mucoid and turbid character of the contents of the intestine, and there is the more reason to suppose that this was the case, since the German pathologists, whose investigations are characterized by the greatest care, found it more frequently than it was observed, either in this country or in France. Thus, Reinhardt and Leubuscher † state that, " in the ileum, and particularly in the lower part of it, the villi were often infiltrated with a finely-granular substance, consisting of oil globules and proteine molecules, frequently to so great an extent as to be quite opaque. We leave it undetermined whether the substance was chyle only, or in part an effusion of finely-granular exudation into the tissue of the villi. We have sometimes seen in those who have died in the algide stage, large patches of the

* Die Kranke darmschleimhaut in der Asiatischen Cholera. Berlin, 1838.
† Op. Citat., p. 482.

mucous membrane of the lower part of the ileum infiltrated with a solid, whitish, amorphous exudation, which occupied the superficial layers of the membrane, and so far encroached upon and enclosed the villi that they were no longer distinguishable."

Virchow[*] directed particular attention to these diphtheritic effusions, and to the subsequent necrosis of the tissues in which they occurred. They were not observed by Briquet and Mignot; and M. Leudet, in his communication to us, says, " I have looked in vain, in the coats of the intestine, for that particular effusion described by the pathological anatomists of Berlin."

The villi of the duodenum were in several instances whitish and opaque, from a collection of oil globules in their interior. This appearance was first noted by Böhm; it is an unimportant as well as infrequent change.

The further morbid appearances of the small intestines are thus described by the German and the French pathologists. According to Reinhardt and Leubuscher[†], "the mucous membrane of the small intestines was constantly of a rose tint, depending upon a fulness of the smaller veins. This venous hyperæmia extended for the most part over the whole length of the small intestines, gradually increasing from the duodenum to the cœcum, being most marked in the lower part of the ileum. Together with this less marked and more venous engorgement we almost always found intense capillary hyperæmia, distinguishable from the former by the brightness of its tint, and associated with more or less extensive ecchymosis into the tissue of the mucous membrane. This capillary injection was sometimes limited to a few spots of the large and small intestine, and to this extent was always present; but sometimes the mucous membrane, especially in the ileum, was, for several feet, of a bright scarlet color, from extreme capillary congestion, and extravasation of blood.

" The tissue of the mucous membrane was infiltrated with serous exudation, the folds (valvulæ conniventes) were enlarged and swollen, and the villi often appeared distended and prominent as at the time of active digestion."

Out of 32 cases, examined by Briquet and Mignot[‡], in 11 the mucous membrane of the jejunum was of a violet color, depending upon congestion of the vascular rete of the submucous tissue (?). This congestion, which was also apparent from the peritoneal surface,

---

* Medicinische Reform, No. 19.   † Op. Cit., p. 480.   ‡ Op. Cit., p. 401.

had its seat in the capillary veins, from which it could be traced, step by step, to the principal mesenteric trunks. In 5 other cases the same condition existed, but in a less intense degree; the vascular ramifications larger and ·less crowded, leaving the intestine of its natural color in their interstices. Conjointly with these traces of venous engorgement, in 10 instances (one-third), we found isolated patches of injection having a decidedly inflammatory character (?).ˉ The redness was in striæ, and in points of a vermillion tint, becoming more distinct by washing and pressure. In many cases the mucous membrane was stained by the sanguinolent fluid in which it was bathed. In the 16 remaining cases the valvular portion of the intestine (jejunum) was of a remarkable whiteness, marked only by some larger vascular ramifications.

In 22 cases (out of 32) there was venous congestion of the mucous membrane of the ileum throughout its whole length; being most marked near the ileo-colic valve. In four-fifths of the cases, together with this venous engorgement, there were scattered patches of punctate, inflammatory (?), injection. In three cases the inflammatory (?) congestion was alone apparent.

" The coats of the intestines, gorged by this afflux of fluid to them and infiltrated by an endosmosis of their contents, presented an increased thickness of their walls, and gave a remarkable feeling of softness to the touch. This condition was most marked on the prominent parts of the valvulæ conniventes. It was present in almost every case, particularly when the disease was fatal in the algide stage."

M. Leudet says, " The color of the mucous membrane of the small intestine, was carefully noted in 33 cases in which death occurred in the algide stage." The following Table gives the results:—

Mucous Membrane		pale throughout	10
,,	,,	pale rose tint	4
		uniform reddish grey . .	2
	,,	yellowish white	3
	,,	pale superiorly, and rose tint below	3
	,,	white, with livid patches .	5
	,,	rose tint, with violet patches . . .	4
	,,	red above, violet below	1
,,	,,	spots of very dark color	1

Glands of the small Intestines. The glandular structures were the seat of changes similar to those observed in the mucous membrane itself. The solitary glands were almost universally distinct, especially in the lower part of the ileum; their prominence and general increase of size being for the most part due to the œdematous state of the tissues in which they were contained. When they had acquired a considerable size they more commonly appeared as compact firm grains; in this state the enlargement depended upon an infiltration of a solid granular fibrinous exudation, which was not confined to the glandular structures, but extended more or less into the surrounding tissue. The fluid evacuated from the follicles by puncture contained merely the normal glandular elements, namely, cells, nuclei, and granules.

The solitary glands were prominent in 31 instances out of 32 examined by Briquet and Mignot. In 24 they were pale and translucent; in 7 slightly roseate. In an infant a fortnight old, the attack being very acute, the intestines presented numerous agminated patches, but the solitary glands were not visible.

Amongst the cases tabulated and appended to this report is one of a man aged 25, who died after 21 hours of severe symptoms. On examination the solitary glands were scarcely visible, even at the lower end of the ileum. Such exceptions were rare, and in favor of the general agreement on this point, we may add the following table from M. Leudet's communication :—

"*Seat of the Follicular Enlargement in the Small Intestines in the Algide Stage.*"

Throughout the small intestines	.	2 cases.
In the inferior $\frac{1}{2}$	.	5 ,,
,, ,, $\frac{1}{3}$	. . .	4 ,
,, ,, $\frac{1}{4}$	. . .	13 ,
,, ,, $\frac{1}{5}$	.	2 ,
,, ,, $\frac{1}{6}$	. . .	1 ,
,, ,, $\frac{1}{8}$	. . .	2 ,
Close to the valve only	. . .	4 ,
Scarcely visible .	- - -	- ..
Not visible	. . . .	1 ,,

Dr. Gairdner[*], in his report on the morbid appearances in 89 cases of cholera, says, "The most frequent of all the abnormal conditions of the mucous membranes, was the prominence of the intestinal glands, both of the aggregated and solitary, but especially of the latter. This condition, the 'psorenterie' of some French writers, was found in about two-thirds of the cases."

      [*] Monthly Journal of Medical Science, July, 1849.

Pirogoff* gives several illustrations of the appearances presented by these structures. In one case, fatal in the algide stage (Plate v A), they were surrounded by an areola of a bright red color, and their summits were yellowish from effusion of pus. This form of the disease, he designates *cholera dysentery*.

The duodenum was the seat of great hyperæmia in the algide stage, and the glands situated in this division of the intestines were often much enlarged. Instances fell under our notice where this enlargement was very remarkable, and was the more striking, inasmuch as the glandular structures of this division of the intestines are rarely so much affected in any other disease. Reinhardt and Leubuscher state, as the result of their observations, that in the duodenum "Brunner's glands were sometimes swollen, and on microscopical examination the acini were more opaque than usual, containing besides their normal cells and nuclei, a greater or less quantity of a finely-granular molecular substance."

The patches of Peyer. The changes in the patches of Peyer were similar to those occurring in the villous surface of the mucous membrane generally, and in the solitary glands. They were often thickened and prominent from infiltration of serous fluid, and the included glands, when visible, presented the conditions found in the solitary glands of the mucous membrane elsewhere. There is no evidence that they were the seat of morbid changes, peculiar to them in kind or degree. They were in some instances more hyperæmic than the other parts of the intestine, but more frequently, by their opacity and paleness, they contrasted with the dark color of the surrounding membrane. Both these conditions were occasionally found in adjacent parts of the same intestine. The appearances presented by these structures are thus described by Reinhardt and Leubuscher† : "The patches of Peyer were almost constantly altered and most remarkably so in the lower part of the ileum, immediately above the ileo-cœcal valve ; sometimes they were the seat of intense capillary hyperæmia, which either included the whole group or only a part. More commonly such hyperæmia did not exist, and the patches were remarkable for their whiteness. In many cases, we observed a more or less prominent swelling of the separate follicles, without thickening of the intervening mucous membrane. The patches had then a granular appearance, and the separate follicles could be

* Anatomie Pathologique du Cholera Morbus. Atlas, St. Petersburg, 1849.
† Op. Citat., p. 484.

c 2

distinguished. These had undergone the same changes as the solitary glands. More commonly there was found a moderate infiltration of the two structures of the patches (glands and mucous membrane), with a white solid exudation, which, as Böhm has particularly described, extended to different depths into the submucous cellular tissue. The patches then formed more or less prominent areas, of a round, elongated, or irregular form. The surface was in general smooth, but sometimes the mucous membrane was raised into folds and rounded masses. The exudation in all these cases was solid, and appeared under the microscope, as an amorphous finely-granular mass, becoming transparent under the action of acetic acid and alkalies." These authors also describe a reticulated appearance which they attribute in some cases, as Virchow* does in all, to a post-mortem imbibition of fluid into the cavity of the glands, leading to their rupture. They, however, express their belief that this explanation will not universally apply, and that occasionally such reticulation is the result of loss of substance and infiltration of the textures during life.

Briquet and Mignot†, in their report, write as follows:—" The patches of Peyer were observed in the valvular portion (jejunum), of the intestine, in 17 cases out of 32; of these 17, in 15 they were greyish, pale, and prominent, but to a less degree than those situated at the termination of the ileum; in the other two cases they were slightly reddened. In the non-valvular portion (ileum), in the same subjects, Peyer's patches were noted in 31 instances. In 20 they were grey and pale, in 8 reddened by the sanguinolent fluid in contact with them, or by slight injection. In 3 they were ulcerated." Of these latter, one had phthisis, one was attacked with cholera whilst laboring under typhoid fever, and the other had had fever six weeks previously, and died of cholera in the stage of convalescence."

M. Leudet gives the following table:—

Development of Peyer's Patches, in the Algide Stage.

In the inferior ⅓ of small intestine	5 cases.	
" " ¼	4	..
" " ⅕	3	
" " ⅙	2	
Near the valve	6	,
	——	
	20	

* Medicinische Reform, No. 10.   † Op. Citat., p. 405.

He also adds, " The patches of Peyer were white and prominent, but never ulcerated, and without any such affection of the submucous cellular tissue as occurs in typhoid fever. The mucous membrane often appeared thickened and soft, especially inferiorly, where it had an uneven granular aspect from enlarged and confluent follicles."

The lesions of the mucous membrane of the intestines in cholera, are thus described by Virchow (" Medicin. Reform," Nos. 10 and 12). His observations extended over 120 cases. " The changes in the intestines consist essentially in a uniform affection of the whole mucous membrane, and not of the intestinal glands. The solitary glands are indeed for the most part affected, and sometimes Peyer's likewise, but neither of them so constantly as the mucous membrane. As regards the bursting of the follicles of Peyer's patches, it would appear, that this is merely a post-mortem phenomenon, since it is not seen when the examination is made soon after death, and it may be produced artificially by laying the intestine in water. It depends upon an imbibition of fluid into the cavities of the follicles and a maceration of their walls. The changes in the mucous membrane are similar to those produced by the different gradations of catarrhal and diphtheritic inflammation. The latter begins with intense hyperæmia, which is quickly followed by extravasation into the tissue of the gut, and into its cavity (hence the bloody stools) ; subsequently there follows an exudation into the superficial layers of the mucous membrane, at first small in quantity and of a greyish white color, but becoming more opaque as it augments, and acquiring a yellowish tint by the imbibition of bile. Examined microscopically it appears as a granular amorphous deposit in the cellular tissue. The parts thus affected soon begin to undergo disorganization, leaving an eroded or superficially-ulcerated surface. The best examples of it were found in the lower part of the small intestine, sometimes extending from four to six feet." This observer states, that " the diphtheritic inflammation of the intestinal mucous membrane was not always equally frequent or equally extensive. It reached its greatest intensity (in the Berlin epidemic) in the first week of September (3rd–10th), then it almost entirely disappeared, and again towards the end of the epidemic showed itself in isolated spots, particularly affecting the large intestine."

Mesenteric Glands. In 34 examinations after death in the algide stage, the results of which are given in the tabulated report, in 23 the mesenteric glands are not named, in 5 they are stated to have been small, pale, and bloodless, in 3 small and reddish, from which it may be concluded that in 31 no obvious morbid changes existed, in the remaining three cases they are thus described : in one, " not enlarged, but congested and ecchymosed ;" in the second, " large, some of them containing pultaceous substance, not injected ;" and in the third, " large and white."

According to Virchow[*], " the mesenteric glands were always affected, for the cases where a change was not very obvious may be referred to special conditions.   The lesion consisted in a moderate hyperæmia, followed by an infiltration into the gland of a whitish granular exudation, which subsequently invaded its whole substance, giving it, on section, a whitish, homogeneous, smooth appearance, as Grüber remarks, like the milt of a herring.   This was quite characteristic, especially as the glands principally affected were those belonging to the duodenum.   In old persons, whose tissues in general are less susceptible of distension and swelling, and in all persons where the mesentery contained much fat, this appearance was less marked or altogether absent."

Reinhardt and Leubuscher[†] write as follows :—" The mesenteric glands appeared more or less swollen.   They were either of a reddish grey color, and rather acutely hyperæmic ; or more commonly pale or yellowish white.   The loss of color generally began at the periphery and extended inwards towards the centre.   In the glands entirely without color a microscopical examination discovered a large quantity of fine molecules, in addition to the normal and unchanged parenchyma —and lymph corpuscles."

Briquet and Mignot[‡] say no more than this : " the mesenteric glands, so far as we observed, always appeared white and without increase of size."

Pirogoff gives two plates (Tab. i. A. fig. 3 ; Tab. ii. fig. 2) exhibiting a remarkable enlargement of the mesenteric glands of the ileum.   In one they are pale, in the other greatly injected, the adjacent portion of the intestine being of a dark color from venous engorgement, and Peyer's patches and the solitary glands prominent.

Large intestine.   The large intestine was more rarely affected with hyperæmia and ecchymosis than the small intestine. In many instances it presented nothing abnormal beyond a greater distinctness of the solitary glands.   The following table gives the result of 34 cases.

* Med. Ref., No. 10.   † Op. Citat., p. 491.   ‡ Op. Citat., p. 399.

No traces of hyperæmia 24
Slight traces 4
Slight traces with spots of ecchymosis . . . 3
Intense venous engorgement of cœcum . . 3

The mucous membrane was often rather pulpy and thickened (œdematous), but much less so than in the jejunum or ileum. In one instance, where the acute symptoms had lasted 63 hours, and the patient died in asphyxia with partial reaction, there was, in the descending colon and rectum, extensive and irregular superficial ulceration with vascular injection of the edges, probably the result of diphtheritic exudation. In a second case, fatal in collapse at the beginning of the fourth day, there was slight granular exudation and patches of punctate injection in the transverse and descending colon; and superficial ulceration to a limited extent near the sigmoid flexure, leaving the solitary glands unaffected and spreading around them. In two others there were a few minute ulcers in the rectum.

The solitary glands. In only 4 out of 34 cases were the solitary glands prominent throughout the whole extent of the large intestine; in 11 others they were slightly enlarged about the cœcum and ascending colon. They were often translucent from distension of their cavities with serous fluid; sometimes this distension had been followed by rupture, producing an appearance of small rounded ulcerations.

After recording the morbid appearances in the small intestine, Reinhardt and Leubuscher * continue thus:—" The veins of the large intestine were commonly congested, not, however, equally so over the whole surface as in the ileum, but rather in isolated patches. The cœcum and rectum were the parts more particularly affected." They add (page 485), " In the majority of cases we found the solitary glands enlarged, but not so constantly, nor to so marked a degree as in the small intestine. They were round, more or less strongly prominent elevations, from the size of a millet seed to that of a hemp seed, sometimes surrounded by a circle of injected vessels, and very commonly marked at a point corresponding to their orifice, with a dark spot, which depended upon extravasated and altered blood. In certain cases the superficial layer of mucous membrane on the prominent part of the glands had exfoliated, producing a cup-shaped or lenticular de-

* Op. Citat., p. 480.

pression, but entire destruction of them in this stage was never observed."

Briquet and Mignot[*] report as follows: "The large intestine was the seat of general venous congestion in 9 cases (out of 32 examined), in only half of these was it very intense. In 4 it was limited to some points of the mucous membrane, and had the characters of inflammation. For the most part the mucous membrane was pale and very coarsely congested.

"In half the cases there was an abnormal prominence of the crypts (solitary glands). In 3 the mucous membrane was obviously softened.

"In no instance was there gangrene, or any appearance which in the least resembled such a change, although certain authors, and especially M. Bouillaud, mention that they have sometimes met with it in their dissections."

M. Leudet writes as follows: "The lesions of the large intestine were less frequent than those of the small intestine. The mucous membrane was generally pale, or, when reddened, it was in patches. The follicles were enlarged in 11 cases out of 38, and sometimes ulcerated."

The following table exhibits the general results of his examinations.

Color of the mucous membrane of the large intestine.

Universally pale	22 cases.
Uniform pale rose	2 ,,
Pale with rose patches	2 ,
Pale with violet patches	5 ,
Pale with black spots . . .	3 ,
Red with violet patches	1 ,,

Pirogoff mentions "a peculiar affection of the mucous membrane of the large intestine, principally of the descending colon, sigmoid flexure, and rectum;" illustrations of which are given in his fifth plate. It consists in a large extravasation of blood into the mucous membrane and submucous tissue, leading to gangrene. As the eschars separate during the period of reaction, the muscular coat is exposed, leaving irregular ulcerations. The morbid changes in these cases were remarkably rapid, and more frequent where diarrhœa of some days' standing had preceded the development of the algide stage.

* Op. Citat., p. 106.

Evacuations. The general appearance of the evacuations in cholera is well known.

Their reaction was alkaline or neutral.

The specific gravity of the clear fluid left after the subsidence of the flocculi was from 1006 to 1010; rarely higher than this.

No change, or only a slight opalescence, was produced by boiling.

The mean of six observations, the details of which are given by Dr. Parkes[*], is as follows:—

Water	.	.	.	.	987·95
Solids	.	.	.	.	12·05
					1000·

The solids consisted of—

Organic matter and insoluble salts (earthy phosphates)	3·9
Soluble salts (chlorides, phosphates, and sulphates of soda and potash)	8·1
	12·

The amount of organic matter varied with the stage of the disease, being at a minimum in the large effusions of the algide stage, and greatest as the symptoms of reaction set in.

Dr. Dundas Thomson[†] gives a table of three analyses of cholera evacuations, in which the quantity of the organic matter was much beyond the mean amount stated above, viz.—

	Sp. Grav.	Organic matter.	Salts.	Water.
Case D	1021	59·	8·	933·
,, E	1010	20·98	7·35	971·67
,, K	——	52·5	——	947·5

In case D the supernatant fluid, when exposed to a temperature of 212°, "coagulated into a mass in a manner corresponding with the serum of the blood, and yielded a similar odour; thus exhibiting the presence of a large amount of albumen." It was, however, very rare that the effused fluids carried off so large an amount of organic matter.

The alkalinity of the fluid, and probably also the physical condition of the albumen, allied more to albuminose, prevented its ready recognition by heat; yet that the principal part of the organic

* On the Intestinal Discharges in Cholera, London Journal of Medicine, 1849.
† Medico-Chir. Transact., vol. xxxiii. p. 88.

matters thrown out was albumen, or allied to it, is shown by the fact stated by Dr. Thomson that, " on evaporation in vacuo, a yellow residue was obtained, which, on being treated with water, yielded a solution coagulating on boiling, and by the addition of acids; and usually," he adds, " the fluids as evacuated, when allowed to settle, yielded by boiling, or, on the addition of an acid, distinct evidence of the presence of albumen."

Dr. Parkes [*] particularly noted the small amount of the so-called extractives, or incoagulable organic substances thrown out in cholera, a circumstance which seems to indicate a suspension of the proper excreting function of the mucous membrane during the algide stage. This observation is important as bearing upon the pathology of the disease. The following table, given by him, exhibits the amount of extractive matter, albumen, and salts in the cholera fluid.

Period of the disease in which the stool was passed.	Sp. Grav.	Albumen in 1000 parts.	Extractives in 1000 parts.	Soluble Salts in 1000 parts.	Total Solids in 1000 parts.
Diarrhœal period	1012·9	0·466	3·846	9·04	13·9
,, ,, ...	...	0·29	6·82	5·99	13·1
Early algide stage	1009·	2·4	1·27	10·98	14·65
Developed and intense algide stage....................	1009·5	1·18	·55	9·14	10·87
,, ,,	...	2·186		7·52	9·706
Developed and moderate algide stage	1008·3	0·27	2·33	8·33	10·83
,,	1005·8	3·2		5·827	8·947
Commencement of reaction	1014·	20·84		6·34	27·18
,, ,, ...	1008·91	1·48	6·055	9·055	16·62
Relapse	1017·83	0·855	17·355		18·21
,, ...	...	not weighable	4·589	3·881	8·47

He further adds, " As in the algide stage, the excretion of the extractives is arrested, so also in great measure is that of the earthy phosphates which are thrown out so largely by the healthy intestinal surface. In some cases there has been hardly a trace of the phosphate of lime; in others it has existed in diminished quantity. In no case has it nearly equalled the healthy standard or approached to the excessive increase which occurs in the stools of typhoid fever."

[*] On Intestinal Discharges, &c., London Journal of Medicine, p. 134.

Occasionally the cholera dejections became of a pink or rose tin when nitric acid was added in small quantity (Schmidt, Parkes), a result probably due to the presence of biliary matter.

Both Schmidt and Garrod agree upon the absence of urea from cholera fluid. According to the former, this is owing to its rapid decomposition into carbonate of ammonia, the presence of which often produces slight effervescence when nitric acid is added.

In one analysis very faint traces of uric acid were observed by Garrod, but in general no indication of its presence could be made out.

Three complete analyses of the soluble salts, taken from Dr. Parkes's paper, give the following results :—

	1st.	2nd.	3rd.	Mean.
Chlorides of Sodium .⎫ ,, Potassium⎭	5·188	⎰4·013⎱ ⎱ ·791⎰	2·038	4·31
Phosphate of Soda .	1·059	·326	1·80	1·061

Other Salts, with Car-⎫
  bonate and Sulphate⎬
  of Soda . . . .⎭
	2·893	3·20	1·602	2·565

	9·140	8·33	6·34	7·936

For comparison, we subjoin the following table of the proportions in which these soluble salts normally exist in the blood itself :—

	Blood.	Cholera Fluid.
Chlorides of Sodium and Potassium	5·95	4·31
Phosphate of Soda	·3	1·061
Carbonate and Sulphate, &c. . . .	1·68	2·565
	7·93	7·936

Microscopical appearances. The membranous shreds and loose flocculi examined by the microscope, presented the following appearances. They were homogeneous, translucent, and indistinctly striated, and contained :—

1st. Amorphous granular matter and larger granules (fibrinous) often very abundant.

2nd. Minute bodies having the general characters of nuclei.

3rd. Finely-granular cells (exudation cells?) Some of these were large.

4th. Occasionally a few scattered blood corpuscles, generally not in sufficient numbers to produce any tinge of colour, but when the cold stage was severe and prolonged, the quantity of blood was often large, and so intimately mixed with the masses of shreds and flocculi as to give the evacuations a remarkable appearance, especially when the amount of fluid was small.

5th. Columnar and scaly epithelium, rarely to any amount, and even generally not readily discoverable. On this point our investigations confirm the observations recorded by Dr. Parkes[*] in opposition to those of Böhm during the last epidemic, and whose accurate descriptions apply rather to the contents of the intestines after death, than to the evacuations during life.

6th. On evaporation by exposure to the air, a large number of crystals of chloride of sodium in cubes and octohedra, and occasionally also some crystals of urate of ammonia and urate of soda, and, when decomposition had commenced, prisms of triple phosphate.

Spleen.   The state of the spleen is noted in 23 cases fatal in the algide stage. Of these, in 3 it was of the natural size, in 18 it was small, or very small; namely, in 2 it weighed but two ounces, in 2 others two ounces and a half, and in 3 three ounces, &c. In most cases there was no obvious change in the tissue, beyond that arising from a want of blood, giving its capsule rather a wrinkled appearance, and enabling it to resist laceration, the texture being often described as pale, firm, and dry. Of the above 23 cases, in one the tissue was mottled by effusions of blood, and by dark red congested portions; and in one only is it stated that the white corpuscles were distinct.

Niemeyer[†] found the spleen small, flaccid, and bloodless in 19 out of 20 cases, the exception occurring in a person who had ague.

According to Reinhardt and Leubuscher[‡], "The spleen presented no constant change in respect to volume; sometimes, particularly in old persons, it was very small, but in the majority of cases it was normal in size. There were cases in which it was very notably increased. . . . . The capsule was sometimes, especially in children and young individuals, smooth and distended, but for the most part it was more or less wrinkled. The tissue was normal in color and consistence, the white corpuscles in most cases distinct. In one instance where the spleen was of very large size, they were equal to hemp-seeds, of a yellowish white color, and of such consistence as to admit of isolation from the surrounding splenic tissue.   . In those who

---

[*] Op. Cit., p. 150.   [†] Medicin. Reform, No. 19.   [‡] Op. Cit., p. 495.

died in the cold stage, it was not rare to find spots of hyperæmia and solid exudation, of a reddish brown, or blueish red color from extravasated blood. These masses (hæmorrhagic infarctions) were of different sizes, from a hazel nut upwards. Under the microscope they presented amorphous fibrin and blood corpuscles. . . . . In the later stages of the disease these infarctions were either in the condition here described, or were more or less changed as follows: they commonly retained their consistence, but lost their color, becoming yellowish red or yellow. Not rarely the exuded matters, after losing their color, softened, to a variable extent, into a greasy puriform mass from a detritus of broken up fibrin and blood corpuscles. In one instance these nodulated masses were very firm, compact, dry, and obviously contracted, the surface of the spleen over them being drawn in."

Briquet and Mignot* report as follows :—" The spleen is mentioned in 25 of our observations ;—seven times we noted a slight ramollissement, and six times it seemed voluminous, and perhaps hypertrophied. In the other cases there was on the contrary a state of atrophy (?) the organ being shrivelled like the surface of a fruit when the juices have evaporated. The consistence of the splenic tissue was increased ; it had a tint of lighter red disposed in patches of irregular size upon a violet ground. In one subject there were spots of apoplexy."

Rüle† found enlargement of the spleen only twice in 16 postmortem examinations.

Leudet says,—" The spleen was generally small, the mean length was 123 centimetres (4·8 inches), the breadth 73 millimetres (2·8 inches), and the thickness 13 millimetres (½ inch). I generally found the tissue firm, exsanguine, and tough. Sometimes the corpuscles of Malpighi were apparent. In only one case was there interstitial apoplexy."

In a report of 70 cases examined by Virchow‡ he states that he arrived at no definite results as to the morbid changes in the spleen. He found acute enlargement of this organ in so many instances, and under such variable circumstances, that he could not refer it to mere accident. During life he had repeatedly, by percussion, been able to determine that it was decidedly enlarged ; and in some cases patients had complained of pain in the left side. In old persons no enlarge-

* Op. Cit., p. 410.   † Medicin. Reform, No. 15.
‡ Ibid., No. 10.

ment was ever observed; but in almost all other cases the spleen was so flaccid and shrivelled that one was obliged to admit a previous enlargement, or rather so recent and rapid a reduction of volume, that the capsule had not yet accommodated itself. The change of color in the tissue, from altered blood, led him to infer a previous hyperæmia.

Liver. After death, in the algide stage, the liver was generally diminished in bulk, the tissue flaccid, and the capsule finely wrinkled. The larger veins, both the hepatic and the portal, but especially the latter, were often full of dark viscid blood. The lobular appearance of the secreting structure was indistinct, and the whole tissue of rather a lighter red than usual. Exceptions were not, however, wanting to this general rule; thus in a male, æt. 23, who died in collapse, after severe symptoms of 21 hours' duration, the liver was of the natural size, but very full of blood; its structure distinct, firm, and of a dark color. In another case, a girl aged 8, who died very rapidly, the whole duration of the attack not being more than nine hours, "the hepatic tissue was dark on section, with much blood in the large vessels, especially in the hepatic veins. Injection around some of the lobules, apparently portal." In a third case, a male aged 34, who died after about 20 hours of acute symptoms, the liver is reported to have been of natural size and structure, with some dark parts in which the centres of the lobules were black with blood.

The secreting structure on a microscopical examination presented nothing abnormal.

Briquet and Mignot[*] report as follows :—"In general the parenchyma of the liver appeared reduced, rather than increased in volume. On section but a very small quantity of blood escaped from the tissue; this chiefly depended upon its coagulation and density. In 8 cases out of 32, a certain degree of venous congestion was obvious, from the violet tint of the hepatic tissue."

According to Reinhardt and Leubuscher[†], "The liver was, in the first stage of the disease, devoid of blood. . . . . The consistence of the parenchyma was normal. It was pale yellow, or yellowish brown; and the so-called red substance either not at all, or only faintly visible. In the latter stages of the disease this became again evident, and the liver was dark and more full of blood than usual."

Niemeyer[‡] states, as the result of 20 post-mortem examinations,

* Op. Cit., p. 409.   † Op. Cit., p. 493.
‡ Medicin. Reform, No. 19.

the greater number of the subjects being young and strong soldiers, " that the liver on section appeared bloodless ; the larger vessels contained thick and dark blood. The gall bladder was always distended, and contained mostly dark bile of variable consistence."

Leudet writes thus,—" The liver presented no change of volume, 12 times in 26 its color was very deep, the texture uniform, without the appearance of yellow granulations (yellow substance of lobules) ; capillary congestion was very rare. I found in one case only a little blood under Glisson's capsule. The biliary vessels were empty."

Virchow * says, " The liver was but little altered ; it was for the most part pale and flabby. Only the large vessels contained blood. Not rarely the volume of the organ appeared to be diminished. The parenchyma was deeply colored with bile."

Gall Bladder. The gall bladder was usually distended with dark bile, generally viscid, but sometimes more watery than natural. In most cases, the gall ducts were not obviously affected. The mucous membrane of the gall bladder and ducts was healthy, except in some rare cases, where it was the seat of morbid changes, similar to those occurring in the intestinal mucous membrane. For example, in one case occurring under our observation, a male, æt. 41, who died in collapse, after 22 hours of acute symptoms, " the gall bladder was distended to three times the natural size. It contained four ounces of semi-transparent, slimy, pale orange-colored fluid, sp. grav. 1007, rendered turbid by boiling, and by nitric acid. It contained cylindrical epithelium, free nuclei, and blood discs. The ducts were full of thin, colorless, mucous fluid." In the following section on the morbid appearances found in the secondary fever, it will be seen that the gall bladder and ducts were occasionally the seat of diphtheritic exudation, like that described above as occurring on the intestinal mucous membrane.

According to Briquet and Mignot †, " The gall bladder was for the most part distended with a large quantity of bile, the excreting ducts being, however, always free. In one case, the lining membrane of the gall bladder was inflamed (?) and covered by a yellow purulent (?) fluid. The color of the bile was variable, its density apparently increased."

Reinhardt and Leubuscher ‡ state, that " with rare exceptions, in patients who died during the cold stage, the gall-bladder was distended

* Med. Ref., No. 12.　　　† Op. Cit., p. 410.　　　‡ Op. Cit., p. 493.

with bile, and by gentle pressure the contents could easily be made
to flow into the intestine. The bile was in general watery and
brownish, but in some cases, where the cold stage had been of long
duration, it was greenish."

Kidneys.   The kidneys were of the natural size, their surface was
mottled by arborescent venous injection, and, on section,
the same venous hyperæmia gave a dark color to the cones. The
secreting structure rarely presented any obvious morbid change.
In one case, that of a girl æt. 8, who died very rapidly, the whole
duration of the attack not being more than nine hours, the kidneys
were of a reddish brown color, and the larger vessels full of
blood. On a microscopical examination, the epithelium of the
tubules was for the most part normal in form, but exceedingly
granular. At different points there were irregular masses, consisting of yellowish granules, and transparent oval globules (exudation
cells and nuclei ?).

The contents of the pelves were mostly turbid with exfoliated
epithelium and free nuclei. The mucous membrane was generally
pale, but in some instances it presented patches of venous injection.

The urinary bladder was empty, or contained but a small quantity
of turbid fluid like that in the pelves of the kidneys, coagulable by
heat. The mucous membrane was occasionally hyperæmic.

According to Reinhardt and Leubuscher *, " The kidneys had frequently, even in the first stage of the disease, undergone a change.
They were not much increased in volume. The vessels, especially
the veins, were slightly hyperæmic, but there was never the same
extent of capillary engorgement as in the latter stages. Even in
those who died in the asphyctic (algide) stage, we not rarely found
portions of the secreting structure whitish or yellowish white from
an exudation into the tissue. This change, as Virchow has proved,
began at the apices of the pyramids, and extended thence towards
their bases. The papillæ, and a greater or smaller section of the pyramids, were compact and of a whitish color. Before the infiltration
had become extensive, similar changes usually began in the cortical
portion, sometimes near the surface, but more commonly at the
bases of the pyramids, thus surrounding them with a layer of a grey
or whitish yellow color. The exudation did not follow a continuous
course from the apices of the papillæ to the periphery of the organ,
but took place simultaneously in the pyramids and in the cortical

* Op. Cit., p. 496.

substance. The other parts of the parenchyma were of the natural color, but had commonly rather a brighter tint. As the disease advanced, the infiltration of the renal structures became more extensive, and particularly affected the cortical substance, which was increased in thickness, of a light grey color, and easily lacerable. On stripping off the capsule the surface was left uneven and granular. . . . . The enlargement of the kidneys accompanying these changes was variable and occasionally very remarkable. . . . . The epithelial cells of the uriniferous tubes in the discolored parts, adhered more firmly together than in their normal state. . . . . They were also more opaque than natural, in part from an increased quantity of granular matter in them, and in part from a finely-granular exudation upon the epithelial surface. In certain cases, even where the patients had died very rapidly, but more frequently if the cold stage had been prolonged, we found solid exudation into the tubes, particularly at the apices of the pyramids. This was sometimes in the form of very long fibrinous cylinders, or cylindrical granular fragments, containing epithelial cells and blood corpuscles, or tinged by the coloring matter of the blood. These appearances were more extensive and more distinct in those who died of typhoid symptoms in the latter stages. In the further course of the disease a deposit of fat in the secreting cells was very frequent. In the early stages, the finely granular matter expressed from the uriniferous tubes was entirely soluble in (weak) acids and alkalies, and the outline of the cell was distinct ; but in the latter stages, there were numerous dark fat granules insoluble in these reagents, but soluble in æther. They obscured the outline of the cell, and, in extreme cases, the enlarged and distended uriniferous tubules became opaque from their aggregation. The parts in which this infiltration of fat had proceeded to the greatest extent were obvious to the naked eye, by their yellow color. The fatty matter was originally contained in the secreting cells (at least for the most part), ... but when the affection of the kidney had continued for any length of time, the cells burst, and their contents were thrown free into the cavity of the tubules." These authors add that in one case, fatal in the cold stage, and in several in the typhoid stage, or with complications after reaction, they found limited hæmorrhagic infarctions of the cortical structure.

Although these remarks are not exclusively applicable to the changes occurring in the algide stage, yet it seemed best to give the report of these authors as it stands in their own words, referring to it again when enumerating the conditions found in the latter periods of the disease.

Briquet and Mignot[*] report as follows:—" We examined with much attention the lesions of this system of organs (the urinary) in 35 cases. In 8, we noted a state of hyperæmia common to the two structures (the cortical and tubular). In these cases the kidneys were increased in volume, of a violet-red tint, and on section gave out a considerable quantity of blood. There were 19 in which the hyperæmia and augmentation of volume particularly affected the tubular substance, the apices of the pyramids being the points at which the redness was most marked. This almost constant hyperæmia of the mamillary portion was many times obscured by opaque white lines running in the course of the tubuli uriniferi from the apices of the cones into the cortical substance—an appearance due to an accumulation of a peculiar turbid and dense fluid in the tubes of Bellini (tubuli uriniferi of the cones). On pressing the mamillary processes between the fingers, these lines disappeared, and the red color became distinct. . . . . There were also other spots of an ochrey or yellowish color, which did not disappear on pressure; they presented the appearance of isolated points, or radiating lines, spreading out upon the surface, and throughout the thickness of the tubular substance. In one case all the cones would be affected, in another only a few of them. . . . . Our friend, Dr. Boulland, an expert microscopist, who at our request examined this substance, found it to consist of crystals of uric acid, and a chemical analysis led us to the same conclusion. . . . . We observed these deposits in the tubuli uriniferi in 13 out of 35 cases.

" The pelves usually presented well-marked venous congestion."

Virchow[†] states, as the result of 120 post-mortem examinations, that he almost constantly found in the urinary passages (including the pelves of the kidneys and the urinary bladder) the results of recent catarrhal irritation with increased epithelial exfoliation. "The kidneys were sometimes in a state of venous congestion, with morbid changes passing from the papillæ outwards. These changes were as follows: first, hyperæmia of the papillæ, extending by degrees into the pyramids; and, secondly, the parts thus affected gradually lost their colour and acquired a whitish homogeneous appearance. The microscope showed that this arose from a granular exudation into the uriniferous tubes."

Lendet writes as follows:—" In general the kidneys had undergone no obvious change of volume. Yet even in the algide stage I often observed an increased thickness of the cortical substance, with some slight punctate redness, accompanied with delicate yellow striæ following the course of the uriniferous tubules in the pyramids of Malpighi. In the subsequent stages the kidneys were often swollen; this change, if not the commencement of Bright's disease, was certainly closely allied to it,—a consideration which leads me to speak of the urine. I have often found it to contain albumen, and more often in the algide stage than during reaction; at the same time it was rather deep in colour, a circumstance which may perhaps induce us to refer the albumen it contained to the congested state of the kidneys. The pathological anatomy of these organs in cholera is still, in my opinion, a subject for discussion."

The urinary passages, as we have mentioned above, were, in some cases, the seat of morbid changes similar to those observed in the intestine; and this observation is confirmed by the continental pathologists. Thus, Reinhardt and Leubuscher * report as follows:— " The urinary passages were commonly, even at the beginning of the attack, the seat of a more or less extensive catarrhal affection. The pelves of the kidneys often exhibited hyperæmia, although only to a moderate extent, and commonly contained a yellow puriform matter, composed of epithelium, mucus, and pus (?). The catarrhal condition of the mucous membrane covering the apices of the cones led to the hyperæmia and infiltration of the tubuli of the subjacent parenchyma, the exudation process extending from the mucous surface to a certain distance into the glandular tissue. The cortical portion, during the further course of the disease, was in itself the seat of lesions, independent of the origin here indicated. The ureters also contained puriform fluid, consisting principally of exfoliated epithelium, in larger quantity than was normal.

" The urinary bladder was, in the cold stage, almost constantly contracted, and without urine; sometimes hyperæmic, especially about the neck, and covered with a layer of exfoliated epithelium. This catarrhal condition not rarely acquired a greater intensity in the latter stages of the disease."

According to Briquet and Mignot †, " In the algide stage the bladder was, for the most part, contracted and empty; twice only it contained an abundant turbid fluid. In 2 cases the mucous

* Op. Cit., p. 418. † Op. Cit., p. 501.

membrane was much injected, and covered by a yellowish puriform
mucus, presenting the appearance of the first stage of cystitis (?).
In 8 instances there was general venous congestion, and in 6 others
this condition existed only at the posterior part."

Female Sexual Organs.   The state of the female sexual organs is not named
in any of the reports we have received. The appear-
ances they occasionally presented are, however, worthy of attention,
and have been carefully noted by the Berlin pathologists. Thus
Reinhardt and Leubuscher [*] state that " the genital organs of the
female were, next to the intestines and the kidneys, the parts which
had most commonly undergone structural change. . . . . In the cold
stage the uterus exhibited the following appearances: its contents
were mostly sanguineous, sometimes mucus tinged with blood, and
sometimes blood only, either fluid or coagulated. The capillaries
and larger vessels of the mucous membrane were very frequently
hyperæmic. The hyperæmia was sometimes universal, but more
frequently, when intense, it was limited to certain parts, namely, the
fundus, the upper part of the body, and the neck, from the os exter-
num to the middle. In these parts, there were spots of ecchymosis,
varying from the size of a pin's head to a hemp-seed, but often of
much greater extent. . . . . The extravasation was generally confined to the mucous membrane, but not rarely the subjacent parenchyma of the uterus was infiltrated, the infiltration extending through
the whole tissue to the serous membrane. . . . . Several times,
under the normal or slightly hyperæmic mucous membrane, there
was extravasation of blood into the subjacent tissue. . . . . When
the mucous membrane was acutely hyperæmic, its tissue was always
somewhat swollen and thickened, although never to any great extent,
and rarely as loose and protuberant as at the menstrual period.
When this happened, the whole organ was congested, and a large
flattened Graafian follicle, full of blood, was found in the ovary;
this was not met with in the other cases of hyperæmia and extravasation occurring in the uterus.

" In those who died in the typhoid stage, the uterus was sometimes
in the state above described, or, more commonly, these lesions had
progressed, the mucous membrane being universally hyperæmic, with
extravasations of blood of variable extent, or still more commonly
the whole organ was uniformly infiltrated with blood. Occasionally
the superficial layer of the mucous membrane was of a dirty yellowish-

* Op. Cit., p. 503.

green color, as observed in other mucous membranes at the beginning of diphtheritic exudation; but we never saw in the uterus extensive diphtheritic infiltration into the deeper parts of its tissue."

These authors also remark upon the occurrence of sanguineous discharges from the uterus in cholera. Such discharges were rare in the first stage of the disease, but during reaction, and particularly in the typhoid stage, they were not uncommon, lasting from two to nine days. They occurred under conditions of the system, and at such ages, as to show clearly that they were hæmorrhagic, and not due to the menstrual function, since not unfrequently persons labouring under amenorrhœa, and others over 60 years of age, were thus affected. The amount of discharge was never very great.

" In those who died in the algide stage, it was not rare to find more or less extensive hyperæmia of the mucous membrane of the vagina, with generally some amount of extravasation into the mucous and submucous tissues. The seat of these changes was generally the deeper parts of the vagina, near the os uteri, which was also sometimes implicated; commonly, also, the entrance of the vagina, and the labia, &c. During the further course of the disease, the hyperæmia of these parts increased in intensity, and was followed, as in the intestine, by diphtheritic exudation. The mucous membrane and subjacent tissue became more or less extensively infiltrated with a yellowish or yellowish-grey exudation, which subsequently disintegrated, and left an uneven surface, which, so soon as all the exudation was thrown off, had the ordinary appearance of a common ulcer of the mucous membrane. This last condition was rare. The diphtheritic inflammation commonly began in the neighbourhood of the os uteri, or even upon it, and afterwards in the other parts of the vagina. It was in the former, therefore, that it had proceeded furthest. In one case extensive diphtheritic inflammation was observed at the entrance of the vagina, whilst there was none near the orifice of the uterus. A fluor albus, of a thin purulent kind, commonly attended these changes in the vagina. Apart from any menstrual condition, even in the cold stage, the ovaries were often hyperæmic in different degrees, with hæmorrhage into the tissue and into the Graafian follicles, the peritoneal covering being also ecchymosed. In the latter stages of the disease these extravasations had in some cases, undergone changes of color. No other morbid changes were observed in the ovary."

" Nothing abnormal was observed in the male organs of generation."

Virchow * states that, according to his observations, "the genital organs presented no constant morbid condition. In women there was very commonly a menstrual (?) condition of the ovaries, and of the lining membrane of the uterus; in the ovaries, recently-flattened follicles with effusion of blood; and in the uterus, great swelling and hyperæmia of the mucous membrane with enlargement of the uterine glands; but, apart from the menstrual period, it was not rare to find numerous extravasations under the peritoneal covering of the ovaries, giving them a mottled and purple aspect."

M. Leudet informs us that he found nothing abnormal in the genito-urinary organs. The uterus sometimes contained recent coagula, but it was doubtful whether they were to be referred to hæmorrhages of a morbid character.

Lungs.   In the majority of cases fatal in the algide stage, no other morbid change existed than engorgement of the lower and posterior parts of the lungs with dark blood. In some instances this was so complete as to cause portions of the pulmonary tissue to sink in water. The anterior and superior parts were drier than natural. In only one case reported to us was there any degree of œdema. In certain cases the pulmonary tissue throughout was full of dark blood.

The bronchial tubes were normal in appearance, or their mucous membrane was congested. They contained a small amount of frothy serum, sometimes tinged with blood.

The pleura was healthy, or sometimes covered with a trace of a slimy albuminous secretion, as on the peritoneum.

According to Reinhardt and Leubuscher†, "In those who died in an early stage, the lungs were found for the most part much contracted. On the pleura pulmonalis, and also on the pleura costalis, there were commonly small ecchymoses and extravasations; in some cases, these were extensive. The pulmonary tissue was in general dry and anæmic, especially in the upper lobes; on section, a small quantity of blood oozed from the larger veins. The lower lobes were in general full of dark blood. Occasionally, in old persons, the pulmonary tissue was much inflated. In 2 instances well marked interlobular emphysema was observed, a condition also noticed by Virchow. When the cold stage had been unusually prolonged, œdema of the lower lobes sometimes occurred. In one case fatal in asphyxia, there were numerous small hæmorrhagic exudations into the parenchyma.

* Med. Reform, No. 12.   † Op. Citat., p. 506.

" On removing the sternum," says Virchow[*], " the lungs in general collapsed to the spine, except when there existed bronchial catarrh or œdema. The lower lobes were for the most part much congested. In 7 cases (of 120) there was rupture of the air passages, giving rise to interlobular emphysema, which, in 2, extended to the mediastinum and under the diaphragmatic pleura. These patients had all suffered from severe dyspnœa. On the pleura pulmonalis there were commonly small extravasations of blood, and almost constantly slight albuminous exudation."

Briquet and Mignot[†] state that they found " the lungs in general flaccid. On opening the thorax, they were contracted to the spine. The anterior parts were in all cases free from engorgement. In two there was serous infiltration, accompanied by extreme congestion of the posterior parts. The pulmonary tissue had sometimes a bright red color, but on section no vascular injection was obvious, and only a few drops of blood escaped. This almost constant state of anæmia was very striking when contrasted with the hyperæmia of the other principal viscera. The posterior parts were, however, frequently the seat of a certain degree of engorgement; this was noted in 16 cases, but in only 6 was it well marked. . . . . In 2 instances some spots of apoplexy were found of the size of a hazel-nut."

" The injection of the pleuræ was not so distinct as that of the peritoneum, nevertheless it was sufficiently apparent on those parts which cover the diaphragm and the ribs. On the pleura pulmonalis there were sometimes spots of ecchymosis, unaccompanied by vascular arborescence. In general the serous membrane was dry; in 2 instances only did the pleural cavity contain a drachm or two of serum."

" The bronchi had the aspect of the adjacent portion of the lung tissue."

Leudet writes as follows :—" The lungs were commonly healthy; in 2 instances there was pulmonary apoplexy; frequently hypostatic congestion. . . . . Larynx healthy. . . . . Bronchi congested."

Pericardium, Heart, &c.   In the cases reported to us, the pericardium generally contained a small quantity of serum varying from a drachm, to half an ounce, or an ounce. The color of the fluid was mostly a pale straw, or citron, but in some instances it was decidedly sanguinolent. On the adherent pericardium, about the base of the heart, small ecchymoses were not infrequent.

* Med. Reform, No. 12.   † Op. Citat., p. 415.

The endocardium was stained in 2 instances. This probably depended upon an imbibition of the coloring matter of the blood post mortem. In one of these cases, fatal in the cold stage with asphyxia, this membrane was found of a deep purple color; the examination was made very early after death, and the body was still warm. In the other case two or three spots of ecchymosis were found on the mitral valve, which was thickened and opaque from old disease.

Briquet and Mignot [*] observed venous injection of the pericardium similar to that existing in the other serous membranes. According to their observation, " the pericardium contained serous effusion more frequently than the pleura or the peritoneum ; very commonly a drachm or two of a slightly-viscid fluid, of a citron color, could be collected. In one case the effusion was turbid and sanguinolent with a flocculent fibrinous deposit." . . . .

In 12 cases the muscular tissue of the heart broke down under slight pressure. In 10 others it was apparently softened, and in 5 it was in that pathological condition designated by the term *chairs cuites* (sodden ?). The color of the tissue was altered in a corresponding degree, in 16 cases; instead of the redness, which it presents in a state of health, it was of a light yellowish brown color (*coloration feuille-morte*). In the others, although the color was normal, its brightness was diminished.

According to Virchow [†], " The pericardium, when overlapped by the inflated lungs, had become dry, but otherwise it commonly contained a small quantity of concentrated albuminous fluid, occasionally acid. In the majority of cases there were numerous extravasations of blood on the close pericardium about the base of the left ventricle.

" The muscular tissue of the heart, like the voluntary muscles (?), was pale, of a dull red, strongly contracted, and with well-marked rigor mortis. The muscular fibres under the microscope were colorless, but not otherwise changed.

" Into the cellular tissue beneath the endocardium of the left ventricle, near the aortic valves, there were in many cases superficial ecchymoses."

Reinhardt and Leubuscher [‡] write as follows:—" In those who died asphyxic (in the algide stage), the heart presented the following appearances :—The pericardium contained but a small quantity of serous fluid. There were commonly small ecchymoses in the

* Op. Citat., p. 417.   † Med. Ref., No. 12.   ‡ Op. Citat., p. 508.

adherent layer, especially at the posterior part of the base of the left ventricle. The muscular substance was firm, well contracted, and of a dull red color. There were small ecchymoses on the endocardium, in some cases. The right auricle, and ventricle, were distended with blood. The left contained, in proportion, but a small quantity.

Blood. The physical condition of the blood in the cavities of the heart and large vessels varied with respect to the degree and mode of coagulation, but most observers admit, that it was more commonly dark and fluid, or less coagulable than in other diseases. Of the cases fatal in collapse, which are tabulated and affixed to this report, the state of the blood is noted in 36: in 11 it was dark and fluid: in 5 fluid, with some imperfect fibrinous clots: in 11 it formed soft coagula: in 8 there were dark coagula and fibrinous clots. In nearly half the cases, therefore, the blood was fluid, either entirely so, or with but a few masses of fibrin. In less than one-fourth of the cases did the coagulation approach the normal condition. This nearly accords with the observation made by Dr. Parkes [*] upon his Indian cases; thus in 34 cases reported upon by him, the results were as follows:—" In 12 cases there were large polypi or fibrinous coagula in the right cavities of the heart; and in the majority of these, there were smaller coagula in the left auricle, and more infrequently in the left ventricle. In 7 cases there were small, loose, and generally dark coagula on the right side only. In 7 cases there were no coagula in any of the cavities of the heart, but the blood from the right side coagulated with greater or less firmness on removal. In 8 cases there were no clots in the heart or elsewhere, and the blood taken from the different parts remained absolutely incoagulable when removed from the body; in other words, in a little less than a quarter of the whole number of cases, the presence of fibrin in the blood was not indicated by coagulation either in or out of the body. In some cases blood from one part coagulated when it did not from another. I have seen it coagulate from the jugular veins when it did not from the pulmonary artery."

Dr. Gairdner [†], on the contrary, in his summary of the morbid appearances, states that " the blood is much less affected in its physical characters than is usually supposed to be the case. Its coagulation within the vessels takes place much as in other diseases. In the majority of instances firm clots are found within the heart, more or

[*] Researches into the Pathology and Treatment of the Asiatic Cholera, p. 31.
[†] Monthly Journal of Medical Science, May, 1849.

less completely decolorised, and the serum, or non-coagulated portion, contains the greater part of the blood corpuscles. The color of
the blood presents nothing unusual, the epithets 'dark' and 'venous'
being in no degree more applicable to cholera blood after death than
to that of every ordinary form of fatal disease."

Notwithstanding this excellent authority, the facts above quoted
are sufficient to prove, that, in a large number of cases, the coagulable
property of the blood was lessened, to which it must be added, that
the blood drawn during life in the cold stage was notoriously viscid
and tar-like, a change, as will hereafter be seen, depending upon a loss
of its water, and imperfect oxidation arising out of venous retardation.

According to Virchow [*], "The heart, especially the right, was always
distended with dark blood. When death had been rapid, the blood
was fluid as in other cases, but when not, it formed a loose coagulum like a thick syrup of whortleberries. In these cases there were
always more or less fibrinous coagula extending from the right ventricle into the pulmonary artery, and from the left ventricle into the
aorta. There was constantly a great increase of the colorless corpuscles, forming, on the under surface of the fibrinous coagula, a smooth,
granular, or mulberry-like layer of considerable thickness, in which
they were so abundant, that the largest part of the coagulum was
opaque, whitish, and often like coagulated pus.

" The change in the red corpuscles was too trifling to make evident
any trace of 'blood disintegration' (*blutserstsung*). Their anatomical appearance also showed no important loss of water. With respect to the distribution of the blood, it was obviously accumulated in
the veins and their ultimate ramifications, whilst the arteries and capillaries were empty. The venous hyperæmia of the small intestines,
contrasted with the paleness of the stomach and large intestines, was
remarkable, and not to be explained on mechanical principles. In the
hyperæmic villi the injection was shown by the microscope to be
always in the veins."

Reinhardt and Leubuscher [†] observe that " the blood contained in
the cavities of the heart was, in the majority of cases, coagulated into
a dark homogeneous mass, with fibrinous coagula extending into the
large vessels. Virchow's statement, that these coagula contained a
large number of colorless corpuscles, was confirmed by our own observations. The large venous trunks, and the veins of individual
organs, were full of blood, whilst the arteries and capillaries were

* Med. Ref., No. 12.   † Op. Cit., p. 509.

for the most part empty. This fulness of the veins was more marked in cases where death followed quickly upon the commencement of reaction after the cold stage."

The state of the blood in the cavities of the heart, venæ cavæ, aorta, and pulmonary artery was carefully noted by Briquet and Mignot : " In 23 cases the blood contained in these cavities presented a considerable quantity of fibrin, either forming pale cylindrical masses or enveloping dark coagula. The right side of the heart and pulmonary artery were the principal seats of these depôts of fibrin, which were sometimes considerable, interlacing with the chordæ tendineæ, and occasionally extending even to the subclavian veins and to the ultimate divisions of the pulmonary artery. In 12 instances, the blood was dark and loosely clotted, and in this state ordinarily combined with the fibrin, which also formed a pale layer over it. In 14, the blood was partly or entirely liquid. In 6 it was grumous and red as in typhus fever (fièvre typhoide)."

With respect to the chemical constitution of the blood, we were unable to institute any new series of observations, as the disease rapidly subsided after the appointment of this sub-committee. The subject was, however, elaborately investigated by Dr. Carl Schmidt [*] and by Dr. Garrod [†]. Schmidt's work is valuable, not only for its contents, but as being a model for similar investigations in a future epidemic. The following are the conclusions arrived at by these two observers.

According to Schmidt, the effect of the abnormal transudation of fluid from the capillaries of the intestine in cholera, upon the remainder of the circulating fluid may be thus summed up.

First.—The density of the blood, and of its morphological elements (blood cells and intercellular fluid), is increased in proportion to the duration of the process of exudation from the intestinal capillaries. It reaches its maximum in 36 hours (III.), and then falls again as water is reabsorbed (I.).

* Characteristik des Epidemischen Cholera, Leipzic, 1850.
† London Journal of Medicine, May, 1849.

		Sex.	Age.	Date of blood-letting.	Sp. Grav., ... in ..., ... = 1.			
					Duration of transudation.	Circulating blood.	Blood cells.	Inter-cellular fluid.
Normal ... (Contemporary.)	I.)	Male	25	14/2 Nov.	0	1·0599	1·0666	1·0512
Cholera . {	VII.)	—	23	16/4 Oct.*	4 hours	1·0728	1·1025	1·0519
	II.)	—	45	22/10 Aug.	7 „	1·0670	1·0055	1·0551
	VI.)	—	71	15/3 Sept.†	9 „	1·0712	1·1027	1·0471
Normal ... (Contemporary.)	II.)	Female	30	6 Oct. / 24 Sept.	0	1·0563	1·0666	1·0209
Cholera . {	V.)	—	20	13/1 Sept.	18 hours	1·0609	1·0961	1·0222
	III.)	—	20	24/12 Aug.	36 „	1·0656	1·0913	1·0248
	I.)	—	35	22/10 Aug.	48 „	1·0601	1·0927	1·0298

Second.—The solids of the blood and of its morphological elements, left after evaporation at 248° Fahr., are relatively increased in a marked degree, according to the time from the commencement of the exudation of the saline fluid from the intestinal capillaries. They reach, after about 36 hours, nearly one-half more than the normal proportion (III.), and afterwards sink as fluid is again absorbed.

		Sex.	Age.	Date of blood-letting.	Solids per 1000 parts of water.			
					Duration of transudation.	Circulating blood.	Blood cells.	Inter-cellular fluid.
Normal ... (Contemporary.)	I.)	Male	25	14/2 Nov.	0	267·89	467·07	109·24
Cholera . {	VII.)	—	23	16/4 Oct.*	4 hours	338·13	547·59	162·69
	II.)	—	45	22/10 Aug.	7 „	314·24	501·94	144·55
	VI.)	—	71	15/3 Sept.†	9 „	341·77	569·29	163·39
Normal ... (Contemporary.)	II.)	Female	30	6 Oct. / 24 Sept.	0	212·79	453·73	93·79
Cholera : {	V.)	—	20	13/1 Sept.	18 hours	281·09	532·24	121·79
	III.)	—	20	24/12 Aug.	36 „	317·15	501·17	134·69
	I.)	—	35	22/10 Aug.	48 „	241·34	480·98	115·79

* Previous diarrhœa.   † Relapse.

Third.—This increase relates only to the organic constituents (albuminates) of the blood and of its morphological elements, and not to the inorganic salts, the absolute quantity of which, although, indeed, increased directly after the onset of severe symptoms, appears to be subsequently diminished.

The degree of concentration of the organic constituents, resulting from the exudation of the saline fluid from the intestinal capillaries, regularly rises according to the interval from the beginning of the attack, and reaches the highest point 36 hours from the onset, after which, even in fatal cases, a re-absorption of fluid occurs (III., I.) The increase of the inorganic salts at the beginning of the disease, owing to the large amount of fluid poured out, reaches its maximum after four hours; they afterwards, within a few hours, fall to the normal quantity; after 18 hours, sink much below it; and after 36 or 48 hours, are still further diminished, according to the time which has elapsed (II., V., III., I.)

		Sex.		Date of blood-letting.	Duration of transudation.	Per 1000 grains of water.					
						Organic substances.			Inorganic substances.		
						Circulating blood.	Blood cells.	Intercellular fluid.	Circulating blood.	Blood cells.	Intercellular fluid.
normal..	L.)	Male	25	14/2 Nov.	0	257·90	456·39	99·81	9·99	10·68	9·43
cholera {	VII.)	—	23	16/4 Oct.*	4 hours	325·68	534·30	153·29	12·45	13·29	9·34
	II.)	—	45	22/10 Aug.	7 „	305·30	492·65	135·95	8·94	9·29	8·61
	VL.)	—	71	15/3 Sept.†	9 „	331·09	575·82	153·40	10·68	13·47	8·99
normal...	II.)	Female	30	6 Oct. ‒‒‒‒ 24 Sept.	0	202·34	440·71	84·61	10·45	13·02	9·18
cholera {	V.)	—	20	13/1 Sept.	18 hours	269·46	522·14	113·42	9·15	10·10	8·55
	III.)	—	20	24/12 Aug.	36 „	307·95	491·30	126·33	9·20	9·87	8·55
	L.)	—	35	22/10 Aug.	48 „	233·53	472·71	108·51	7·81	8·27	7·46

Fourth.—The mean proportion of the albuminates, &c., to the inorganic constituents is—

In blood . . .	25 to 1
In blood cells . .	40 „ 1
In intercellular fluid	10 „ 1

In the fluid transuded from the intestinal capillaries during an attack of Cholera the proportion is, on the contrary, 1 to 2, or at most 1·5 or

* Previous diarrhœa.   † Relapse.

2 to 2. If, therefore, no fluid be absorbed, the proportion of the albuminates (in the morphological elements and in the blood still continuing to circulate) is increased according to the duration of the transudation, and by induction from these data we obtain the following comparative results :—

Blood	34 to 1
Corpuscles	58 ,, 1
Intercellular fluid	20 ,, 1

that is, the proportion of the albuminates to the inorganic constituents is increased by one-half in the blood cells, and to double in the intercellular fluid.

		Sex.	Age.	Date of blood-letting.	Duration of transu-dation.	Inorganic constituents to 1000 parts of organic.		
						Circu-lating blood.	Blood cells.	Inter-cellular fluid.
Normal ... (Contempo-rary.)	I.)	Male	25	14/2 Nov.	0	3·87	2·84	9·45
Cholera . {	VII.) II.) VI.)	— — —	23 45 71	16/4 Oct.* 22/10 Aug. 15/3 Sept.†	4 hours 7 ,, 9 ,,	3·84 2·93 3·06	2·49 2·01 2·34	7·79 6·63 4·20
Normal ... (Contempo-rary.)	II.)	Female	30	6 Oct. 24 Sept.	0	5·16	2·96	10·71
Cholera . {	V.) III.) I.)	— — —	20 30	13/1 Sept. 24/12 Aug. 22/10 Aug.	18 hours 36 ,, 48 ,,	3·40 3·01 2·96	1·94 1·89 1·75	7·43 6·77 6·67

Fifth.—During capillary transudation the solids are retained in the vessels with more force than the water, the organic solids (albuminates, &c.) with more force than the inorganic (salts), the phosphates with more than the chlorides, and the salts of potash with more than the salts of soda.

* Previous diarrhœa.   † Relapse.

		Age	Date of blood-letting.	Duration of transudation.	500 parts water.	Inorganic constituents to 100 of organic.	100 parts of inorganic constituents contain			
							Potash.	Soda.	Phosphoric acid.	Chlorine.
	Transuded fluid (vomited and dejected) Intercellular fluid			10 hours	9·51	129·6	6·23	34·80	2·53	48·61
I.)	Male	25	14/2 Nov.	0	109·24	9·45	3·69	40·09	4·96	41·58
VII.)	—		16/4 Oct.*	4 hours	162·63	7·79	6·08	39·66	6·00	34·91
VI.)	—		15/3 Sept.†	9 „	192·39	4·90	9·56	34·54	7·02	39·16
II.)	Female	30	6 Oct. / 24 Sept.	0	93·79	10·71	3·96	37·82	6·44	43·47
V.)	—	20	13/1 Sept.	18 hours	121·97	7·43	5·56	34·89	7·67	39·82

Sixth.—In the secondary exosmosis of the contents of the blood cells into the intercellular fluid consequent upon the disturbance of balance by the previous loss of fluids, the solids are retained in the corpuscles with more energy than the fluids, and the organic solids with more than the inorganic, also the phosphates with more than the chlorides, and the salts of potash with more than the salts of soda.

		Sex.	Age	Date of blood-letting.	Duration of transudation.	Solids in 1000 parts water.	Inorganic constituents to 100 of organic.	100 parts of inorganic constituents contain			
								Potash.	Soda.	Phosphoric acid.	Chlorine.
I.)		Male	25	14/2 Nov.	0	467·07	2·34	42·45	6·45	19·73	24·03
VII.)		—	23	16/4 Oct.	4 hours	547·59	2·49	36·35	15·15	17·51	13·66
VI.)		—	71	15/3 Sept.	9 „	589·29	2·34	43·22	1·66	25·52	14·92
II.)		Female	30	6 Oct. / 24 Sept.	0	453·73	2·96	39·79	18·25	11·53	18·12
V.)		—	20	13/1 Sept.	18 hours	532·14	1·94	46·84	9·77	15·62	19·06

Seventh.—The two currents (the primary of the intercellular fluid through the walls of the capillaries, and the secondary from the blood

* Previous diarrhœa.　　　　　　　† Relapse.

cells into the intercellular fluid) may be thus characterised. At the onset of the disease, the water and the salts transude through the capillary wall in the proportion of 1000 to 4. The intercellular fluid (liq. sanguinis), thus deprived of its water, reacts upon the blood cells and draws out a portion of their fluid. In the intercellular fluid and in the cells the salts appear to be absolutely increased, although, in portion to the organic constituents, they are relatively diminished. When there is no reabsorption from without, the amount of the salines continues to decrease according to the duration of the effusive stage of the disease. The chlorides of the alkalies, being less important for cell function, are diffused into the cellular fluid in equivalent proportion to those poured out from the latter. The relative amount of the phosphates and potash salts is increased according to the duration of the effusive stage at the expense of the chloride of sodium so largely thrown off.

Dr. Garrod commences his paper * by giving the details of investigations made on the blood in the epidemic of 1831-2, and which, according to him, admit of the following conclusions:—

" 1. That in cholera, the physical characters of the blood are altered, and that its tendency is to become thicker, tar-like, and less coagulable.

" 2. That the proportion of water is much diminished.

" 3. That the specific gravity of the serum is very high, which is due to the increase of the solid portion of the serum, and especially of the albumen; and that this fluid also tends to become less alkaline in its reaction.

" 4. That with regard to the salts of the serum, some doubt exists as to their excessive diminution.

" 5. That urea sometimes exists in cholera blood."

The review of the results of his own inquiries is as follows:—

" *Physical Condition of Cholera Blood.*—As far as this point is concerned, all recent observations agree with those formerly made, and indicate, that from the commencement of the disease, this fluid becomes more tenacious, of a darker color, with less disposition to coagulate, and that its specific gravity is very greatly increased. It will be found by reference to the tables, giving the results of Becquerel and Rodier's examination of the blood of men and women, that the maximum specific gravity in the male is 1062, in the female 1060. Now, in our cholera cases, we have found the specific gravity in adult males to be, in round numbers, 1076 and 1081, and in females 1068, 1074, and

* London Journal of Medicine, May, 1849.

1076; also, in children under ten years of age, in whom the blood probably has a specific gravity not exceeding 1045, we have found it as high as 1076 in one case, and in the second it was doubtless even higher (for it contained more solid matter), although the small quantity of the blood did not allow it to be accurately determined. We have thus proved, that, in cholera, this property of the blood is greatly altered.

" *Water and Solids.*—Of course, the watery portions of the blood experience a diminution nearly corresponding to the increase of the specific gravity of the fluid, and the solids a corresponding increase. In the table above referred to, the maximum amount of solids in males was 240, and in females 227 parts in the 1000 of blood; in children it is very much less. In our cholera cases we have found that the numbers representing the total solids were 251, 260, 271, 275, 282, 284.

" *Blood Globules.*—These we have also found to be increased in quantity, in the case in which we have been enabled to separate them from the albumen; and in place of 140 parts in the 1000 (which is considered a very high healthy average), we have found them to form 166 and 171 parts.

" *Fibrine.*—In the case (Worts), where the blood coagulated pretty firmly, 2·61 parts of fibrine were obtained in the 1000 parts of blood; in Dr. Parkes' case 0·88; but I remarked that the fibrine in Worts' case, although exceeding in quantity the normal average (2·20), was yet much less consistent than natural in character. After death, the blood of this man did not coagulate at all, and I think it is probable that in cholera this element of the blood undergoes changes of quality, rather than of quantity, and that as long as it can be ascertained correctly, analyses do not indicate any marked deficiency; after a time, however, it can no longer be collected.

" *Serum.*—As to the specific gravity of this portion of the blood, our observations were only two in number, and these were obtained from the blood of the same patient, at different times; both of them tend to confirm the results previously found; namely, that this fluid becomes much heavier, from the large increase in the amount of its solid constituents; healthy serum being of specific gravity 1028, we found it in cholera to be 1039 and 1041.

" *Albumen.*—This constituent of the serum was only estimated in 2 cases, and in these amounted to about 125 parts in the 1000 parts of serum, and to 103 parts in the 1000 of blood; so we see that it

E

is increased in both fluids. This we might naturally expect, when we take into consideration the character of the stools in this disease; for in them, we find that, compared with some of the other ingredients of this fluid, the albumen is thrown out in very small proportions; and although the ratio between the serum and clot is diminished, yet the decrease in the water more than counterbalances the loss which the albumen sustains.

" *Salts of the Blood and Serum.*—On this point our results have far from accorded with those obtained by Dr. O'Shaughnessy, and upon which so much stress has been frequently laid; we will therefore dwell a short time to consider the facts which have been elicited. Becquerel and Rodier found that the maximum amount of soluble salts in the 1000 parts of blood was, in the male 7·4, the minimum 4·3, the mean 5·6 parts; in the female, maximum 7·0, minimum 6·0, and mean 6·8 parts. We have found in our cholera cases, that, where the soluble salts were separately estimated, they were represented by the numbers 10·7, 7·54, 7·5, 6·15, 6·02, and 5·72 parts in the 1000 parts of blood; every number exceeding the mean, and many the maximums obtained by Becquerel and Rodier from the healthy blood both of males and females. The analyses were performed in the same way. Again, with regard to serum in health, in Lecanu's standard we find 8·1 parts in 1000; in a specimen of healthy serum (analysed by myself for the purpose of comparison), 9·34 parts; and in Becquerel and Rodier's table, when estimated in 1000 parts of serum, from about 6 to 8 parts. In the serum of cholera we observe 8·12 and 7·43 parts; in neither case less than the mean of numerous analyses of healthy serum; and it should be borne in mind, that when the specific gravity of the fluid is high, from the increase of the albumen, as happens in cholera, the estimation of the salts in the 1000 parts of *serum* or *blood* is scarcely correct (for we should rather find the ratio existing between the *water* and soluble salts); if this is done, then, from our experiments, the amount of salts, instead of being *decreased*, as supposed by Dr. O'Shaughnessy, will be found always *increased*. It is curious to remark the composition of the blood in Cases I. and II.; the subjects were children under ten years of age, in whom the disease proved rapidly fatal. In both specimens of blood, the soluble salts were very greatly increased; in that from the younger child, they were nearly twice the amount found in health. I should have been almost inclined to doubt the accuracy of these analyses, as they were made on very small quantities of blood, but on looking into my note-book, every step appears to have been correctly performed, and, to confirm their accuracy, the third analysis made on the top portion of the blood (much more fluid being used in the operation), showed a still greater increase of these salts, due to the presence of a larger quantity of serum in a given weight of blood. It would have been extremely interesting to have known the composition of the stools passed by these children, to have seen whether or not the ratio between the water and soluble salts was increased. In Dr. Parkes' paper on ' Intestinal Discharges in Cholera,' it will be observed, that the stools passed by children, 10 and 11 years of age, contained in the 1000 parts a smaller amount of the salts than those discharged by adults; and it is possible that there may exist some difference in the mode of action of the poison in children and adults : a difference in the symptoms certainly does exist.

" It was noticed in the cases now referred to, as well as in the previous epidemic, that the blood often became neutral, in some cases even acid. Dr. O'Shaughnessy considered this as depending on the blood losing its carbonate of soda, to the presence of which its normal alkaline reaction was referred. At the present time, however, the existence of this salt, even in healthy blood, is denied by many ; and certainly many of the properties of the serum, formerly ascribed to it, depend on the tribasic phosphate of soda, which, when it contains two atoms of fixed base, possesses an alkaline reaction, and has the power of holding carbonic acid in solution. That this alkaline salt is not deficient, even when the blood shows a decided acid reaction, was clearly proved by our finding that the ash from such blood or serum exhibited alkaline properties, quite as strong as that obtained from these fluids in health.

" The nature of the acid which existed in such blood was not made out ; but it certainly was not volatile. Though we have found no diminution of the salts in the blood of cholera patients, yet, of necessity, the total amount in the system must be decidedly lessened, but so also is the total bulk of the blood.

" Urea.—It was stated by observers in the last epidemic, that urea had been detected in the blood and other fluids in cholera; but in most cases its amount was not estimated, and no relation between the quantity of this principle and the stage or intensity of the disease was observed : to this point we paid some attention, and I think that the results obtained will prove interesting. In Cases II. and III. (Tooting children), no urea was found, and certainly it did not

exist in the blood to any large extent. Still, from the small amount
of blood examined, a quantity greater than in health might have
escaped discovery; and that such was the case, we have some
evidence in the increased amount of uric acid, which, when suspension of the urinary excretion takes place, is found in excess in the
blood along with the urea, and can be more easily discovered, not
being so liable to suffer decomposition; still the urea was not in
large excess. In these cases, death took place during the stage of
collapse. In Case III. it will be also observed that no urea was
found, but Dr. Parkes remarks, that it may have been present in
small quantities, but certainly *not in large excess*. The blood in
Case IV. was not examined for this principle. In Case V. urea
was sought for twice: first, when the patient was in a state of
partial collapse; next, in the blood obtained from the large vessels
after death; and it will be seen, that in the collapse stage (not
intense), 1000 parts of blood contained 0·38 part of urea; after
death (partial reaction having taken place), as much as 0·92 part
was found in the same quantity of blood. In Case VI., where the
blood was taken after death, the patient having had partial reaction,
and then becoming semi-comatose, 0·65 part of urea was obtained
from the 1000 parts of blood; and, lastly, in Case VII., where reaction had been restored, and the patient was suffering considerably
from head symptoms and fever, the 1000 parts of the serum of the
blood taken during life, yielded 1·14 part of urea. So we find that
the urea gradually increases in amount, from the cold stage to that of
febrile reaction. The explanation of this phenomenon is, I think,
exceedingly simple; for I should imagine, that in intense and sudden
collapse not only is the function of the urinary excreting organ
diminished or suppressed, but also the vital metamorphoses, and
therefore the formation of urea, are likewise nearly suspended. This
would account for the small amount usually found in the collapse,
and probably the quantity varies inversely with the intensity of this
state; but when partial reaction ensues, and the vital changes take
place with greater activity, should the function of the kidneys not be
at the same time restored, urea must accumulate in the blood, and
the amount must depend on the degree of the reaction (febrile or
not), and the extent of suppression of the urinary secretion. This
view is certainly supported by the results which have been as yet
obtained, not only recently by ourselves, but also in the former epidemic by Dr. O'Shaughnessy and others.

" CONCLUSIONS.

" In comparing the recent analyses with those made during the last epidemic, it will be seen, that as far as concerns the physical properties of the blood, the diminished amount of water, and the consequent increase of the solid portion, also the high specific gravity of the serum, and its tendency to become less alkaline, our own conclusions perfectly agree with those previously made ; and, therefore, that conclusions 1, 2, and 3, before given, are thus far confirmed. With regard to (4) and (5), concerning the salts and urea, our conclusions must be—

" 4. That, in cholera, the saline constituents of the blood are not only not decreased in amount, but sometimes exist even in increased proportion, and that the diminution of its alkaline reaction is not due to the loss of salts, but to the impeded excretion of organic acids, which are constantly being formed in the system.

" 5. That urea usually exists in increased quantities in cholera blood, but that the amount differs considerably in the different stages of the disease ; being but small in quantity in the intense stage of collapse, increasing during reaction, and in excess when consecutive febrile symptoms occur."

Encephalon. The sinuses, and veins of the meninges, were more or less loaded with dark blood. In most cases this was the only morbid appearance. In 3 instances there was sub-arachnoid effusion ; thus in a male, æt. 64, who died in collapse, an hour and a half after the injection of a saline solution into the veins, the whole duration of his severe symptoms being 16 hours, the brain was watery and soft, with several drachms of fluid in the ventricles, and also great sub-arachnoid effusion. Again, in a male, æt. 56, who died in collapse, with asphyxia, after 18 hours' severe symptoms, the superficial veins between the convolutions were much distended with dark fluid blood ; and a large quantity of serous fluid was effused beneath the arachnoid ; each lateral ventricle also contained about half an ounce of clear fluid. In the third case, a female, æt. 53, who died suddenly in collapse, the vessels of the pia mater were moderately full of blood, with slight œdema of the tissue. In addition to these cases, 2 others were reported, in which there was effusion into the lateral ventricles ; death took place in collapse, the duration of the severe symptoms being in one 30 hours, and in the other 12 ; in both, " the lateral ventricles were dilated and full of serum."

The brain substance was normal, except that it often presented on section numerous red points, from fulness of the smaller veins. In one of the cases noted above, and in 2 others, the tissue was rather moist.

The results given by Briquet and Mignot[*] are drawn from 22 cases : " For the most part the sinuses of the dura mater and the large vessels were full of blood.   In 20, a fine injection of the capillary vessels of the pia mater gave a purple color to the surface of the hemispheres, more marked on the convexity than at the base of the brain. . . . . In 5, a general opalescence of the arachnoid was noticed, with patches of a milky whiteness.   In 5 there was adhesion (?) of the pia mater to the cerebral substance ; and in 10 sub-arachnoid effusion. . . . .

" The grey substance was dark colored, and the white dotted with points from the engorged vessels.   The surface of the ventricles was frequently of a roseate tint.   In 5 cases the ventricles contained a considerable quantity of serous fluid, slightly tinged with blood.   The cerebral substance had the normal consistence.   In some cases, the flattening of the convolutions seemed to indicate a certain amount of turgescence."

Virchow [†] observes that he met with no structural changes in the brain and spinal cord.   " There was well-marked venous hyperæmia, with œdema of the pia mater, and sometimes a slight increase of fluid into the ventricles."

Reinhardt and Leubuscher [‡] report as follows :—"After death in the algide stage, we always found the veins of the meninges more or less congested, together with œdema of the pia mater in different degrees.   The cerebral substance was healthy, occasionally rather vascular.   In the ventricles nothing abnormal, except venous congestion of the plexus choroides."

---

[*] Op. Cit., p. 420.   [†] Med. Reform, No. 12.   [‡] Op. Cit., p. 509.

MORBID APPEARANCES WHEN DEATH OCCURRED AFTER REACTION.

THE mucous membrane of the stomach was either natural
Stomach. in appearance, or presented scattered patches of hyperæmia at different parts, especially at the greater cul-de-sac, and along the lesser curvature towards the pylorus. In a male, æt. 29, who died on the ninth day of consecutive fever, the mucous membrane of the stomach was of a dark color, from congestion, with numerous minute spots of ecchymosis. In a female, æt. 37, who died on the seventh day of the disease, "there was general and intense injection of the mucous membrane of the stomach, most marked along the lesser curvature and posterior surface; the injection was striate and punctate, the tissue not softened." Again, in a male, æt. 39, who died on the eighth day, "there was punctate injection in different parts of the stomach, and at the cardiac end a slough as large as a split pea nearly through the coats. The surface of the mucous membrane was covered with bloody mucus." In a fourth case, a male, æt. 45, death occurring on the third day with partial reaction, the stomach was "much contracted, the mucous membrane hyperæmic along the lesser curvature and near the pylorus, the ridges of the rugæ being of a dark color, from vascular injection. About three or four inches from the pylorus there were two ulcers, the larger being about half an inch long; the edges were sharply defined and minutely injected.

Reinhardt and Leubuscher [*] observe that, "in the latter stages of the disease, the hyperæmia of the stomach was much less marked or altogether absent. Fibrinous exudations upon the surface of the mucous membrane were not observed."

Briquet and Mignot describe the morbid appearances occurring during the period of reaction under four distinct sections:—

1st. As observed after death from asphyxia, reaction being incomplete.

[*] Op. Cit., pp. 186, 192.

2nd. From cerebral congestion.

3rd. From meningo-encephalitis.

4th. From thoracic inflammation.

The following is a summary of their observations upon the gastric mucous membrane as recorded under these different sections. It was examined in 35 cases, in 23 of which there was some amount of congestion. This was greatest in the 5 cases contained in the first section, and which obviously belonged rather to the cold stage than to the period of reaction; in all the others it was but trifling.

This accords with the observations of others, that during the period of reaction, the congestion of the gastro-intestinal mucous membrane which characterized the algide stage, was lessened or entirely removed.

In a few of their cases these authors speak of softening of the mucous membrane, principally limited to the greater curvature, and never extensive. It was probably, from its seat, a post-mortem change, in confirmation of which probability they state that, in some cases, the softening was gelatiniform.

Small Intestine, &c. The mucous membrane of the small intestine was generally pale or only slightly hyperæmic, and the pulpy œdematous condition of the tissue and intestinal glands, occurring in the algide stage, had much diminished or entirely disappeared. There were, however, some exceptions to this tendency to resolution of the previous hyperæmia, and restoration of the tissue to its normal condition; those parts of the mucous membrane which during the cold stage had been most affected by vascular injection, being occasionally subject, during reaction, to progressive diphtheritic effusion, which subsequently led, as described below, to disintegration of the tissue.

The glandular structures were not the seat of any special secondary affections. When they were in a morbid condition, which was rare, it was in common with the general mucous surface adjacent; but inasmuch as, at this period of the disease, the lesions of the first stage were receding, so the patches of Peyer and the solitary glands were either quite normal or less swollen and œdematous than in the cold stage.

The following are the particulars given by Reinhardt and Leubuscher, of the morbid appearances found in the intestinal tract in this stage :—" In one series of cases of which the numbers were small, the changes in the mucous membrane previously observed in the cold stage were either receding or had entirely disappeared. The hyperæmia of the capillary veins in particular had lessened or was no longer perceptible, and only the larger ones were here and there congested. Corresponding to this change, the membrane, instead of being of a bright red, was of a dull grey or slate color. The solitary glands and Peyer's patches were now only slightly enlarged or quite normal. The contents of the canal fæculent. The intestinal tract often presented no further morbid appearances either when death had occurred in the typhoid stage, or when accidental complications had supervened. . . . . In a second and more numerous series of cases, some parts of the intestine were in the condition above described, whilst others presented, to a greater or less extent, appearances having the closest similarity to dysentery.

" The mucous membrane, and also the submucous tissue in the severer forms of the affection, were deeply reddened, vividly injected, and also infiltrated to a greater or less extent with extravasated blood. In the large intestine the affected parts were commonly in the form of longitudinal or oblique folds, or irregular bosses and protuberances, arising from œdema of the submucous cellular tissue; when incised and compressed, the serous fluid was discharged, and they collapsed. In the small intestine, the hyperæmia was mostly on the ridges of the transverse folds (valvulæ conniventes), which were also swollen from serous exudation. In only one of the cases of this series, where death occurred quickly upon reaction, were the changes in the large and small intestine such as are here described; in all the others the congested parts were infiltrated to a greater or less extent with a solid exudation, which, after Virchow, we would designate ' diphtheritic.' This exudation contained but little water, was of a greyish or yellowish-white color, and under the microscope was amorphous. It was rendered translucent by acetic acid and caustic alkali, but resisted the action of the former for some time. The deposit began in the superficial layers of the mucous membrane, and was mostly confined to the membrane itself, but in certain parts it extended somewhat beyond, as in the small intestine, where it filled up the spaces between the villi, fusing them together into a continuous mass, in which, by the aid of the microscope, the outline and tissue of some of the villi could occasionally be distinguished. The infiltration gradually extended from the superficial to the deeper layers of the membrane, and not rarely to the submucous tissue.

The deeper layers were never affected, whilst the superficial remained free, but the converse was frequent. The surface of the diseased parts was generally of a dirty yellowish-brown, from imbibition of the coloring matter of the bile, and hence it was easily distinguishable; it was in those rare cases only where the intestine contained no bile, that the exudation had its proper yellowish white color. The extent of the effusion varied extremely; in some cases it was slight and only on a few of the hyperæmic patches, in others it infiltrated the swollen mucous membrane and the submucous tissue over a wide extent, and in some places to the depth of two or three lines. These changes were found in both the large and small intestine, either in the one or the other only, or in both at the same time. Those parts where the hyperæmia had been most marked in the cold stage were principally affected. In the small intestine the ileum was the principal seat of the diphtheritic inflammation, particularly the vicinity of the ileo-cœcal valve, from which point it extended, lessening in intensity, to a variable distance upwards into the ileum or even into the jejunum. Very frequently the infiltration was limited to the swollen valvulæ conniventes, the intervening portion of the mucous membrane being free; adjacent to the ileo-cœcal valve large tracts of the intestine in its whole circumference were not rarely affected. In the large intestine the cœcum and rectum were the seat of this lesion, whilst the intervening parts were in a much less degree prone to it. In 2 cases through the whole length of the large intestine there was acute hyperæmia with diphtheritic exudation, producing an appearance precisely like dysentery, and diminishing in intensity from the rectum upwards. During life there had been numerous watery dejections containing mucous flocculi tinged with blood. In the other cases the evacuations presented no obvious change, and had not the characters met with in the first stage of dysentery. This was probably owing to the small extent and the slow development of the diphtheritic exudation.

" The exudation, without undergoing any degree of organisation, gradually softened, and the tissue in which it was contained softened with it. This process of disintegration commenced on the surface, and by extension to deeper parts produced a loss of substance of variable extent; subsequently having the characters of common ulceration. In general, however, the cases were fatal before the diphtheritic matter was fully thrown off."

Liver, &c.   The morbid appearances presented by the liver when death occurred in the consecutive fever, were by no means distinct. They often differed but little from the normal state, and were probably due in great part to the condition of the venous system at the time of death. There was no increase of volume. On section, the secreting structure was of a dull reddish brown color. The secreting elements, examined microscopically, appeared to be normal.

The gall bladder and ducts were in general healthy, and the bile contained in them often dark and viscid; there was, however, no uniformity either in the quantity or physical qualities of the secretion. In several instances the gall bladder and the larger ducts contained a turbid watery mucous fluid, either colorless or tinged with bile; the lining membrane being at the same time hyperæmic, and in parts roughened by granular fibrinous exudation. The following cases, quoted from the tabular report, may serve as examples:—A female, æt. 37, was in collapse for 24 hours; during the consecutive fever there was great tenderness over the gall bladder: death occurred on the sixth day of the disease. On a post-mortem examination the liver was pale. The gall bladder was distended, and contained about 2¼ ounces of greenish thin turbid bile. The mucous membrane was minutely injected and roughened and opaque from exudation. . . . . A male, æt. 39, was in partial collapse for more than 36 hours, followed by moderate reaction, during which the urine was albuminous. Death occurred on the sixth day of the disease. The liver was rather small and pale, the gall bladder full of turbid yellowish serum, and the lining membrane of a pale grey color, with adherent mucus; in the contents examined by the microscope were found granules, granular nuclei, blood corpuscles, and oily particles.

It is probable that this morbid condition of the gall bladder and ducts begins during the cold stage, in common with the affection of the mucous membrane of the duodenum, and that it is not to be regarded as any new action set up in the consecutive fever.

Pirogoff (Plate XIV., fig. 4) gives a sketch of this diphtheritic affection of the lining membrane of the gall bladder, which he obtained from Professor Himmelstern, of Dorpat, together with the following history:—" The patient was a male, æt. 56, admitted into the hospital 12 hours after the commencement of the attack. He then complained of a very severe pain in the region of the liver, accompanied with the principal symptoms of the cold stage of epidemic cholera. After 24 hours the severity of his symptoms lessened, but the pain in the hepatic region continued, and rather increased in violence; an intense peritonitis set in, and the patient died on the fourth day after admission. On a post-mortem examination there was found recent plastic exudation upon the surface of the peritoneum. The base of the gall bladder had contracted adhesions to the colon, and was perforated by a small ulcer. The internal surface was of a reddish-brown color, over which were scattered yellowish exudations, irregular in form, and of several lines in extent. The mucous membrane beneath was much injected, and completely deprived of its epithelium. In the intestinal canal the villi were observed to be swollen, and the patches of Peyer and the solitary glands affected with the cholera process."

Reinhardt and Leubuscher, and Briquet and Mignot, record similar observations upon the occasional occurrence of inflammation of the gall bladder and ducts, with diphtheritic exudation upon the surface of the mucous membrane. Respecting the hepatic tissue they observe, that it in general presented nothing remarkable, except being more full of blood than in the cold stage.

Spleen.   The spleen was small and shrivelled, but its texture normal. The morbid appearances occasionally observed in it, such as mottling of the tissue, from partial congestions and fibrinous effusions, have been described in the former section, since they had their origin in the collapse of the algide stage. The morbid hypertrophy of the spleen, and the various alterations of its tissue, which occur in miasmatic and low-lying districts, in which also cholera prevailed, are to be considered apart from any influence of the choleraic poison.

Kidneys.   The kidneys in this stage were frequently enlarged, the structure coarse, and presenting traces of venous hyperæmia. The state of the urine during life indicated a condition similar to that occurring after scarlet fever, and the morbid appearances of the secreting structures of the kidney were not dissimilar to those that are met with after that disease. The following instances may be taken as illustrations:—

J. J., æt. 30, was in collapse for 32 hours—this was followed by consecutive fever, and he died on the tenth day. During the collapse the urine was altogether suppressed. In the consecutive fever, the secretion was very small in quantity, of the color of coffee, and coagulable by heat. It contained blood corpuscles, exudation cells, free nuclei, and epithelium. On a post-mortem examination the kidneys weighed 15½ ounces. The capsules were not adherent. The secreting structure was pale, œdematous, and easily lacerable. The Malpighian bodies injected. The tubules contained finely-granular epithelium, with oil globules and free nuclei.

J. B., æt. 45. Stage of collapse well marked, duration 30 hours, followed by moderate reaction. On the third day about an ounce of urine of a dark brown color was drawn off by the catheter. It was coagulable by heat and nitric acid; and contained blood and exudation corpuscles in large numbers. The patient lay in a drowsy state, with contracted pupils; death occurred on the evening of the fourth day. The kidneys weighed 9¼ ounces. The capsules separated readily. The surface was marked by stollate venous injection. The cortical substance was slightly increased in thickness, and pale; but so far as the naked eye could discover, not otherwise abnormal.

J. W., æt. 39, in well-marked collapse for 24 hours, followed by slight signs of reaction. As he was passing into collapse, a small quantity of urine was voided. It was acid and albuminous. On the fourth day about an ounce of dark alkaline and very albuminous urine was secreted; it was otherwise nearly suppressed. He died on the seventh day. The kidneys were rather large, capsules adherent, surface granular and injected.

Speaking of the progressive morbid changes in the kidney, which had their origin in the cold stage, Reinhardt and Leubuscher * add, " As the disease advanced, the infiltration of the renal structures was more extensive, the cortical substance being principally affected. It was increased in thickness, of a pale color, and easily lacerable. On stripping off the capsule the surface was left uneven and granular. In the tubular structure the infiltration extended from the apices of the cones towards their bases, portions of which often retained their normal appearance whilst the cortical substance adjacent was swollen and of a greyish-white color. It is worthy of remark, that the degree of hyperæmia which led to these exudations was slight. In the further course of the disease there was a deposit of fat into the epithelium of the uriniferous tubules, and a production

* Op. Cit., p. 497.

of granule-cells. The deposit of fat often began so early as the fifth or seventh day of the disease."

According to Briquet and Mignot[*], out of 24 cases, fatal in the stage of reaction with cerebral complications, in 15 the kidneys were increased in volume with well-marked hyperæmia of their tissues. In these cases the urinary secretion had been scanty and albuminous. The mucous membrane of the bladder was congested in half the cases. In one case the ureter and pelvis of one of the kidneys contained coagula; the patient having passed bloody urine just previous to death.

Lungs. The appearances presented by the lungs varied according to the mode of death. In general the whole pulmonary tissue was full of blood, and, the posterior parts in particular, subject to hypostatic engorgement, in some instances so extreme that the portions thus affected were entirely devoid of air. The bronchial membrane was reddened, and the tubes were full of frothy mucus. Where the symptoms of reaction had been decided, pneumonia of a low form supervened in the posterior and inferior parts of the lung, the portions thus affected presenting all the gradations from mere engorgement with œdema to red or reddish-grey hepatization. In some rare instances the anterior parts were affected with lobular pneumonia.

Recent fibrinous exudations upon the pleura, with some amount of fluid effusion into the cavity, were not uncommon, but rarely extensive.

Reinhardt and Leubuscher[†], speaking of hæmorrhagic exudation into the pulmonary tissue during the cold stage, go on to state that, "in the latter stages of cholera, these were more frequent, and sometimes of considerable extent. They presented various appearances, being at first of a dark venous color, afterwards becoming grey, compact, and solid, and, when more advanced, softening in the centre into a puriform fluid. When pneumonia existed it constantly had its seat in the lower lobes, the hepatized parts being firm and compact. In one case there was extensive bronchitis, with tracheitis and œdema glottidis. The inflammation extended in parts to the finest bronchi, and was complicated, with lobular pneumonia. In one instance the mucous membrane of one of the larger bronchi was infiltrated with diphtheritic exudation."

[*] Op. Citat., pp. 443, 444.   [†] Op. Citat., p. 507.

Dr. Budd[*], writing on the last epidemic, states that he found pneumonia in 4 out of 6 cases where the patients had lived 45 hours after the attack.   In one of these, which was fatal at the end of the above period, the pneumonia was partial, interlobular (?), and confined to the lower lobe of the right lung.   In 2, fatal at the end of 96 and 138 hours respectively, the lower lobes of both lungs were in a state of red hepatization.

Pericardium.   Traces of pericarditis were found in a few instances, but it was among the more rare complications of the secondary stage.   In one case which occurred to ourselves, there were rough and firm deposits of fibrin about the base of the ventricles, and in another the cavity contained four ounces of turbid fluid, with fibrinous flakes.

Heart, Blood, &c.   In many cases nothing was observed worthy of note, either in the cardiac tissue itself or in the general condition of the blood in the different cavities, but not rarely the muscular substance was flaccid and soft, and, according to some observers, altered in color.

Briquet and Mignot[†] found the muscular tissue of the heart soft and friable in 11 cases out of 23, fatal in the typhoid stage, with cerebral complications.   With this alteration a change of color was also noted, the tissue being pale or yellowish in five cases, and in one of a violet tint.   These authors also observe that the interior of the heart and large vessels was frequently stained by imbibition.

The degree of distension of the cavities and the state of the blood, whether coagulated or not, depended very much upon the mode of death.   When the cases were fatal with symptoms of asthenia, the blood more frequently remained fluid, or formed only a soft coagulum; but when the cause of death was pulmonary obstruction, the right cavities and the large vessels contained fibrinous coagula and firm clots, having the usual appearances.

Brain, &c.   The morbid appearances in the brain and its membranes were generally indistinct, and were principally venous hyperæmia and serous effusion, varying in degree and amount according to the duration of the symptoms and the mode of death. The pia mater was often œdematous, and the lateral ventricles in some instances contained an excess of fluid.   The cerebral substance was either natural or rather watery, but not altered in consistence.   Plastic

* Library of Medicine—Article, Cholera.   † Op. Cit., pp. 434, 444.

fibrinous effusions were very rare. These observations are confirmed by Reinhardt and Leubuscher, who state that, "in those who died in the typhoid stage, they found no obvious morbid condition of the brain besides venous congestion, which was in general less than in the cold stage. Not rarely there was œdema of the pia mater, and sometimes an increased quantity of serum into the ventricles, and the brain substance itself was slightly œdematous." They further add, that "all these appearances were observed by them in persons who died with other complications, as pneumonia, &c., and when there had been no symptom of cerebral affection."

Briquet and Mignot in their report * state that, of the cases coming under their notice, 17 sank with symptoms of cerebral congestion after complete reaction. Of these, 11 were examined post mortem, and the state of the nervous centres particularly investigated. On an average, the patients lived four days and a half after reaction was established. There were bright red patches on the dura mater in one case. In 3, an opalescence of the arachnoid with serous effusion beneath. In 4, the sinuses and large veins were gorged with blood, and the smaller vessels of the pia mater injected. This latter condition was well marked in 10 cases, and in two-thirds of these more so on the convexity of the hemispheres than at the base. In 8 cases there was thickening and œdema of the pia mater, the infiltrated fluid being generally limpid and colorless, but sometimes sanguinolent. In 3 cases there was firm adhesion of the membranes to the grey matter. In 8, the cortical substance showed an active state of congestion, being of a rose tint with numerous red points. In 7, a similar condition of the white substance was well marked. The surfaces of the ventricles had frequently a tint of redness more or less vivid, and their contents were faintly colored with blood. In one instance there was a rather abundant effusion of a citron color.

They also give the details of 13 cases fatal with symptoms of meningo-encephalitis, the mean duration from the period of reaction being about six days. In 11 of these there was intense injection of the small vessels of the pia mater, and in 5 sub-arachnoid effusion. In only 3 instances was there plastic effusion on the surface of the arachnoid. The cerebral substance, both grey and white, was injected in 12 cases; in 6 of these the injection was very marked, especially

* Op. Citat., p. 480.

in the white matter. The interior of the ventricles had a rose tint, and contained a few drachms of slightly-sanguinolent fluid in 7 cases; in only one was it so abundant as to distend the cavities. The cerebral substance seemed rather softened in 2 cases, and in 4 the convolutions were flattened, indicating a decided turgescence of the whole mass.

Case.	Sex and Age.	Duration of severe symptoms.	Death in		Mucous Membranes.			Intestinal Glands.		Mesenteric Glands.	Spleen.
			Collapse.	Reaction.	Stomach.	Small Intestines.	Large Intestines.	Solitary.	Aggregate.		
1	Male 45	20 hours.	Collapse.	...	Increased vascularity.	Increased vascularity, especially at lower part of ileum, with spots of ecchymosis.	Increased vascularity, with large spots of extravasation at commencement.	Enlarged throughout small intestine, especially at lower end.	Enlarged throughout, chiefly at lower end.	...	...
2	Male 34	12 hours.	Collapse.	...	Increased vascularity, with thick coating of epithelium.	Increased vascularity, especially towards end of ileum.	No vascularity.	Enlarged throughout whole of ileum, especially at lower end.	Enlarged throughout ileum, chiefly at lower end.	...	...
3	Female 35	32½ hours.	...	Partial reaction.	Healthy.	Increased vascularity, especially at end of ileum.	Slightly vascular.	Enlarged near ileocecal valve, very few in large intestines.	Enlarged throughout ileum, chiefly at lower end.	Enlarged.	...
4	Male 35	21 hours.	Pulse never returned to wrist. Coma.	...	Highly congested, with numerous spots of ecchymosis.	Slight congestion of duodenum, none at upper part, very great at lower part of ileum.	Healthy.	Numerous and prominent in small intestine, few little enlarged in large intestine.	...	Slightly enlarged.	..

Case	Liver	Gall-bladder and ducts	Peritoneum	Kidneys and Urinary Passages	Female Sexual Organs	Heart and Blood	Lungs	Membranes	Brain Substance	Ventricles	Remarks
1	Contained less blood than normal.	Loaded.		Slightly congested.		Blood dark and thick, not coag., large fibrinous clot in right ventricle.	Empty, sometimes slightly congested posteriorly.	D. M. unusually adherent, vessels and sinuses loaded with blood.	Numerous vascular points.	Dilated, full of serum.	Slight puckering of apex of one lung, atheroma in aorta. Dr. Whyte Barclay.
		Large quantity of dark bile.		Congested.		Heart flabby. Blood dark, thick, fluid, fibrinous clot in right ventricle.	Slightly congested posteriorly.	D. M. rather adherent, vessels and sinuses loaded with blood.	Numerous vascular points, substance soft.	Dilated, full of serum.	Old pleuritic adhesions. Dr. Barclay.
3		Ful		Slightly congested. Capsules adherent.		Heart flabby. Blood pitchy, large fibrinous clot in inferior cava.	Much congested posteriorly. Bronchial membrane of right lung congested.	D. M. rather adherent, vessels and sinuses loaded with blood.	Blood vessels congested.	Small quantity of serum.	Dr. Barclay.
4		Full of dark blood.		Slightly congested.		Heart flabby, containing large, black, soft coagula.	Very slightly congested. Cretaceous deposit at right apex.	...	Rather dry, numerous vascular points.	Empty.	Dr. Barclay.

| Case. | Sex and Age. | Duration of severe symptoms. | Death in | | Mucous Membranes. | | | Intestinal Glands. | | Mesenteric Glands. | Spleen. |
			Collapse.	Reaction.	Stomach.	Small Intestine.	Large Intestines.	Solitary.	Aggregate.		
5	Female 19	3 days.		No reaction, delirium and coma.	Healthy.	Slight congestion at commencement of ileum.	Healthy.	Few enlarged at end of ileum, none visible in large intestine.	Throughout, very distinct.		
6	Female 63	Diarrhœa, a month, sickness and vomiting 4 days. Died 18 hours after admission.	Collapse.		Healthy.	Increased vascularity, especially at lower end.	Healthy.	Enlarged at end of ileum and in large intestine.	Enlarged throughout.		
7	Male... 5	No history, died 5 hours after admission.	Collapse.		Increased vascularity.	Patches of congestion in jejunum and ileum.	Healthy.	Few enlarged at end of ileum, none in large intestine.	Throughout prominent with intensely congested capillaries.	Much enlarged.	
8	Female 1.25	26 hours.	Collapse.		Increased vascularity.	Increased vascularity throughout.	Healthy.	Enlarged at end of ileum.	Only two patches prominent.		

Case.	Liver.	Gall-bladder and Ducts.	Peritoneum.	Kidneys and Urinary Passages.	Female Sexual Organs.	Heart and Blood.	Lungs.	Membranes.	Brain Substance.	Ventricles.	Remarks.
5		Full		Healthy.	.	Heart covered with fat, white patch on surface. Blood coagulated, large discoloured clot in left ventricle.	Slight congestion of inferior and posterior part of left.	D. M. rather adherent, vessels and sinuses loaded with blood.	Rather dry, numerous vascular points.	Scarcely any fluid.	Dr. Barclay.
6				Granular, atrophied. Capsules adherent.		...	Healthy.	...	Rather moist.	Small quantity of fluid.	Apoplectic clot of some standing in cavity of arachnoid. Some atheroma in aorta. Dr. Barclay.
7		Distended.		Congested.		Blood dark, fluid, with sweetish smell.	Healthy.	Head not examined.			Vena cava and renal veins much distended. Portal almost empty. Dr. Barclay.
8		Loaded with dark bile.		Healthy.		Blood dark, coagulated.	Emphysematous: cretaceous deposit.	Head not examined.			Dr. Barclay.

№	Sex and Age	Duration of severe symptoms	Death in		Mucous Membranes.			Intestinal Glands.		Mesenteric Glands.	Spleen.
			Collapse.	Reaction.	Stomach.	Small Intestines.	Large Intestines.	Solitary.	Aggregate.		
9	M. 44	8 hours.	Collapse, conscious to the last.		Increased vascularity, with thick coating of exfoliated epithelium.	Increased vascularity, with thick coating of mucus.	Healthy.	Few enlarged at end of ileum.	None prominent.		
10	Male 7	Death third day.	Collapse, with coma.			Increased vascularity; ulceration at lower end of ileum.	Increased vascularity.	...		Much enlarged.	
11	Female 30	death ...	Semi-comatose.		Increased vascularity, especially to the pylorus.	Increased vascularity with thick adhesive mucus.	Increased vascularity with adhesive mucus.	Few enlarged at end of ileum.	None prominent.		
12*	...	...			Intensely vascular.	Intensely firm duodenum to upper end of ileum.	Healthy.	Few thit at end of ileum.	None prominent.		Atrophied.
13	Male.. adult.	12 ...	Life.		Bloody mucus at the pylorus; great hyperæmia of the mucous membrane; numerous small spots, partly at the fundus.	Distended with effusion, injection in extensive patches in jejunum and ileum, but most marked in lower part of ileum.	Great hyperæmia, much swollen with dark spots at spaces.	Enlarged, Brunner's glands enlarged.	Enormously enlarged. Infiltrated with white bodies.	Notably enlarged and moderately infiltrated with white (molecular) bodies.	Enlarged 5¼ in. long, 2¼ " broad, ¾ " thick. Tissue flaccid,...white bodies distinct.

* NOTE.—In the above autopsies of twelve fatal cases, those organs only are particularized which most usually indicate deviations from health in cholera; the other organs, serous membranes, &c., are supposed to be in their normal condition, except when mentioned at the head of "Remarks."

Case.	Liver.	Gall-bladder and Ducts.	Peritoneum.	Kidneys and Urinary Passages.	Female Sexual Organs.	Heart and Blood.	Lungs.	Membranes.	Brain Substance.	Ventricles.	Remarks.
9	..	Loaded with dark bile.		Slightly congested. Capsule adherent.		Blood dark,... brown,...fluid.	Slightly congested posteriorly.	Head not examined.	Head not examined.	...	Dr. Barclay.
10	Liver large and congested.	...		Much congested.	Uterus atrophied.	...	Healthy.	Congested,... sinuses loaded with fluid blood.	Soft, watery, rather vacular.	Small amount of serum.	Dr. Barclay.
11		Contained small quantity of bile....not distended.		Healthy.	Cysts in both ovaries.	Blood dark and pitchy, with imperfect coagula. Heart flabby.	Cretaceous deposit in left lung.	Head not examined.			Dr. Barclay.
12		Distended with bile.				Blood dark, quite fluid.	Somewhat congested.	Congested, sinuses loaded with dark fluid blood.	Vascular points numerous.		Dr. Barclay.
13	Less blood than normal, slightly fatty.	Ducts distended with catarrhal secretion. G. bladder distended, bile dark green, fluid.	Covered with slimy secretion.	Slightly mottled. No change of substance.		Pericard. empty. Heart flaccid,dark coagula and fluid blood in right ventr., no fibr. coagula.	Emphysematous, inf. lobes congested.				Reinhardt and Leubuscher. Case vi.

Case.	Sex and Age.	Duration of severe symptoms.	Death in		Mucous Membrane.			Intestinal Glands.		Mesenteric Glands.	Spleen.
			Collapse.	Reaction.	Stomach.	Small Intestine.	Large Intestine.	Solitary.	Aggregate.		
14	Male... 41	13 hours.	Collapse.		Distended with rice-water fluid; glands near pylorus much swollen.	Duodenum much congested, hyperæmia extending throughout the small intestine, gradually increasing in ileum. Extensive extravasation of blood into the mucous membrane of the lower part of ileum.	Hyperæmia in small patches with small extravasations; glands but slightly swollen.	Brunner's glands much swollen; solitary glands throughout remarkably enlarged, infiltrated with solid matter.	Much enlarged; infiltrated, and whitish.	Much swollen, of a reddish grey color.	Slightly enlarged. 5½ in. long, 3 " broad, 1 " thick. Slightly shrivelled, in upper bluish-red, hæmorrhagic infiltration. White corpuscles distinct.
15	Female 68	60 hours.	Collapse.		Moderately distended, ridges of the rugæ hyperæmic.	From pylorus to end of ileum, well-marked hyperæmia. In upper part glands prominent, in lower ulcerated. In the transverse folds of the lower part of ileum intense hyperæmia with mucous and extensive extravasation, with diphtheritic exudation particularly on applying the transverse folds.	Cæcum much congested, surface raised into irregular patches with diphtheritic exudation upon them and infiltrating the tissue. The lower part of the rectum dotted with slightly raised congestion and hyperæmic.	Enlarged, and in lower part of ileum ulcerated.	Enlarged.	Moderately swollen.	Spleen of normal size. White corpuscles not distinct.

Case	Liver	Gall Bladder and Ducts	Peritoneum	Kidneys and Urinary Passages	Genito Urinary Organs	Heart and Blood	Lungs	Membranes	Brain substance	Ventricles	Remarks
16	Much drained of its blood.	...	A quantity of adhesive secretion over the surface.	Congested, not enlarged. The tissue normal, in the pelvis acute catarrh,.... small ecchymoses in muc. membrane.	...	Fluid is pericardium small in quantity, ecchym. on post. part, and towards apex of heart. Distension of right ventr. and auricle. Blood dark, imperfectly coag.; small fibrinous clot. Bothy, on the endocard. of left ventricle. Left side constricted, nearly empty.	Lungs anaemic, some of bronchi normal.	Great venous congestion of all the membranes. Œdema of pia mater.	...	Rather a large quantity of serum in the ventricles.	Traces of old contraction at apex of lung. Reinhardt and Leubucher. Case vii.
15	Pale, anaemic.	Distended.		Not obviously enlarged. Cortical substance pale, of a greyish red. Tissue soft and lax. Fibrinous casts in the tubes. Moderate catarrh of the pelvis. Bladder empty.	Uterus with bloody mucus, lining membrane hyperaemic and ecchymosed. Similar patches in vagina.	But little fluid in pericardium. Small ecchymoses at the base of the heart. Blood perfectly coagulated, quantity of fibrin small.	Lungs anaemic.				Traces of old contraction at apices of lungs. Reinhardt and Leubucher. Case viii.

Case.	Sex and Age.	Duration of severe symptoms.	Death in Collapse.	Death in Reaction.	Mucous Membranes. Stomach.	Small Intestines.	Large Intestines.	Follicles of Small Intestine. Solitary.	Aggregate.	Mes. Gl.	Spleen.
16	Female 54	54 hours.		Hydrocephalic symptoms.	uln distended with gen ld. Muc. th. on-, especially at the fundus, dark and ish adherent mue. Glands enlarged.	Beginning of dd. infiltrated with yellow m. In-tensely ed in pah-mic with pro-mnt fol d. In some parts	Old cxlr in descending lon. Solitary gls en-lg.	Enlarged.	Slightly enlarged.	Swollen and infil-r ted with hi.	Spots of re-cent hy-mosis; me. as large as a l lut. Tissue om-pact and full f dd. Wte cor-l les id-cl.
17	Me... 33	8 da/s.		Typhoid.	Muc. membrane of a slate ish a mll bou the ciia.	D'um dwith fl id, osts of a slate-grey color,...about the middle of mll in-test, dark red om-gestion. Gts yellowish-green,... fld, faeculent.	Below the valve conge-di, extravasa-ion of dd, and t rsfinl dd. Small m-scribed patches of diphtherite.	Enlarged.			Rith-rs, rd l ra, td Full of dd.
18	M... 37	7 d.		Bm with cm.	fgtion f the fundus, ish mall extrav ih.	Of a greyish-red dor distended with fluid, veins com-tgd, villi swollen, mll well-defined ul-cers from exfoliation of sol. glands. Diphth. exudation.	tled. tlj. Solitary glands tegd.	Brunner's glands swol-len. Solitary glands much enlarged.	Moderately enlarged.	Enlarged and pal.	Small, with spots of hemorrhagic congestion.

Case	Liver.	Gall-bladder and Ducts.	Peritoneum.	Kidneys and Urinary Passages.	Spinal Cord.	Heart and Blood.	Lungs.	Membranes.	Brain Substance.	Ventricles.	Remarks.
16	Not enlarged, ... congested.	Distended with bright yellow bile.	...	Cortical substance congested and swollen, and in many parts infiltrated with grau. matter. Apices of pyramids white.	Normal.	Ecchymosis at base of left ventricle. A large quantity of watery fibrin in right ventricle. Left contracted and empty.	Œdema of lower lobes. Ecchym. on pleura. Upper lobes dry and anæmic.	Superficial veins congested.	Medullary structure mod. congested, soft.	Very small quantity of fluid.	Reinhardt and Leubuscher. Case ix.
17	Liver pale, anæmic.	Moderately distended with dark-green ropy bile.		Numerous points of hæmorrhagic engorgement, extending deep into the tissue, dark brown or yellowish. In one point this infiltrat. had softened. Pelvis of kidney hyperæmic, with catarrh of the membrane. Not enlarged. Cortical subs. and pyramids in many parts pale.		Pericardium empty. Adhesions at anterior part of left ventricle. No ecchymosis. Tissue of heart soft,	Congestion and distension of the upper lobes. In middle and lower spots of apoplec. engorgement. Numerous small ecchy. on pleura.	Veins of surface congested. Œdema of the pia-mater.	Grey matter, pale. White, normal.	Bloody serum in lat. ventricles.	Ibid. Case xv.
18	Anæmic.	Catarrh of the ducts. G. B. much distended with clear watery fluid. Mes. mem. acutely congested. Diph. exud. ...slight ulceration.				Ecchymosis on base of heart. Fibr. coag. in both ventricles.	Apoplectic engorgement of post. lobes, with ecchymosis.	Veins of surface congested, subarachnoid effusion.	Moderately vascular, consistence normal.	Increased quantity of fluid.	Ibid. Case xvi.

Case	Sex and Age	Duration of severe symptoms	Death in		Mucous Membranes			Intestinal Glands		Mesenteric Glands	Spleen
			Collapse.	Reaction.	Stomach.	Small Intestines.	Large Intestines.	Solitary.	Aggregate.		
19	Male... 45	5 days.	...	Reaction, followed by gradual exhaustion.	Color, slate-grey, covered with tough mucus.	In lower half of ileum the val. conniv. much congested, and on the ridges diphth. exudat. The other portions of a slate-grey.	Muc. memb. of ascending colon and caecum raised into folds and botches by oedema of submuc. tissue with diphther. exudat. Here and there ulcerations.	Enlarged.	Enlarged.		Small, white corp. visible.
20	Male... 28	8 days.		Mild typhoid sympt.	Pharynx vascular. Diphth. ulcerat. Muc. memb. of oesoph. suffused with blood, and deprived of epithel.; diphth. inflamt. extending to mb-muc. tissue, in the lower third, surface at this part reticulated by small superficial ulceration. Stomach congested, with spots of extravasation. Glands swollen.	Duodenum congested. But very trifling vascularity of small intestines.	Spots of congestion and superficial diphth. exudat.	Brunner's glands enlarged. Sol. glands of ileum very slightly enlarged.	Not altered.		Rather large. Numerous excrudations of a pale color in the tissue.

Case	Liver	Gall Bladder and Ducts	Peritoneum	Kidneys and Urinary Passages	Spleen and Lymph. Glands	Heart and Blood	Lungs	Membranes	Brain Substance	Ventricles	Remarks
19	Pale and anæmic.	Gall bladder mod. full, bile bright green, with numerous floce. of epithelium, mucus, and mucous corpuscles.	…	Slightly swollen, cortical subst. of a reddish grey. Rather bright-colored urine in bladder.	…	Minute ecchymosis at the base. Fibrin, with soft dark cong. in right ventr. Left nearly empty.	Lower lobes hyperæmic and œdematous.	Normal.	Normal.	Normal.	Reichardt and Lembucher. Case xiv.
20	Pale, anæmic.	G. B. distended with a clear serous whitish-yellow fluid.		Rather enlarged and pale. Bladder empty.		Right side distended. Large fibrinous coagul. Some fibr. coag. in left ventr.	Slight œdema of the vocal chord. Diphtheritic ulcer on the pharyng. surf. of aryten. cart. Great congestion of trachea and larger bronchi. Hypostasis to a small extent in right lung.	Venous congestion of dura mater and arachn.	Vascular.	Some fluid in ventr.	Ibid. Case xxi.

Case	Sex and Age	Duration of severe symptoms	Death in		Mucous Mem.			Intestinal Glands.		Mesenteric Glands.	Spleen.
			1 mo.	Reaction.	Sth.	Small Intestines.	Large Intestines.	Solitary.	Aggregate.		
21	Male... 31	14 days.		Typhoid. Exanthem.	Congestion at the cardia and lo er part of œso ph.	Duodenum congested.	Limited patches of hyperæmia in cæcum, colon, and rectum.	Brunner's glands swollen, spots of great congestion and infiltration of blood. Solitary glands enlarged.	Many with small round ulcerations.	Slightly enlarged and pale.	Normal white corpuscles distinct.
22	Female 61	9 days.		Typhoid.	Normal.	Congested, and of a dark greyish co ol.	Congestion of the cæcum and large intestine grad. increasing in intensity from above downwards. The surface of the muc. mem. raised and infiltrated with diphth. exudation, in parts ulcerated. The whole surface of the rectum covered with the same of a brownish color.	Not obviously enlarged. Solitary glands enlarged.	Not obviously enlarged.	Kried and pale.	

Case	Liver	Gall Bladder and Ducts	Peritoneum	Kidneys and Urinary Passages	Female Sexual Organs	Heart and Blood	Lungs	Membranes	Brain Substance	Ventricles	Remarks
21	Full of blood.	G. B. much distended with pale yellow serous fluid containing mucus. Gall ducts distended with similar fluid.		Enlarged, the cortical subst. swollen, flabby, of a whitish grey. Catarrh of the pelves.		Fluid in pericard, Heart fluid, right side distended with partly coag. fluid, partly coag. blood with fibrinous coagula.	Slight ecchymosis on pleura, lungs much distended with air. Lower lobes congested and oedematous, small haemorrhagic spots. Muc. memb. of trachea congested.	Sub-arachnoid effusion. No congestion of veins. Old opacity of arachnoid. Choroid plexus normal.	Pale, rather oedematous.	Small quantity of serum in ventricles.	Reinhardt and Leubuscher. Case xvii.
22	Moderately full of blood.	G. B. distended. Bile brownish yellow.	Covered with an abundant exudation of adhesive fluid.	Enlarged; cort. subst. and pyramids at apices pale. Small extravasation in pelvis, with acute catarrh. Bladder empty.	Cavity of uterus filled with bloody mucus. Extravasation at fundus.	Increased quantity of fluid in pericard. Small ecchym. at the base of the heart. In right side dark fluid blood and fibr. coag., left nearly empty.	Very much distended with air. Lower lobes congested and oedematous, with haemorrhagic infarction. Bloody mucus in bronchi.	Congestion of the veins, subarach. effusion.	Moderately vascular.	But little fluid in ventricles.	Normal in size, small haemorrhagic exudat. into tissue. Ibid. Case xx.

Case	Sex and Age	Duration of severe symptoms	Death in — Collapse.	Death in — Reaction.	Mucous Membranes — Stomach.	Mucous Membranes — Small Intestines.	Mucous Membranes — Large Intestines.	Intestinal Glands — Solitary.	Intestinal Glands — Aggregate.	Mesenteric Glands.	Spleen.
23	Male ... 53	7 days.		Typhoid.	Covered with tenacious, adherent mucus. Congestion of the larger curvat. with spots of ecchymosis.	Muc. memb. of duoden. of a slate color. Congest. of small intest., especially at the lower part.	Much distended, greyish-red. Cæcum congested. Infiltration of the mucous folds of colon, with diphth. exudation several lines thick. Superficial ulceration.... In descending colon and rect. memb. raised by greenish-yellow infiltration. Sub-mucous tissue with white indistinction. Contents of intest. decomposed.	Brunner's glands swollen. Sol. swollen.	Not prominent.	Enlarged.	Large. Thickening and contraction of capsule. Tissue soft.
24	Female 8	Duration of attack 9 hours.			Distended with whitish turbid mucoid fluid, glands near pylorus enlarged.	In first part of duodenum Brunner's glands slightly enlarged, remainder of a faint yellowish-red, not of dark, and aggregate pale.	Muc. memb. of cæcum and ascending colon universally pale. In remainder and... enlarged.	Numerous, white	Large and prominent from infiltration of tissue.		9 § dark red, soft, structure distinct.

Case.	Liver.	Gall-bladder and Ducts.	Peritoneum.	Kidneys and Urinary Passages.	Female Sexual Organs.	Heart and Blood.	Lungs.	Membranes.	Brain Substance.	Ventricles.	Remarks.
23	Fatty.	G. B. distended.	...	Both atrophied and scarred by old contraction.	...	In right side a large soft watery fibr. coag.	Full of air, bloody and frothy serum in upper lobes.	Considerable quantity of sub-arach. effusion. Thickening of membranes.	Grey sub., pale.	Distended with clear fluid.	Reinhardt and Leubuscher. Case xix.
24	Hepatic tissue dark on section. Large vessels, especially hepatic veins, full of blood. Injection around some of the lobules apparently portal.	G. B. contg. 3 ss olive-green bile.		Larger vessels full of blood. Tissue normal.		Right auricle distended, contg. coagula. In right ventricle fibrinous. Mus. subst. healthy.	Fibrinous coag. stretching from right ventricle into pulmonary artery. Lung subst. dense, not normally crepitant, contg. very little serum.	...			Dr. Parkes.

a

| Case. | Duration of severe symptoms. | Death in | | Stomach. | Small Intestines. | Large Intestines. | Intestinal Glands. | | | Spleen. |
		Collapse.	Reaction.				Solitary.	Aggregate.	Mesenteric Glands.	
25	4 days.	Collapse.		Reddish-brown mucous fluid in stomach, muc. mem. slate-grey, with black points. At the fundus, bloody mucus, with spots of extravasation.	Convolut. distended. Congestion of the duodenum at the orifice of the common duct.	Great conges. of cæcum. Transverse colon pale. In descending colon and rectum extravasation and greyish-yellow and greyish-yellow exudation. Sol. glands enlarged, and ulcerated. Contents flocculent.	Much enlarged.	Moderately and uniformly swollen.	Swollen, greyish-red.	Firm, rather corrugated.
26	6½ days.		Reaction with typhoid symptoms.	Surface of muc. memb. covered with white tenacious mucus, intensely injected; most marked along lesser curve and post. surface. Inject. of the muc., capillaries, and punctate. Fib. cor. not reduced.	Muc. memb. of duod. pale, first inch or two yellow,...only very slight reddening of val. conniv. in the lower part of the jejunum. Vivid inject. of upper part of ileum. Contents brownish, fæculent.	Muc. memb. stained yellow. Transverse folds minutely and uniformly injected. Glands of moderate size, slightly injected on their surfaces.		Not visible except in lower 2 ft. of ileum, and then not much enlarged.		Wt. 7 ounces, color dark.

Case	Liver.	Gall-bladder and Ducts.	Peritoneum.	Kidneys and Urinary Passages.	Female Genital Organs.	Heart and Blood.	Lungs.	Membranes.	Brain Substance.	Ventricles.	Remarks.
25	Yellowish brown. Pale mottling. No portal nor hepatic congestion.	G. D. distended. G. B. moderately distended with dark-green tenacious bile.	Covered with slimy secretion.	Right kidney coarsely granular. Bladder empty, firmly contracted.	Extravas. into muc. membr. and muscular tissue of uterus. At fundus and os, and also in the vagina, on the ant. wall greyish-yellow exudation. In left ovary recent extravasation.	Fluid in pericard. Heart flaccid, covered with fat. Right ventr. distended with dark fluid blood, slight fibr. cong. upon tricuspid. Left ventr. contracted and empty.	Midd. and lower lobes œdematous, with inter. lob. emphys. Small hæmoptisic infarction in left. Ecchymosis of pleura at bases.	...	...	...	Bethhursit and Lawbumber. Case xxiii.
26	Wt. 44 ounces. Pale mottling. No portal nor hepatic congestion.	G. B. distended, contg. 3½ ounces of greenish thin turbid bile. Lining membrane injected and roughened, in parts opaque and dull.	Over stomach and small intestine pale.	Wt. without capsule 11½ ounces. Tissue flabby, cortical portion thick (swollen?) whitish, and coarse. Pelvis of right, pale, left slightly injected.	Not named.	Right auricle distended with dark coagula. Large fibrinous clot in right ventricle. Endocardium not stained.	Collapsed. Lobular pneumonia in upper lobes of both lungs. Œdema and congestion of lower lobes.	Rather pale.	Firm, not congested.	Scarcely a drop of fluid.	Dr. Parkes.

Duration of severe symptoms.	Collapse.	Reaction.	Stomach.	Small Intestine.	Large Intestine.	Solitary.	Aggregate.	Mesenteric Glands.	Spleen.
9 days.		Typhoid. Dyspnœa.	Small extrav. at greater curvature.	Of a slate-grey, rather congested, especially the ileum.	Congestion of cæcum, other part of large intest. pale.	But little altered.	But little altered.	Rather enlarged, grey, ish-red and white.	Spleen large, full of blood.
24 hours.	Suddenly in collapse.		Contains several ounces of fluid mixed with the remains of food. Muc. memb. not reddened, rather thickened, but not softened.	Distended of a dark color. Mesenteric veins full of blood. Duoden. of a dark color throughout. The vascularity occupies the villi. Villous struct. of jejun. very distinct, with some prominences. Contents "rice water," of a slight chocolate tinge. Muc. memb. reddened in ileum, generally reddened with ecchymosis, about a foot from termination.	Contracted. Ascending colon pale, in transverse colon slight injection of the mucous folds. Glands not visible.	Numerous, distinct.	Distinct, but not ulcerated.	...	Wt. 8	3. times blood-less.

Case	Liver.	Gall Bladder and Ducts.	Peritoneum.	Kidneys and Urinary Passages.	Female Sexual Organs.	Heart and Blood.	Lungs.	Membranes.	Brain Substance.	Ventricles.	Remarks.
27	Liver moderately full of blood.	G. B. flaccid. Bile dark brown.	...	Slightly increased in size, cort. subst. swollen, greyish red. Apices of pyramids pale. Slight catarrh of pelvis. Bladder full of dark urine.	...	Right side much distended with dark cong. and fibrin. clot.	Small ecchymosis on pleura. Lower lobes congest. and œdem., with hæmorrhagic exudation. Congest. of muc. memb. of trachea.	Congestion of the sinuses and veins, sub-arach. effusion. Choroid plex. full of blood.	Normal.	Some fluid in the lat. ventricles.	Reinhardt and Leubuscher, Case xviii.
28	Wt. 38 ʒ. Very little blood except in portal veins.			Cortical struct. pale, with a few vascular striæ. Thickness normal. A little milky fluid in pelvis. Bladder contracted.		1 ʒ of reddish serum in pericardium. Coronary veins full of blood. Right auricle and ventricle distended, and contg. fibrinous coagul. Dark cong. in left side.	Collapsed, inelastic. Pulmonary tissue bloodless, no œdema in any part. No ecchymoses on pleura. Bronchial tubes without mucus.	But little blood in long. git. sinuses. Vessels of pia mater moderately full, slight œdema.	Not injected. Consist. normal.	Quantity of fluid small.	Dr. Parkes.

Case.	Sex and Age.	Duration of severe symptoms.	Death in		Mucous Membranes.			Intestinal Glands.		Mesenteric Glands.	Spleen.
			Collapse.	Reaction.	Stomach.	Small Intestines.	Large Intestines.	Solitary.	Aggregate.		
29	Female 82	Death at beginning of fourth day.		Moderate reaction.	Flaccid,... large. Coats pale, punctate injection about greater curvature, small quantity of blood on surface, M. memb. of a yellow color.	Distended. Duodenum stained yellow. Lower part of ileum, much congested with ecchymosis. No enlargement of glands. Effusion of granular exud. of a yellow color. Muc. memb. not apparently softened.	Colon moderately contracted. M. m. pale, stained yellow near transverse colon with granular exudation. Patch of congestion in descending colon. Superficial ulceration near sig. flexure, leaving solitary glands undisturbed and spreading around them.	Not enlarged.	Not obviously enlarged, in many parts not visible.		3 ounces, shrivelled.
80	Male... 20	Ninth day.		In conv. fever.	Epith. detached in patches from lower part of œsophagus. M. m. of mix. color, of a dark color from congestion with numerous minute dark spots (ecchymosis).	Sol. glands of duod. enlarged.	Nothing abnormal	None visible in pl; rather prominent in lower part of them.	A little enlarged.		Not esp. healthy.

æ.	Liver.	Gall-bladder and Ducts.	Peritoneum.	Kidneys and Urinary Passages.	Female Sexual Organs.	Heart and Blood.	Lungs.	Membranes.	Brain Substance.	Ventricles.	Remarks.
29	Weight 48 ounces.	G. B. containing 2 ⅛ oz of bile, not id. Duct en- um. full of bile. Liver pale on san, tubular injection.	Covered with slimy album. secretion.	Urinary bladder contracted. Kidneys 8½ ℥. (½ oz inject. of fœs. Pyramids h dkry. M. mb. of pelis pa, ag. tish iñ, cag. of erfol ised th. and fee 1 nlei.	...	Heart flaccid. Right aur. empty. Sall firm les in right ventricle. Large soft black cag. in left ventricle.	Congest. posteriorly. Œdematous at apices.	Slight injection of vessels of dura mater and arach- noid. No œdema of pia mater. No increased vas. of cho- roid plexus.	Consistence good, nume- rous red points.	₃ss straw- colored serum.	Dr. Parkes.
30	Nat. color.	G. B. filled with dark- green bi.		Very large, text. um, softened, of a pale dull red. Capsule not id. Bladder contg. "a large quantity of clear healthy- looking urine."		In pericard. small quantity of hr m. Heart healthy.	Lwer lies on both ides pic, of a dark red, only lshn down, not cling in far, hr half of upper lobe in me s ts.				Dr. Baly.

Case.	Sex and Age.	Duration of severe symptoms.	Death in		Mucous Membrane.			Intestinal Glands.		Mesenteric Glands.	Spleen.
			Collapse.	Reaction.	Stomach.	Small Intestines.	Large Intestines.	Solitary.	Aggregate.		
31	Female 55	52 hours.	Collapse.		Containing 8 ℥ of a greyish pultaceous fluid. M. memb. pale and apparently healthy.	Peritoneal surface dark throughout. Universal venous congestion of muc. memb. most marked in ileum. Ecchymosis and fibrinous exudation about 3 ft. from cæcum. Villi prominent, not vascular.	Glands not visible, except in descending colon. Hæmorrhagic and papilliform injection of cæcum. Ascending colon pale. Transverse and descending colon injected. A few minute uniniform ulcers in rectum.	Slightly enlarged and white.	Prominent in upper part of ileum. Not visible at lower part.	Rather large and white.	Weight 2½ ℥ empty of blood.
32	Male... 36	12 hours.	Collapse.		Containing 1½ pint (from lead?) of dark-brown fluid. Muc. memb. not softened, nor glands enlarged. Congestion at the cardiac end.	Externally of a deep bright pink, except at lower third. Contents of duod. like those of stomach. Glands visible but not much enlarged. Villi very distinct. M. m. of a deep pink. Small intest. contained 40 ℥ of a turbid fluid of a choc. brown colour. M. m. of jejunum deep pink. Villi distinct. Duom. pale.	Contained ½ pt. of dirty white turbid fluid. No trace of epithelium. M. m. white and rather opaque. Sol. glands enlarged throughout.	Not distinct, except at the lower part of the ileum.	Very distinct, thickened, and opaque white.		Very small, retract, normal.

Case	Liver.	Gall-bladder and Ducts.	Peritoneum.	Kidneys and Urinary Passages.	Female Sexual Organs.	Heart and Blood.	Lungs.	Membranes.	Brain Substance.	Ventricles.	Remarks.
31	Wt. 3 lbs. 11 ʒ. Portal and hepatic veins full of dark blood. Secreting structures bloodless. Color and consist. normal.	G. B. extremely distended with dark-green viscid bile.	...	Wt. 7 ʒ. Surface smooth and pale, very slight stellate injection of surface, contr. post. on section pale, pyramids unaltered. M. memb. of pelvis pale, some milky fluid in them. Bladder empty, contracted.	Not named.	Pericard. without fluid, post. coronary veins much distended, ecchymosis beneath serous coat. Right aur. and ventr. distended with large clots. Endocard. and muscular subst. healthy.	Crepitant throughout. Congested post. and inferiorly.	Vessels of pia mater rather full.	Red points on section not numerous. Consist. natural.	Only a few drops of clear fluid.	Dr. Parkes.
32	Nat. size, dark slate color from post-mortem staining. Structure indistinct.	G. B. contained a mod. quantity of thick bile.	"The peritoneum and cellular tissue surrounding the small intest. much congested, blood effused to some extent into the tissue of peritoneum, around duoden."	Very small, of a deep brown color, structure distinct. Bladder contracted.		No fluid in pericard. No ecchymosis. Right side mod. quantity of blood with cong., in left blood fluid. No staining of membrane.	Ant. parts light in color. Post. much gorged with blood, yet everywhere crepitant. No fluid in pleuræ.				Dr. Baly.

Case	Sex and Age	Duration of severe symptoms	Death in		Mucous Membrane			Intestinal Glands.		Mesenteric Glands.	Spleen.
			Collapse.	Reaction.	Stomach.	Small Intestines.	Large Intestines.	Solitary.	Aggregate.		
33	Female 62	36 hours.	Collapse.	Reaction with albuminuria, delirium towards the end of life.	Muc. memb. pale except near pylorus, where there is injection. On larger curvature, near cardiac end, soft granular exudation slightly raised, accompanied with inject of large vessels. Near pylorus several pits produced by loss of substance, edges defined and injected.	General suffusion of large and small intestines, of a pinkish-grey. Injection and extravasation in duod. and commencement of jejunum. Ileum of a pale grey, very small ecchymoses in lower part.	Muc. memb. of cæcum pale grey. Inject. and ecchym. of transverse colon. Sol. glands a little raised in descending colon, not visible elsewhere.	Not apparently enlarged except about 2 feet from cæcum.	Follicles with whitish matter.		Flaccid, light coloured. Weight 3ii.
34	Male... 80	12 days.			Softening (probably post mort.), considerable ecchymosis at cardiac end.	Duodenum stained yellow. Brunner's glands not visible. Some black points at the commencement of duod. on apices of villi. Jejunum pale, rather stained. Ileum of a flesh tint.	Solitary glands barely visible. Muc. membrane stained, of a deep claret color.	Only here and there visible, apparently empty.			Weight 3iv, tissue mottled olive purple.

Case.	Liver.	Gall-bladder and Ducts.	Peritoneum.	Kidneys and Urinary Passages.	Female Sexual Organs.	Heart and Blood.	Lungs.	Membranes.	Brain Substance.	Ventricles.	Remarks.
33	Wt. 61 ℥. Tissue pale fawn color.	G. B. containing 1½ ℥ of dark red-dish-green viscid bile. G. D. full of secretion. Only small quantity of blood in veins.		Wt. 9½ ℥. Slightly granular from old disease. Tub. portion pale. Pelvis of left rather injected.		Vena cava full of dark coagula. Right auricle and ventricle simi-larly distended, containing fibri-nous clots.	Nothing re-markable.	Conside-rable quantity of blood in sup. long. sinus.	Nothing	abnormal	Old disease of mitral. Dr. Parkes.
34	General appear-ance of liver nor-mal. Wt. 56 ℥. Hepatic and portal veins mo-derately full.	G. B. full of bile. Lining memb. na-tural.		Wt. 16 ℥. Capsule readily removed, leaving surface smooth and moist. Cortical substance generally pale.		Right side and large vessels con-tain considerable quantity of dark coag. blood.	6½ ℥ of se-rous effus., tinged with blood in each pleura, ge-latinous fibrin, and recent pleu-ritic adhesions on right. Great con-gestion of post. part of both lungs, with hypo-stasic pneu-monia in the right middle lobe.	Dura mater opaque. Arachnoid, opalescent. Injection and œdema of pia mater. "Nearly ℥i of serum in occip. fossæ."	Grey mat-ter, lighter than normal. Consist. normal. White sub-stance, con-taining less red points than usual, rather wa-tery.	℥iii of slightly reddish serum.	Dr. Parkes.

Case	Sex and Age.	Duration of severe symptoms.	Death in		Mucous Membrane.			Intestinal Glands.		Mesenteric Glands.	System.
			Collapse.	Reaction.	Stomach.	Small Intestine.	Large Intestine.	Solitary.	Aggregate.		
35	Male... 45	63 hours.		Partial reaction with asphyxia.	Much contracted. Contents yellow turbid fluid, from 1 to 2 ounces. Muc. memb. of lesser curvat. congested, also summits of rugæ, near pylorus, with two or three superficial ulcerations, their surface greyish, edges sharp and injected.	Peritoneal surf. of small intest. much injected, particularly at lower part. No ecchymosis. Duod. and small intest. generally contained yellowish turbid fluid mixed with blood. Slight and partial inject. with occasional ecchymosis in duod. In ileum, congestion and ecchymosis, with diphtheritic effusion upon and into the tissue. No ulceration.	Peritoneal surf. of colon pale. In cæcum bloody fluid mixed with fæcal matter. Muc. memb. of cæcum dark, with venous injection. Ascending colon pale. From beginning of descending colon to rectum intense ulceration, irregular, superficial, surface yellowish-grey with vascular points, edges injected. Solitary glands visible, some pale, others injected, near the feet of the ulceration.	Visible in ileum.	But little affected. Diphth. exudation on one of the patches.	Large, "some of them containing pultaceous substance, not injected."	2 ℥ empty of blood.

Case.	Liver.	Gall-bladder and Ducts.	Peritoneum.	Kidneys and Urinary Passages.	Female Sexual Organs.	Heart and Blood.	Lungs.	Membranes.	Brain Substance.	Ventricles.	Remarks.
85	Wt. 49½ ℥. Paler than natural. Very little blood in the vessels.	One ounce of brownish bile in gall-bladder.	Dry.	9½ ℥, stellate. venous inject. of cortical substance pale. Slight inject. of muc. membrane of pelves. Bladder firmly contracted.	...	Spots of ecchymosis under close pericard. posteriorly. Large clot in right auricle and ventricle. Muscular tissue healthy. Two or three spots of ecchymosis on mitral.	No ecchymosis on pleurae. Slight congestion, tissue devoid of air.	Vessels of pia mater moderately distended. "A great quantity of fluid in the meshes." 8 ℥ collected from cavity of arachnoid. Thin layer of plastic exudat. over whole of left lobe of cerebellum.	Minute injection of grey matter of the convolutions. White substance natural.	From ℥ii to ℥iv of reddish serum. Choroid plexus rather injected.	Dr. Parkes.

Case.	Sex and Age.	Duration of severe symptoms.	Death in		Mucous Membrane.			Intestinal Glands.		Mesenteric Glands.	Spleen.
			Collapse.	Reaction.	Stomach.	Small Intestines.	Large Intestines.	Solitary.	Aggregate.		
36	Male... 30	12 hours.	Collapse.	...	Extremely distended. Muc. memb. pale, except at greater curvat. near pylorus.	Small intestines distended and injected. Muc. memb. of duod. pale. Brunner's glands and villi very distinct. Muc. memb. of jejunum and ileum with slight and occasional injection.	Ascending colon diamonded, transverse and descend. Muc. memb. throughout pale. Solitary glands large.	Numerous, enlarged, white.	Peyer's patches prominent, mostly pale, one or two slightly injected.	...	Wt. 3 3, containing but little blood.
37	Male... 84	About 20 hours.	Collapse.		Contents yellow, opaque. Glands prominent near cardiac end.	Duod. uneven, and glandular near pylorus. Stained of a deep yellow at the opening of the duct. Villi very distinct at the termination of duod. and throughout jejunum. Small intest. generally extremely pink, from arborescent venous injec. Muc. memb. in jejm. pale, in ileum congested in patches.	Sol. glands large, white, not punctate, some small, round, oval, or irregular ulceration. Traces of old ulceration.	In jejm. a few sol. glands seen, at end of ileum very prominent.	Pale.	Mesenteric glands pale.	Spleen of nat. consistence, rather pale.

Case	Liver	Gall-bladder and Ducts	Peritoneum	Kidneys and Urinary Passages	Female Sexual Organs	Heart and Blood	Lungs	Membranes	Brain Substance	Ventricles	Remarks
36	Weight 2 lbs. 1 ℥. Tissue cong. but little blood. Very slight, but defined, hepatic congestion. "Vena portæ full of blood."	In G. B. one ounce of thin yellow bile, bile flows from ducts on section of tissue.	...	Right, 4½ ℥. Left, 1 ℥. Minute injection of cortical substance of right. M. m. of bladder pale.		Right side and large veins full of dark coagula. No ecchymosis on pericard. Endocardium pale.	Pulmonary artery full of blood. In bronchial tube reddish frothy mucus. Pulmonary tissue cong. but little blood. Congestion, to a slight degree, in posterior lobes.	Vessels of pia mater moderately filled. Scarcely any serum in meshes.	Cortical subst. natural. Medullary rather congested.	But a few drops of fluid. Choroid plexus not injected.	Dr. Parkes.
37	Nat. in size and struct. Some dark parts, in which the centre of the lobules are black with blood.	G. B. half full of thin greenish-yellow bile.		Kidneys small, caps. adherent from old disease, tissue of a uniform red color, firm. Bladder contracted, containing 1 ℥ of opaque fluid, highly cong. by heat.		2 or 3 ℥ of straw-colored fluid in pericard. No ecchymosis. Large fibrin. clot in right cavities. In left blood liquid, no staining of endocardium.	Congested, particularly the left.				Dr. Baly.

Case.	Sex and Age.	Duration of severe symptoms.	Death in		Mucous Membrane.			Intestinal Glands.		Mesenteric Glands.	Spleen.
			Collapse.	Reaction.	Stomach.	Small Intestine.	Large Intestines.	Solitary.	Aggregate.		
38	Male... 50	12 hours.	Collapse.			Much contracted, of a pale red color. Mucous memb. of same color. Flakes of firm colorless glutinous matter lie on the m. m. Some adherent to it (mucus and epithelium).	Nothing abnormal.		Thickened and whitish, conspicuous in the midst of the generally congested surface.		Small and of nat consistence.
39	Male... 31	Whole duration 12 hours.	Collapse.	Partial reaction. Albuminuria.	Remains of food in the contents. M. m. pale and raised extensively by gas from decomposition.	M. m. generally pale, arborescent venous congestion externally.	Contents watery and turbid, but less so than in small intest. Sol. glands visible.	Generally enlarged in ileum, visible in jejunum.	Pale and prominent in jejunum and throughout ileum.		Pale, flabby, small.
40	Male... 39	7 days.			Much contracted, a slough as large as a split pea nearly through the coats at the cardiac end. Prostate large, surface covered with bloody mucus. Oesophagus much congested, a ring of congested glands in lower part.	Generally congested. In duod. and jejum. contents pulticeous and mucoid. In ileum more watery, and of a greenish color. M. m. in ileum generally pale and thin with some large venous ramifications.	M. m. pale and smooth. Sol. glands scarcely visible. In rect. m. m. a little vascular.	Only just visible.	Pale and thin.	Small and pale.	Very small, red in color and consistence.

Case.	Liver.	Gall-bladder and Ducts.	Peritoneum.	Kidneys and Urinary Passages.	Female Sexual Organs.	Heart and Blood.	Lungs.	Membranes.	Brain Substance.	Ventricles.	Remarks.
38	Flaccid and soft. Color dull red. Texture indistinct.	G. B. full of dark-brown bile, more fluid than natural.	Dry, and deficient in lustre.	Small, contracted (old disease), tissue dark, with arborescent venous injection. Bladder empty.	...	Heart large, flaccid, fat, and full of dark fluid blood, with some fibrinous coagula.	Not examined.	...	...	...	Dr. Baly.
39	Pale, color dull, texture homogeneous.	G. B. full of green bile. Common duct large, orifice into duod. patent and stained green.		Text. close and smooth, of uniform red color, capsule separ. easilv. Bladder contracted, containing ℥ss of turbid urine.		℥j of clear serum in pericard. No coag. in right side, no staining. Left ventr. not contracted.	Congestion of lungs extreme, the left the most so, in great part like pulmonary apoplexy.				Dr. Baly.
40	Rather small and pale, text. homogeneous.	G. B. full of turbid yellowish serous fluid contg. exrud. cells and blood corpus. Lining memb. pale yellow.		Large and congested, especially on the surface. Capsule adherent, subst. granular. Creamy fluid in pelves. In bladder, ½ pint of turbid dark urine, with whitish flocculi.		Rough and firm deposit of lymph on pericard. of base. Firm fib. coag. in right cavities, extending into pulmonary vessels. Left ventr. well contracted, contg. a firm dark clot.	Texture red, but everywhere crepitant. M. m. of bronchi deep red. Ecchymosis in spots on post. part of trachea.	No sub-arachnoid effusion.	Of normal color and consistence.	Containing only a few drops of fluid.	Cerebral oppression. Dr. Baly.

Case.	Sex and Age.	Duration of severe symptoms.	Death in — Collapse.	Death in — Reaction.	Mucous Membranes. Stomach.	Mucous Membranes. Small Intestines.	Mucous Membranes. Large Intestines.	Intestinal Glands. Solitary.	Intestinal Glands. Aggregate.	Mesenteric Glands.	Spleen.
41	Male... 20	21 hours.	Collapse.	...	Distended, pale. Muc. mem. at cardiac end thin and discolored. Veins of pancreas fuller of blood than natural.	M. m. of duod. very much injected, redness deep, punctiform. Brunner's glands distinct. Sol. glands not seen. Contents creamy and yellow. M. m. of jejunum vascular. Contents of small intest. gradually becoming more consistent to the end of ileum, where they are like half-melted glue (epith. and blood corpuscles). M. m. congested and ecchymosed, especially the last 2 or 3 feet of ileum.	M. m. pale. Contents creamy, without color. Sol. glands not very distinct, punctate.	Very prominent in ileum, not seen in jejunum.	Present nothing remarkable.	Not enlarged, but much congested and ecchymosed.	Flaccid, white corpuscles distinct.
42	Male... 24	10 days.		In consec. fever with albuminuria.	Contained a large quantity of turbid yellow bilious fluid. M. m. congest. at the larger cul-de-sac, generally mammillated.	Duod. muc. memb. quite healthy. M. m. of jej. and ileum opaque, villi distinct.	Sol. glands very prominent, with punctate spots at the apices.	In lower part of ileum distinct, pale, large, and prominent.	Not unusually distinct.	Large, but pale.	Nat. size and color.

Case.	Liver.	Gall-bladder and Ducts.	Peritoneum.	Kidneys and Urinary Passages.	Female Sexual Organs.	Heart and Blood.	Lungs.	Membranes.	Brain Substance.	Ventricles.	Remarks.
41	Subst. of liver of a dull red. Centres of lobules congested.	Ducts, even in the middle of the substance, stained yellow from bile. G. B. contains considl. quantity of dark-green viscid bile.	Natural shining appearance.	Small, full of blood. No creamy fluid in pelvis. Bladder contracted, contains only a few drops of turbid fluid, contents caudate, and pavement epithelium with blood corpuscles.		℥ii or ℥iii of turbid brown serum in pericard., some small ecchymoses on post. surface of heart, near base. In right cavit. loose dark coag. Left ventr. not contracted, blood nearly fluid. No staining of lining membrane.	Ant. parts normal. Post. three-quarters very full of blood, everywhere crepitant. Bronch. m. m. stained, of a deep red.	Vessels of dura mater very full of blood. Veins of surface of brain turgid. Arachnoid transparent. No serum beneath.	White substance, dusky grey, darker than normal.	Small quantity of clear fluid.	Dr. Baly.
42	Dull brown, struct. indistinct.	G. B. filled with almost black bile.		Structure uniformly red. Bladder full of urine.		℥iv of brownish turbid fluid in pericard., with fibrinous flukes.	Each pleura contd. about a quart of brown turbid fluid, with flakes of lymph on each side. Pleura pulmonalis of bases covered with recent adherent lymph, pneumonia of lower lobe on left side.				Dr. Baly.

Case.	Sex and Age.	Duration of severe symptoms.	Death in Collapse.	Reaction.	Mucous Me. Stomach.	small Intestines.	Large Intestines.	Intestinal Glands. Solitary.	Aggregate.	Mesenteric Glands.	Spleen.
43	Male... 27	36 hours.	Collapse.		Distended. Rill of a dark greenish-gy fluid, with m-cus envelop ng da-ml. M. m. pæl.	uḃd. containing dmel enveloped m. in Jej. and in externally of a gde red, lower part of ileum mch con-ted. Contents pæ, gradually agring color and more iæ. in lower part of mi.	Contents like those of ileum. Solitary glands very distinct and hi.	In lower part of ileum prominent and white.	Prominent. In lower partof ileum, two or three patches white and swollen with a few round clean cut cavities, apparently due to the falling out of entire folli-cles.	Of uniform pale pinkish color.	Very flac-cid, rather large, softer and paler than ordi-nary.
44	Male... 56	18 hours.	Collapse, asphyxia.			Of a remarkably dark dø, with large turgid in, containing a gruel-like fluid with numerous minute granular dø, M. m. hød, denuded of epith. and rough, "so as to resemble false membrane."	M. m. less congested than in small intes-tine, a chain of ecchymosed patches along the depending parts.		...		Small and very firm, of nat. color.

Case	Liver.	Gall-bladder and Ducts.	Peritoneum.	Kidneys and Urinary Passages.	Female Sexual Organs.	Heart and Blood.	Lungs.	Membranes.	Brain Substance.	Ventricles.	Remarks.
43	Natural size and consistence.	Ducts much dilated. Some filled with yellow- ish matter, of a putty-like consistence. In one branch two lanceolate distomata, G. B. full of dark-green viscid bile.	...	Of natural size, text. full of blood, especially the ... por... ... Nothing remark- able in ... of kidneys.	...	In ... but 1 ℥ of ... ...d, tinged with ... ...d, no ... larity. Staining of ...do- card.(commencing ...on in body). Blood in right cavities fluid.	Very much congested at the posterior parts.	Veins on surface of brain rather full, no fluid under arach- noid.	Normal.	...	Dr. Baly.
44	Of ... ...g, ...d- ...t, ...t, ... indistinct.	G. B. full of dark-green bile.		Size nat., tub. portions congeat- ed, of ...lk color. Creamy matter in pelves, large cyst full of cl...ar fluid at the ...ide of pelvis in left.		...℥ of serum in pe... ...d. R ght ...ntr. ...cid and ...h, containing a ...l, quantity of loose coagula, endocard. stained, of a ...rp purple ...y still warm when examined).	Pale su- periorly, much congested posteriorly, so as to sink in ...r, texture ... ...g.	Superficial veins be- tween ...lutions ...mb ...d ...sh dark fluid ...d. A large q... ...ty of ...am ...b- ...eath the arachnoid.	...fn, ...dy moderately ...gd.	℥is of ...r fluid in ...l. ...si. Old ...t. ...ts, some se- rous cysts on ...g.	Dr. Baly.

Case.	Sex and Age.	Duration of severe symptoms.	Death in		Mucous Membranes.			Intestinal Glands.		Mesenteric Glands.	Spleen.
			Collapse.	Reaction.	Stomach.	Small Intestines.	Large Intestines.	Solitary.	Aggregate.		
45	Male... 25	12 hours.	Collapse.		... ...	Distended, of a pale red color.	Solitary glands remarkably enlarged, and have at their summits grey pellucid points. Evidently filled with a clear fluid, which escapes when they are incised or punctured.	Enlarged, white.	In lower third of ileum thickened and pale (œdematous).	...	Rather small, dark color, nat. consistence.
46	Male... 41	22 hours.	Collapse.		M. m. of stomach generally pale, contains a pint of turbid fluid, much tenacious mucus adhering to the m. m.	Nothing remarkable in the aspect of the exterior. The duod. more congested than other parts of the m. In the ilium congestion of the m. m., and spots of hyperemia, especially along the unattached side of the intestine. Contents turbid and of a pale yellow color.	In ascending colon ecchymosis and some grey spots due to solitary glands, which are open.	Prest firm ? duodenum ? ileum, in the ileum also large open mouths.	In the ileum the majority are slightly thickened, and a few large not minute beyond and are congested, particularly in the lower part of the small intestine.	Small, pale, and reddish.	Small, soft, firm, dry, and pale.

Case.	Liver.	Gall-bladder and Ducts.	Peritoneum.	Kidneys and Urinary Passages.	Female Sexual Organs.	Heart and Blood.	Lungs.	Membranes.	Brain Substance.	Ventricles.	Remarks.
45	Very full of blood, particularly right lobe.	G. B. full of dark watery bile.	Nearly dry.	Very small. Dark, as if deeply stained with venous bld, but when incised but little bld escapes.	...	Heart flaccid, moderately full of fluid blood. No staining of the endocardi m.	...	...	...	...	Dr. Baly.
46	Liver small, of uniform color, texture rather dy.	G. R. id- ned, to 3 nies at size, length 4½ in, contg. 4 ʒ of semi-transparent, slimy, pale orange-co-led id. Sp. g. 1007. Turbid by ڸ, and nitr. id. In the fluid cylindric. epith., free nuclei, and old disc. tBts de, ctg. pale thin mucoid id.		Healthy, pelves contd. a small quantity of watery fluid (pale urine?) ith ittle flocculi. Bl hr contract-ed to size and hardness of a u ts, oats ⅓ in. di, dd. ⅓ ʒ of urine, which, when had, be-came like ilk		Pericard. con-tas an unce of pale m. In right cav. large ztk og, parly 1 ith, smaller, but of the same character, in left.	Tissue paler than usual, a little frothy mucus in bronchi.				Dr. Baly.

Case.	Sex and Age.	Duration of severe symptoms.	Death In		Mucous Membranes.			Intestinal Glands.		Mesenteric Glands.	Spleen.
			Collapse.	Reaction.	Stomach.	Small Intestines.	Large Intestines.	Solitary.	Aggregate.		
47	Male... 31	36 hours.	Collapse, with asphyxia.		Just above cardiac orifice in the œsoph. Many white bodies about the size of glandulæ solitar., similar at the cardiac orifice. Pancreas redder than usual.	Brunner's glands enlarged. Villi very distinct. Intestines externally of a pink color. M. m. of jej; pale and opaque. Ileum mottled with bright red patches. Epith. detached with ecchymosis beneath.	Some arborescent ven. congest, but m. m. generally pale. Sol. glands prominent, punctate at apices.	Greatly developed in last 3 or 4 feet of ileum.	Congested in jejun. In ileum cribriform. M. m. abraded and roughened with traces of old ulcerations.	Pale and small.	Nat. in size and consistence.
48	Female 22	31 hours.	Collapse.		Contents an opaque thin flocculent fluid. M. m. thin and very soft at cardiac end, mammillated in middle, an appearance of white promin. glands near pylorus.	Duod. m. m. glandular, green, staining at orifice of bile duct. Jejunum and ileum of dusky color externally. M. m. smeared with drab-colored mucus, when washed surface appears eroded. Congestion at edges of rugæ and around aggregate glands. Contents fluid of dirty deep drab color with mucus and powdery matter.	M. m. pale in descending colon and sigmoid flexure. Ecchymosis and venous congestion on depending part. Contents pale watery fluid with reddish sediment. Solitary glands prominent.	Large and white.	Not prominent.	Small, rather congested.	Very small and firm, of natural color.

Case.	Liver.	Gall-bladder and Ducts.	Peritoneum.	Kidneys and Urinary Passages.	Female Sexual Organs.	Heart and Blood.	Lungs.	Membranes.	Brain Substance.	Ventricles.	Remarks.
47	Tissue dark. Centre of lobules congested.	G. B. distended with dark-green viscid bile.		Tubular portion somewhat congested, whole tissue moister than usual. Bladder contg. ʒ3 of urine, loaded with albumen.		Pericard. contains a tea-spoonful of citron-colored fluid. Ecchymosis at apex of heart. Soft dark coag. in right side, extending far into pulmonary vessels.	Lungs much congested, crepitant.				Dr. Baly.
8	Large, pale. Lobular struct. distinct, in the centres of some an appear. of ecchymosis.	G. B. full of green bile.		Medullary portions and veins about pelvis full of blood. Cort. natural. Capsule easily detached.	Blood in cav. of uterus. Abrasion of os uteri. In right ovary a cyst as large as a hen's egg, full of gelatinous clot and bloody watery fluid.	In pericard. 1 dr. of clear citron-colored fluid. Heart large and flabby, ecchymosis at base posteriorly. Slight staining. Large coagula in right ventricle, partly fibrinous.	No fluid in pleura. Both lungs much congested posteriorly, but everywhere crepitant, a few small tubercles in summit of right. Bronchial glands not enlarged.				Dr. Baly.

Case.	Sex and Age.	Duration of severe symptoms.	Death in		Mucous Membranes.			Intestinal Glands.		Mesenteric Glands.	Spleen.
			Collapse.	Reaction.	Stomach.	Small Intestines.	Large Intestines.	Solitary.	Aggregate.		
49	Male... 64	16 hours.	Collapse, about 1½ hour after saline inject. into veins, restlessness, coma.		M. m. of cardiac extremity of a greyish tint and softened, in the parts in r nd, me mucus being sur pylo m.	M. m. of duod. of a dark e grey color, which grad. fades towards the jejun, orange-yellow staining around orifice of gll du. Brunner's glands much developed. In jejun. general tor of m. m. grey, ght phys. under mucous es. cG-tents reddish-grey "rice water."	End of ileum and cœcum not examined. In ascending colon sol. glands white and surrounded with greyish ring, punctate. M.m. greyish-red. In descending colon and sigmoid flexure great congestion, with ecchymosis.	Scarcely visible.	In jejunum Peyer's patches thickened and distinct by their whiteness. In the ileum not thickened.	At the surface pale, almost white, at the centres of a darkish-grey color.	Small and of natural consistence.
50	Male... 58	3 days.	Colapse int ... tense, died in the stage of r ... va, the pulse being no more than 80.		Pancreas dark from congestion. Contents of a much fluid dirty opaque yellow, some open mouths of glands near cardiac end.	M. m. of duod. s ained yellow with bile. M. m. in jej. presents nothing remarkable, in eüm tand of a yellowish-green.	In cœcum and colon solitary glands very numerous, large, and prominent.	In eüm all, prominent and hi, distinct by their opacity.	In ileum distinct, white, not much thickened, follicles open.		Small and shrivelled, of nat. color and consistence.

Case.	Liver.	Gall-bladder and Ducts.	Peritoneum.	Kidneys and Urinary Passages.	Female Sexual Organs.	Heart and Blood.	Lungs.	Membranes.	Brain Substance.	Ventricles.	Remarks.
49	Small, tissue rather redder than natural.	G. B. half full of greenish-yellow bile.	Having the natural shining appearance.	Texture natural, not congested. M. m. of pelves of nat. appear. Contents creamy, examined by the microscope, found to consist of epithelium.	...	Pericard. contd. a small quantity of serum, tinged with blood. Right side of heart very flaccid, contents fluid.	Ant. part of upper lobes pale, post. lobes on both sides much congested. M. m. of trachea and large bronchi congested, contg. opaque thick yellowish mucus.	Sub-arachnoid effusion in large quantity.	Watery and soft.	Several drachms of fluid.	Dr. Baly.
50	Nat. size, struct. dull red, homogeneous, lobules not easily distinguishable.	G. B. distended with dark-green liquid bile.		Kidneys full of blood, moist, texture uniform red. Ecchymosis on outside of capsule on one side.		℥i of clear dark serum in pericardium. A few small spots of ecchymosis on posterior part of base. Blood fluid. Staining of endocard. of right ventricle.	Very much gorged. On right side, lower ⅔ of lower lobe solid, pale red, and easily broken down. Patches of extreme congestion in left.	Vessels of dura mater turgid, veins on surf. of hemispheres not fuller than natural. No serum beneath arachnoid.	No obvious congestion.	Contains ½ ℥ of rather turbid fluid.	Dr. Baly.

Case	Sex and Age	Duration of severe symptoms	Collapse	Reaction	Mucous Membranes. Stomach.	Small Intestines.	Large Intestines.	Intestinal Glands. Solitary.	Aggregate.	Mesenteric Glands.	Spleen.
51	Male 33	12 hrs.	Collapse.		M. m. at cardiac end softened, pulpy dark brown (effect of digestion?)	M. m. of udd. pad Villi. ept. St. glands not much enlarged. Some m. of os gest in ci. Contents of jej. homogen. of a dull reddish tint with numerous dark sh e ds; in ilm more obc.	Contents, liquid, whitish, turbid. Numerous grey or black spots with small ulcerations (solitary glands?). Superficial ulceration in rectum. Interspersed with the black spots are enlarged white solitary glands.	Sol. glands enlarged throughout, most so at the lower extremity of the ileum.	Visible in jejun., gradually becoming more thick and prominent in ileum, where they are in contrast by their whiteness with the congested m. m.	Small and reddish.	Capsule speckled by white deposit. Texture mottled with spots of coag. blood and some large dark red masses.
52	Female 45	8		Imperfect reaction.	Coats of dull purplish dor. M. m. not add.	Duodenum glandular, yellow tining mr orifice of bile ia. Jejunum and ileum distended with gas. Gigedin of venous ramidha. M. m. not altered.	Not noted, except as being distended with ag.	In a all intestines not ht.	Only distinguished by paleness in midst of congested ems etc.	Small and pale.	Small, flexible, tough, of pale brown color.

Liver.	Gall-bladder and Ducts.	Pancreas.	Kidneys and Urinary Passages.	Female sexual Organs.	Heart and Blood.	Lungs.	Membranes.	Brain substance.	Ventricles.	Remarks.
Rat. in size, of a dark dull red (from decomposition?)	G. B. half full of opaque, dark-green, rather thin bile.		Rather small. Fine arborescent venous congestion of whole substance. Creamy matter in pelves. Bladder collapsed, containing 3ᵢ of slightly turbid urine.		3ᵢ of citron-colored and clear serum in pericard. Heart flaccid. Soft black coag. in right side. Some staining of pul. art. and valves. In left, blood almost fluid. No staining.	Everywhere crepitant, of dark red color throughout, much blood oozing on section.				Dr. Baly.
Of normal size, color, uniform dull red, lobular struct. indistinct, soft.	G. B. full of clear watery fluid, with pale greenish tinge, and a little mucus.		Left large, of pale dmb color, especially the cortical portion. Capsule adherent. 3 ounces of urine in bladder.	In cavity of uterus some coagulated blood. In right ovary two cysts of size of peas. One containing recent blood, the other clear watery fluid.	In pericardium a mere trace of fluid. Ventricle firmly contracted. Coagula in right ventricle firm and partly fibrinous. In left, soft and dark.	Both lungs firm from œdematous infiltration, and of deep red color throughout, a small portion in centre of right being in state of red hepatization; no tubercles. Bronchial glands not enlarged. Bloody froth in bronchi.	Sinuses and veins of surface of hemispheres turgid. Arachnoid transparent, slight œdema of pia mater.	Hemispheres of natural consistence, vascularity not remarkable. No softening of walls of ventricles.	3 or 4 drm. of clear watery fluid in lateral ventricles.	Dr. Baly.

51

Case.	Sex and Age.	Duration of severe symptoms.	Death in — Collapse.	Death in — Reaction.	Mucous Membranes. Stomach.	Mucous Membranes. Small Intestines.	Mucous Membranes. Large Intestines.	Intestinal Glands. Solitary.	Intestinal Glands. Aggregate.	Mesenteric Glands.	Spleen.
53	Male... 14	12 hours.	Collapse.	...	Loss of epith. in the interior of the œsoph. M. m. partly red, rugose, mammillated. White solid particles scattered over cardiac extrem. Pancreas healthy.	Sol. glands in duod. very large and prominent. Small intest. throughout of a pale red or pink, especially in upper half. Contents like vermicelli.	M. m. generally pale. Solitary glands transparent with opaque outline. Contents like fine gruel or arrowroot.	Promin. in cardiac end of stomach in duod. and in ileum.	Much thickened and rugose in jejum, and in ileum, where they are redder than the surrounding m. Most enlarged at the lower end of ileum.	Healthy.	Rather pale, small, firm, and fleshy.
54	Female 24	12 hours.	Collapse.		Contents like thin gruel, but of reddish-brown color. M. m. smeared with reddish mucus. Very numerous solitary glands near pylorus.	M. m. of duodenum reddish and glandular. M. m. of jejunum thick, white, and opaque. Villi very large. Venous network of ileum congested. M. m. hyperæmic. Villi of large size. No apparent abrasion or ecchymosis. Contents like thin gruel.	M. m. smooth, shining, and pale. Contents of consistence of thin gruel, but whiter than those of small intestines.	In ileum very distinct and white. In colon visible, but not enlarged.	White and opaque, but not much thickened. Some spots of deep redness beneath them.	Very small.	Half the nat. size, soft, and mottled in color.

Case.	Liver.	Gall-bladder and Ducts.	Peritoneum.	Kidneys and Urinary Passages.	Female Sexual Organs.	Heart and Blood.	Lungs.	Membranes.	Brain Substance.	Ventricles.	Remarks.
53	Nat. in size, structure red, fleshy, and homogeneous.	G. B. full of dark-green treacly bile.	...	Generally congested, especially tubular portion. Bladder firmly contracted.	...	Fluid in large vessels, some small coag. in right ventricle, blood mostly fluid. Left ventr. firmly contracted, no staining.	...	Dura mater very vascular. Veins of surface of hemisphere turgid. No fluid under arachnoid.	Congested blood oozing in dark drops from cortical and medullary substance.	Plex. choroid full of blood, ventric. fluid small in quantity.	Dr. Baly.
54	Of normal size and color. Lobular structure tolerably distinct, rather soft.	Half full of dark-green bile, of natural consistence.	Healthy.	Not enlarged. Capsules partially adherent. Creamy matter (epithelium) in pelvis of right, cortical portion pale; of left cortical portion deficient, and of dark red color. Bladder quite empty, but not firmly contracted.	Blood and mucus in the cavity of the uterus. Os uteri ulcerated. Coverings of ovaries thickened and congested. Cysts in one ovary.	In pericardium 1 dr. of clear citron-colored fluid. Heart small and flabby, valves healthy, no staining, no coagula.	No fluid in pleuræ, partial adhesion of left lung. Both lungs everywhere crepitant, texture throughout red and full of viscid blood, no tubercles. Bronchial glands healthy.				Dr. Baly.

Case.	Sex and Age.	Duration of severe symptoms.	Death in — Collapse.	Death in — Reaction.	Mucous Membranes — Stomach.	Mucous Membranes — Small Intestines.	Mucous Membranes — Large Intestines.	Intestinal Glands — Solitary.	Intestinal Glands — Aggregate.	Mesenteric Glands.	Spleen.
55	Male... 32	30 hours.	Collapse.	...	Containing brown opaque liquid, with some portions of food. M. m. pale and firm.	External appearance of intestines of a dark rose-red color. Duod. contains bilious liquid. In jejun. m. m. generally opaque and pale, at lower part some congest. and ecchymos. opposite mesentery. In ileum congest. of muc. memb. general with ecchymosis, especially at the lowest part, where the surface of m. m. is uneven and abraded. Contents of small intest. an opaque creamy dull red fluid.	No congestion. Solitary glands distinct.	Distinct in lower part of ileum, not large, open.	In jej. few, small, white, opaque. In ileum thick, white, and reticulated; follicles open.	Very small, white.	Small, flaccid, rather pale, of nat. consistence.
56	Male... 36	3 days.	Collapse, stupor. (Inject. of saline into the veins was practised, but without good effect.)		M. m. generally pale, some congest. at cardiac end.	Externally of a pale red, empty and contracted. M. m. congested throughout. Surface covered with mucus and exfoliated epithelium.	In caecum and colon sol. glands very distinct, punctate, with a grey circumference.	Throughout ileum promin. and white, especially at lower part. M. m. generally pale.	In lower part of ileum thickened, in some parts of ileum and jejun. redder than the surrounding memb., reticulated; follicles open.		Small, but otherwise healthy.

Case.	Liver.	Gall-bladder and Ducts.	Peritoneum.	Kidneys and Urinary Passages.	Female Sexual Organs.	Heart and &c.	Lungs.	Membranes.	Brain Substance.	Ventricles.	Remarks.
55	Small, color dull brown, text. homogeneous.	G. B. half full of dark-green bile.		Small and flaccid, uniformly red. Not contracted, but collapsed, containing about a tea-spoonful of milky fluid. Slight injection of m. m. but tint gone.		Fluid blood in right auricle and ventricle, some g. in latter. No staining.	Throughout full of dark blood.				Dr. Baly.
56	Of a uniform dull red. Struct. indistinct.	G. B. full, bile dissive, dark, and page.	No remarkable	Of nat. size, of deep red, tubular tems almost black. quite empty.		Presents nothing remarkable.	Much gorged with blood in posterior half, everywhere pitant.				Dr. Baly.

Case	Sex and Age	Duration of severe symptoms	Death in		Mucous Membrane.			Intestinal Glands.		Mesenteric Glands.	Spleen.
			Collapse.	Reaction.	Stomach.	Small Intestines.	Large Intestines.	Solitary.	Aggregate.		
57	Male... 25	21 hours.	Collapse.	...	Pancreas healthy. M. m. of stomach firm, of an opaque white color.	Contents fluid, of a bright yellow color, containing abundance of flakes. M.m. generally of an opaque white. Villi not very distinct.	M. m. of a dull dusky color. Contents small in quantity, like thin gruel.	Not very distinct.	Distinct, but not swollen.	...	Nearly double the normal size, texture firm, of a dark slate color.
58	Female 26	2 days 10 hours.	Collapse.		M. m. not altered. Contents greenish-yellow, opaque, fluid.	Duodenum healthy. Contents of a deep yellow color, pultaceous. Jejunum m. m., some patches of superficial ecchymosis. Contents, a yellow liquid of consist. of gruel with streaks of blood. In ileum, opposite to mesentery, a line of small patches of venous congestion and ecchymosis, increasing towards coecum. Blood in venous network quite black. In last 5 feet of ileum m. m. of dull grey tint, soft, and beginning to disorganise (dead). Contains the same as those of jejunum.	Colon m. m. generally healthy, two or three patches of a grey color with ecchymosis, at these parts here and there superficial ulceration with scalloped borders. In rectum the same state of m. m. without congestion or ecchymosis. Contents, a dirty yellow, turbid, watery fluid in large quantity.	In ileum not enlarged or prominent.	In upper half of ileum distinct and white, not thickened; in lower half obscured by the congest, ecchymosis, and disorganisation of the m. m.		Small, and moderately firm.

Case.	Liver.	Gall-bladder and Ducts.	Serous Membranes.	Kidneys and Urinary Passage.	Female Sexual Organs.	Heart and Blood.	Lungs.	Membrane.	Brain Substance.	Ventricles.	Remarks.
57	Nat. size, very full of blood. Struct. distinct, firm, of a dark color.	Gall bladder quite collapsed, contg. about a teaspoonful of very thick bile.		Of the normal size, of a dark-brown color, cortical subst. rather deficient, caps. not adherent.		½ ounce of straw-colored serum in pericard. No ecchymosis. Fibr. coag, in right side of heart.	Very intensely congested, everywhere crepitant.	...		...	Dr. Baly.
58	Dark red, text. fleshy, mottled, centres of lobules congested.	G. B. full of dark watery bile, with flakes of mucus.		Of normal size. Capsules adherent firmly at one or two parts. Cortical portion mottled, pale and dark dull red, natural fine mottling not seen, hard in consistence. Creamy matter in the pelvis. Bladder firmly contracted, containing 1 dr. of turbid urine.	Os uteri nearly obliterated, passage through cervix too small to admit a probe. Ovaries enlarged and adherent to surrounding parts, their structure altered.	In pericardium no fluid. Much fat on heart. Valves healthy, no staining. Large fibrinous clots in right cavities, black clots in left.	Old adhesions of right upper lobe. Both lungs crepitant throughout. Texture redder and drier than natural				Dr. Baly.

PATHOLOGY OF CHOLERA.

THE first unequivocal symptoms of Cholera indicate that the gastro-intestinal mucous membrane with its ganglionic nervous centres is the focus of the morbid action.

Whether there be a primary absorption of poison * into the blood or not is not at present known, though our knowledge of the laws by which many deleterious agents produce their effects renders the former hypothesis highly probable. But in our ignorance of the substantial cause of the disease and of the channels through which it reaches the body, whether through the skin, pulmonary membrane, or intestinal tract, we must expect that different views will be entertained by different observers, according to their speculative ideas on the nature of disease in general, or the theory they may have formed of the Cholera poison.

Pathology of the cholera-process in the intestines. The morbid appearances characteristic of Cholera are most marked in the small intestine, duodenum, and stomach, and the general symptoms indicate an early and severe depression of the ganglionic nervous centres of these parts.

The principal phenomena which arrest attention are the œdematous state of the mucous membrane, and the more or less extensive patches of capillary and venous hyperæmia, and ecchymosis. These, together with the character and amount of the fluid effused, demonstrate an important lesion of the circulation through the affected parts. How this is produced can at present be no further elucidated than by the hypothesis of a specific poison, acting upon the ganglionic nervous centres, or upon the mucous membrane itself. The former appears to us the more probable supposition, from being more in accordance with some other phenomena of the disease, as the profuse sweating and the sudden and severe collapse, which, as will be seen hereafter, is not in a necessary and constant relation to the discharges from the mucous membrane. Either would, however, suffice

* Since it is convenient to employ some short term to designate the cause of Cholera so as to avoid the tediousness of paraphrase, we have used the word "poison," and have spoken of the "Cholera poison;" thereby, however, intending no more than a general reference to the cause, without any theory of its nature.

to explain the altered condition of the circulation, since it is well known that if one of the agencies in operation in the capillary circulation be abnormal, there will be a corresponding change in the ease and rapidity with which the blood is sent through the tissue. In this respect nearly the same result is produced, whether the blood be unfitted to stimulate and nourish, or the nutritive operations in the part itself be perverted or defective, or the vessels be deficient in nervous supply. We no longer look for mere mechanical causes of vascular retardation, and whatever light may hereafter be thrown upon this stage of Cholera, it will no doubt come from a more intimate knowledge of the pathology of the capillary circulation.

These morbid changes in the first stage of Cholera are of the simplest kind;—the tissue is infiltrated, and the glandular follicles are distended with the same watery fluid as escapes into the cavity of the intestine;—the epithelium, by this maceration, readily separates after death, and to a certain extent during life, but not so largely as Böhm supposed. Exfoliation of the epithelium appeared to this excellent observer to constitute an essential part of the primary morbid action, but further investigations show that during life it occurred to only a very limited extent, and was in itself an unimportant change. The coats of the capillaries and smaller veins are often ruptured, giving rise to ecchymosis;—this and the punctate and stellate character of the hyperæmia denote a want of tonicity in the vessels.

As death occurs only when the phenomena reach their greatest intensity, and when the circulation in the venous system generally is much retarded, the ramifications of the intestinal veins in particular are often distended with dark blood.

An examination of the fluids effused from the mucous membrane gives no evidence of active plasmatic changes taking place in them. On the contrary, the large amount of fluid thrown out, its low specific gravity, and its other physical characters, indicate an almost passive exosmosis as through a dead membrane. Some observers have referred the morbid changes to a *catarrhal condition*, others have regarded the disease as a form of *serous hæmorrhage*, and the Berlin pathologists, whose attention was particularly arrested by the occurrence of amorphous granular fibrin in and upon the affected surface of the mucous membrane, designate it a *destructive diphtheritic inflammation*. We believe that, for the present, such generalizations, however plausible, are of little value, and that we arrest inquiry by their adoption. The depression of the capillary power—the extreme exhaustion of the great ganglionic nervous centres in the abdomen—the passive character of the lesions of the mucous membrane,—its normal action being reversed to a fatal exosmosis—are peculiar to Cholera, and give it an individuality which forbids our merging it for the present in any general category.

Although the intestinal tract is the principal seat of the morbid actions, they are not limited to it.

The kidneys, at an early stage, are sometimes affected; the urine having been found albuminous prior to its suppression, and the secreting tissue and the lining membrane of the pelvos occasionally presenting after death lesions of the same character as those observed in the intestine.

In the female the uterine organs were similarly affected, the lining membrane of the uterus and vagina being frequently much congested and ecchymosed, with commencing diphtheritic exudation upon it.

The liver is free from disease, except in some rare cases, where the lining membrane of the ducts and gall-bladder is the seat of the cholera-process, their contents being then of the rice-water character.

The distension of the gall-bladder with bile is nearly constant, but cannot be referred to as a pathological indication of any moment, as such a condition is common when the digestive function is long interrupted, and indicates a passive rather than an active state.

There is a hypothesis regarding the nature of Cholera based upon the supposition of a suppression of the hepatic secretion, and consequent congestion of the liver; this is altogether unsupported by anatomical facts. The absence of bile from the evacuations is not a necessary phenomenon of the early stage of Cholera. In a large proportion of cases the diarrhœa ceases to be bilious, only when the more intense symptoms set in, and even then, the "rice-water" fluid often gives, with re-agents, distinct evidence of the presence of bile, but when it is no longer passed in the evacuations, the secretion is not altogether suppressed, as shown by the contents of the gall-bladder and ducts after death. The hepatic function does not appear to be subject to any further derangement than that which naturally *follows* *upon* the retardation of the circulation during the stage of collapse.

It would have been unnecessary to advert to this hypothesis had it not widely influenced the treatment of the disease. Dr. Ayre, the great advocate of the administration of calomel, gives the following rationale of the cholera-process. He says, " Now there is one condition which is uniformly and conspicuously present in malignant

Cholera, and is, indeed, characteristic of it; namely, a suppressed or suspended secretion of bile, as shown by the diminution, and at length the total disappearance of it from those watery discharges which are poured so profusely from the stomach and bowels. As a consequence of this cessation of the hepatic function, an accumulation," he adds, " will take place in the liver, of venous blood, and an impeded circulation result from it, producing a congested state of that organ, and subsequently, by a retention of the blood in its course through them, of those abdominal organs whose circulation is associated with it. Now the congestion thus produced in the portal venous system of the liver and its associated organs, constitutes the stage of collapse, and under various modifications and grades of intensity, whose real nature and amount are unknown, forms the essence of it in all."

Such a train of reasoning is unsupported by any evidence. The serous, rice-water character, of the Cholera stools, is obviously due to special pathological changes in the mucous membrane, and not to any merely mechanical congestion of a secondary kind, as here stated. What these pathological changes are, we have endeavoured to show, and have referred them to a specific action of the Cholera poison operating through the blood; a more minute account we are unable to give.

The appearances after death in the chest and cranium show that the viscera in these cavities were not primarily affected. The occasional emphysema of the lungs, their emptiness of blood, except at the posterior and inferior parts, and the inelastic compressed character of their tissue observed in some cases, are explicable by the state of the respiration and circulation in the last stage of life.

The congestion of the veins, and the effusions under the membranes and into the ventricles of the brain, are referable to the same cause.

Although the blueness of the skin in many cases may be in part due to a general retardation of the venous circulation, it is, we believe, more commonly owing to a condition independent of such a cause, and appears to be a pathological indication of a loss of tonicity in the capillaries and capillary veins.

The intensity of the colour is not in proportion to the loss of fluids. Slighter degrees of it are, in severe cases, discoverable about the upper lip, alæ of the nose, and around the eyes, before any large amount of fluid has been lost, or the propelling power of the heart is greatly diminished. This colour may be produced in its intensest degree, upon the healthy skin, by exhausting the capillary tone by sparks of electricity drawn from any part of the surface. In the skin of young children this effect readily takes place. The blue tint in such a case is obviously independent of inspissation of the blood, or of a diminution in the propelling power, since it follows slowly after the application of the stimulus, and the effects are transient.

Many of the symptoms of the cold stage evidently depend upon the loss of fluids from the blood, and consequently have been removed in a sudden and remarkable manner in those cases where saline injections have been successfully thrown into the veins.

Cholera has been classed amongst zymotic diseases, but its clinical history and morbid anatomy are opposed to the theory of its being due to a zymosis, in a strict sense of the term. In a zymotic disease, the ζυμη induces certain plasmatic changes, from which results its augmentation. In Cholera, we have no evidence of such changes, the alterations in the blood, so far as they are yet known, being referable to the loss of its fluid parts, in accordance with the physical laws of exosmosis. The local morbid action appears to be of a negative rather than of a positive kind. The marked depression of the organic functions, and the morphological characters of the effused fluids, as well as their general physical properties, indicate a passiveness almost peculiar to Cholera. In Cholera, the onset of an attack is frequently sudden, and the effects apparently direct, such as would follow the immediate action of an extraneous poison upon the body. The zymotic process is more gradual, and the symptoms follow a more constant rule with respect to time.

Is Cholera a zymotic or contagious disease ?

Cholera appears to consist of but one single series of actions, which may vary in intensity through every gradation, but, throughout, maintain the same character of passiveness. There is no febrile stage, to which zymotic changes, as ordinarily observed, and the production of a materies morbi may be referred.

The fluid effused from the intestinal mucous membrane has by some been regarded as a materies morbi, possessing the power of propagating the disease. As it is the effect of the morbid action, it is so far a materies morbi, but beyond this we cannot at present predicate anything concerning it.

Dr. Snow has framed a theory of the diffusion of Cholera upon the hypothesis of a contamination of the water-supply of cities and towns by the evacuations, but he gives no facts to prove that they have the power he attributes to them, nor have we any evidence that they can excite the disease.

We can confirm Schmidt's remarks, that those who were occupied

in examining the discharges, and inhaled the effluvia from them, felt
no ill effects. They were also brought into contact with abraded
surfaces with impunity.

They who were engaged in making post-mortem examinations of
Cholera subjects seemed to incur no risk of thereby taking the disease.

Schmidt *, states, that within his own knowledge, a drunken man by
mistake swallowed half a beer glass of the vomited matters, slept
away his drunken fit, and remained well. Many similar facts, he
says, were made known during the epidemic of 1831–32, when
medical men, by way of experiment, swallowed these transudations
without injury; but he adds, "I have not had self-denia. enough to
institute these experiments on myself." Mr. Marshall† remarks,
that the performances here alluded to were limited to *tasting the
vomited matters* only, and did not extend to *swallowing* the *alvine
evacuations.*

Many experiments have been made upon animals with the blood
and effused fluids in Cholera, with the view of determining whether
the disease is communicable by them. Fresh Cholera blood and
filtered " rice-water fluid " have, in different instances, been injected
into the veins of dogs, cats, and rabbits, without producing any effects
that indicate a specific poison, the results being only a temporary depression, and in some cases slight diarrhœa.

The evacuations have also been thrown into the stomachs of these
animals by Meyer‡ and Marshall, but with uncertain results.

In 11 instances no ill effects followed beyond temporary depression
and slight diarrhœa. In 6, death took place in from 24 hours to 5
days. Mr. Marshall observes upon these experiments, that " equivocal
rice-water discharges, bluences, coldness, cramps, tarry blood, and non-
secretion of urine, are not in the catalogue of the effects, and so long
as we know so little as a ground of comparison of the pathology of
natural Cholera in animals, we cannot draw safe conclusions from the
phenomena produced by the administration of the Cholera evacuations."

General   Certain prodromata of a general kind have been
prodromata.   enumerated as occurring prior to the symptoms which
                  arise from the local morbid action in the intestinal
mucous membrane, such as vertigo—headache—general malaise—

* Characteristik der Epidemischen Cholera, p. 81.
† On the Communicability of Cholera to Animals, Med. Chirur. Review,
April, 1853, pp. 390–409.
‡ Archiv. von Virchow und Reinhardt, Band iv. pp. 29. 54.

muscular fatigue—faintings—wandering pains in the limbs—cramps—gripings in the abdomen—sense of weight at the precordia—and nausea. A cursory inspection of such a category suffices to show that, even if generally present, these indications would be unsatisfactory. Many of them arise from mental emotion, so prevalent during an epidemic, and others are not so much premonitory of an attack as the first symptoms of its onset, and the result of the morbid action already begun in the abdomen. It may be worthy of remark, that in several of the communications received the writers state that, without any further symptoms, they suffered from frequent spasmodic pains in the bowels, and cramps in the calves of the legs, during the height of the epidemic; a circumstance also alluded to by Mr. Grainger in his report *. " This peculiar twitching," he says, " was often observed in London during the late and previous epidemic, especially in those districts where the disease was severe. It is an interesting fact pathologically, that these slight cramps, which, like the other symptoms, were not of course always followed by collapse, being indeed most amenable to treatment, often occurred without being preceded or accompanied by diarrhœa, a circumstance which tends to show that the violent cramps and spasms accompanying the profuse discharges in collapse do not depend on these, but rather on the morbid quality of the blood deranging the force of the spinal cord." The pathology of these irregular symptoms here given is doubtful, since they are equally referable to a derangement of the nervous functions from fatigue and the other depressing concomitants of the epidemic.

Briquet and Mignot† made careful inquiry upon the subject of prodromata in 188 cases admitted into La Charité; of these, 88 were labouring under other diseases at the time of the attack of Cholera, and hence any such symptoms, if present, would have been ambiguous; 83 stated decidedly that they had experienced *no feeling of indisposition before the occurrence of diarrhœa ;* 18 had precursory indisposition of variable duration as follows:—

Cephalalgia was observed in	3 cases.
Vertigo and noises in the ear in . . .	1 ,,
General malaise and weariness in .	9 ,
Pains in the stomach in	6 ,,
Loss of appetite in	4 .

* Op. Citat., p. 104.
† Traité Pratique et Anatomique, &c., p. 128.

" In some of these patients, there were at the same time, derangement of sensibility, and a perversion of the digestive functions. The symptoms here enumerated lasted from 8 to 10 days in 3 cases;—from 2 to 4 days in 7 cases;—1 day in 1 case;—several hours in 4 cases;—from a fortnight (!), to a month (!), in 3 cases." It will be seen from this statement, that in only 5 cases out of 100 were the general premonitory indications, including their character and duration, in any degree to be relied on. It may therefore be repeated, that, practically, the earliest signs of the disease are from the gastro-intestinal mucous membrane and its nervous centres.

Premonitory diarrhœa.

In most cases a painless diarrhœa, lasting for a variable time, precedes the more characteristic symptoms. Although all observers admit the frequency of this precursory stage, there has been some difference of opinion and much unfruitful discussion about its pathology, whether it be a part of the disease, and due to the action of the poison, or merely a common diarrhœa, upon which the specific effects may at any moment be engrafted. There are no characteristics which enable us to draw these distinctions, with any certainty.

Experience has abundantly shown, that during the epidemic the stages from a mild and apparently simple diarrhœa to the rice-water purging and collapse are not definable, and that the former, if unchecked, does in numerous instances gradually pass into the latter, with its attendant collapse and fatal results.

There is evidently in some minds a disinclination to regard any case as Cholera, unless it manifests symptoms of marked intensity; but that the diarrhœa which prevails when Cholera is epidemic is due to the same cause as Cholera itself, is to be inferred not only from its clinical history, but also from other circumstances.

The extent to which diarrhœa prevails, and its gradations towards Cholera, are greatly in favour of such a conclusion.

Again, its invariable occurrence with Cholera apart from any influence of season;—for whether Cholera prevails in winter or summer, epidemic diarrhœa is attendant upon it, as a shadow upon substance, and is apparently as independent of these external conditions as Cholera itself.

Frequency of premonitory diarrhœa.

In answer to the fourth query in the circular letter issued by the College, referring to the groups of symptoms preceding the full development of the Cholera attack, numerous replies were received, all serving to establish the frequency of a stage of diarrhœa, lasting from a few hours to several days. Of these we may quote a few which indicate the character of the whole. Mr. Paul, surgeon to the Bermondsey workhouse, says :—

"As a general rule the attack of Cholera was preceded by diarrhœa, at first fæculent, then watery, lasting for 2, 3, or more days, or there was an occasional looseness for 2 or 3 weeks, generally without pain, and giving a sense of relief, which prevented the patients accepting medical aid."

Mr. Hooper of Haggerstone, the Cholera officer of the district, writes as follows :—

"It is known that Cholera has sometimes attacked individuals without any premonitory symptoms whatever. I feel confident however that, in by far the greater number of cases, careful enquiry will elicit the fact of previous ailment, the most general symptom being diarrhœa. My own experience leads me to give the following as the usual group of symptoms preceding the full development of the attack ;—loss of appetite, uneasiness about the præcordia, with more or less pain and oppression, and diarrhœa, at first bilious, with or without pain in the bowels, sometimes but slight in quantity, sometimes profuse, and often lasting for several days before the evacuations became serous."

Dr. George Burrows states—

"Out of 134 cases of Cholera of different degrees of severity which came under my own charge during the present epidemic, I have not met with one where the full development of the attack has not been preceded by some relaxation of the bowels. Of 7 cases which I have attended in private practice 4 terminated fatally, in 3 of these a relaxed state of the bowels existed for some days before collapse occurred. The duration of this state of simple looseness appears to vary considerably : I have known cases where it has existed for 10 days or a fortnight and been almost neglected by the individual. In such cases where the more confirmed symptoms appear, they run rapidly on to a state of profound collapse."

Mr. Tebay of Westminster says :—

"The symptoms have been variable, usually diarrhœa, followed in a few hours, or a day or two, by vomiting and cramps—occasionally diarrhœa, vomiting, cramps, and collapse have come on at once ; in a few cases sudden collapse has supervened, without previous diarrhœa, and carried off the subject in a few hours."

Dr. Bainbridge, medical officer to St. Martin's-in-the-Fields, says :—

"Diarrhœa for several days or hours, almost invariably preceded the full development of collapse. Out of 48 cases of pulseless collapse, I have not seen one without the premonitory diarrhœa. Sometimes the diarrhœa was painless, but in many cases it was accompanied with violent pain and cramps in the abdomen."

Mr. Painter, medical officer to the parish of St. Margaret's, Westminster, says :—

"In the majority of cases the symptoms preceding an attack were diarrhœa, varying in duration from a week to 12 hours, followed by sudden sickness, vertigo, and cramps. I have, however, seen many cases of collapse where there were no promonitory symptoms."

Mr. Frost, of Kensington, says :—

"In four-fifths of the cases there was premonitory diarrhœa, for which no remedies had been administered."

Dr. Burchell, medical officer to the parish of Shoreditch, says :—

"Diarrhœa preceded the attack in every case that came under my notice. It was usually of a more depressing character than under ordinary circumstances."

Mr. M'Clure, surgeon to a corps of Royal Marines at Plymouth, says :—

"I was often astonished at the numbers brought into the hospital in a state of collapse. The men were sometimes so far gone as to be unable to give any account of the commencement of their illness. Upon enquiry, however, from others, it invariably came out that they had been suffering from diarrhœa for at least a day or two previously. I have met with some instances in which it was ascertained that the bowels acted above 20 times within a couple of hours, and in a number of cases this excessive diarrhœa was considered by the men as salutary. Of 300 cases of genuine Cholera, which I have observed, I have never yet met with an instance in which the disease was not preceded by diarrhœa of longer or shorter duration."

Notwithstanding the above evidence, as to the frequency of diarrhœa, it is affirmed by many, and is in accordance with our own experience, that numerous cases occurred where this stage was very short, and the onset of the symptoms remarkably sudden.

Dr. Peacock, who had under his care many of the children from Drouet's Asylum at Tooting, says :—

"It was not easy to obtain satisfactory information as to the previous state of the bowels in the more severe class of cases. In two or three instances, the children were known to have suffered from diarrhœa to a greater or less extent during the night, and the more urgent symptoms supervened at 8 or 9 o'clock in the morning, but in others no complaint was made of any previous indisposition, vomiting first attracting the notice of the attendants. In all these cases, however, the evacuations passed were entirely colourless, and, as the alimentary canal after death presented no appearance of fæcal matter, the severe symptoms must have been preceded by diarrhœa of a longer or shorter duration. The period which elapsed from the first accession of the alarming symptoms to complete prostration was usually very short. In the first three fatal cases, it was stated, that the children sunk into extreme collapse *within an hour*, and, in the fourth case, which I had myself the opportunity of watching throughout, the hands and feet were cold and livid, and the pulse scarcely to be felt at the wrist in less than *half an hour* from the commencement of serious indisposition."

Mr. Guazzaroni, medical officer to Kensington workhouse, says:—

" There was a premonitory diarrhœa in about one-half the cases (I do not here speak from written notes), but I am sure it was not present in more. Many cases had rather confined bowels, good appetite, and were even in good spirits, up to the time of the sudden invasion of the disease."

Dr. Harding, of Golden Square, says :—

" The worst cases of Cholera I have had under my care were preceded by little or no diarrhœa."

Dr. Basham says:—

" Sudden prostration attended by vomiting, and purging of serous discharges, appeared to me to be the most characteristic symptoms preceding a full development of the disease. In some cases they were not of more than 2 or 3 hours' duration before the most hopeless collapse set in."

Dr. Wilson of Haslar describes the attack as sometimes coming on with overwhelming force:—

" Soon after eating a hearty meal in perfect health, the subject has been obliged to be relieved from duty in the ranks, or on deck, becoming in an instant faint and giddy, with a rush of fluid from the stomach and bowels, the features being collapsed, the pulse fluttering, and the surface, tongue, and breath cold. These cases," he adds, " were invariably more fatal than where there had been precursory diarrhœa, or where there had been a gradual, though rapid, progress into collapse."

According to Reinhardt and Leubuscher, "diarrhœa was in the greater number of cases the first abnormal symptom;—it generally lasted ½, 1, 2, 8, or even 14 days before other symptoms set in. In many cases it came on simultaneously with vomiting and cramps, mostly before, sometimes soon after these, and commonly in the night. Where diarrhœa preceded for a long time the Cholera attack, the stools were neither frequent nor copious. In 24 hours, 2, or at most 6; these, sometimes gradually, but more often quite suddenly, without any intermediate stage, became as frequent as 20 in 24 hours, and were very profuse; then set in the other symptoms."

Of 200 cases observed by Briquet and Mignot, 12 gave no precise account of the commencement of their symptoms. Amongst the 188 others, there were 45 in whom the attack was sudden, invading as it were at once all the organs, and developing in the space of from half an hour to an hour, the most intense symptoms; such as vertigo, trembling, vomiting, diarrhœa, loss of expression in the face, falling of the pulse, coldness of the body, &c. In 143, these symptoms were constantly preceded by diarrhœa more or less severe.

In some cases it was difficult to determine the period within which the symptoms of invasion gave place to those of a more marked character. But these observers state, that in general they were able to fix the period definitely. As follows :—

In 3 cases				1 hour.
5 „				2 hours.
3 ,				3 „
6 ,		.	.	4 „
2 „	.	.	.	5 ,
10 „	.	.	.	6 ,
1 ,	.	.	.	8 ,
9 ,	.	.	.	12 „
2 ,		.	.	16 „
24 ,	.	.	.	1 day.
11 .		.	.	1 day and a half.
21 ,	.	.	.	2 days.
14 „	.	.	.	3 „
3 ,				4 ,
3 „	.	.	.	5 „
2 ,		.	.	6 „
13 ,		.	.	8 ,
2 ,		.	.	10 „

The diarrhœa premonitory of the severer symptoms of Cholera was often feculent and bilious, and presented no characteristics whereby it could be certainly distinguished from other forms. There were, however, occasionally some subordinate points of slight diagnostic value. The evacuations were generally more profuse and liquid than usual, but otherwise of a natural appearance, often unaccompanied by pain, and passed without effort, the painlessness and passiveness giving a false security to the patient. It was not until the nervous system began to be depressed, and the feculent character of the stools was lessened or lost, and they became alkaline, watery, and flocculent, that they were distinctive. On this point, the experience of the profession appears to be uniform, and hence we may draw the following important conclusion ;—that during the prevalence of the epidemic every case of diarrhœa arising without obvious cause may be regarded as a probable result of the specific poison.

The following quotations will show the general tenour of the evidence received by the College on this subject.

Dr. Plomley of Maidstone says :—

" I have not observed any distinctive marks by which a diarrhœa about to pass into developed Cholera may be recognised. All the cases I have had the opportunity of minutely observing, have begun with the usual feculent and bilious diarrhœa passing with more or less rapidity into the rice-water discharges."

Dr. Fincham says :—

" I have searched in vain for any distinctive marks. This, however, I can state, that several scores of cases of diarrhœa fell under my care at the Western Dispensary, whilst the epidemic was raging, in many of which the evacuations were thin and colourless and profuse, but in which I had no difficulty in checking the flux."

Dr. Roupell says :—

" I know of no means of distinguishing."

Dr. Shapter of Exeter says :

" Its chief characteristic is its painlessness, and its passing from a light colour and yeasty appearance into the rice-water evacuation."

Dr. Barlow says :—

" I know of none besides coldness of the tongue, shrinking of the

x

eyes, duskiness of the countenance, and shrinking of the skin of the hands."

Mr. Hooper of Haggerstone says:—

"I have not observed any distinctive sign in the diarrhœa which has afterwards passed into developed Cholera, that is, before the stools or vomited matters have become serous."

Dr. Shearman of Rotherham says:—

"In my opinion there is less griping pain in the abdomen about that time."

Dr. George Burrows says:—

"My opportunities of watching cases of diarrhœa, which have subsequently passed into confirmed Cholera, have been few. I have not observed any distinctive characters between the diarrhœa which has been arrested by simple remedies, and that which has preceded confirmed Cholera."

Dr. Wright of Wakefield says:—

"Diarrhœa about to pass into Cholera is distinguished by the evacuations becoming more watery and devoid of feculent smell, with symptoms of approaching collapse."

Mr. Guazzaroni of Kensington says:—

"The diarrhœa about to pass into developed Cholera, is generally unattended with pain, and of a watery character with flocculent deposit. The evacuations are passed without effort."

Dr. Moore of Tunbridge Wells says:—

"I could not say when a diarrhœa was about to pass into developed Cholera, but the absence of fecal characters from the evacuations, the diminution in the bile, and a large amount of fluid would induce me to think that a patient would soon fall into Cholera."

How far collapse depends upon loss of fluids.   The Cholera poison is not known to produce its fatal effects without the characteristic affection of the intestines. Cholera sicca, in a strict sense, does not occur, for although the disease may be fatal without any evacuation, the intestines, after death in such cases, have been found to contain the rice-water fluid. In one instance of this kind which came under our observation, on a post-mortem examination, the large intestines contained healthy feces, whilst in the upper ⅔ of the small intestine the mucous membrane presented the ordinary changes induced by the Cholera process, and the rice-water effusion was abundant.

As many of the symptoms of the stage of collapse depend upon the loss of fluid, it has been too absolutely inferred that the general phenomena of the disease are always in a necessary relation to the amount of these effusions.

In tropical regions, where either the intensity of the poison is greater, or the predisposing conditions of constitution are more favourable to its operation, it appears to be by no means unfrequent for the strongest subjects to fall into sudden collapse, without any very notable loss of fluid. Such facts are authenticated by so many careful writers, as to leave us in no doubt of their occurrence. In temperate regions, such cases, though rare, are not unknown, and in a less marked degree are within the experience of most who have seen the disease in its severer forms. Even when the loss of fluid is very great, it is doubtful whether death is due to it alone, since we often see patients in an apparently equally hopeless state, collapsed, and bloodless, whose tissues, so soon as the nervous system begins to react, recover their elasticity before any amount of absorption could, from the circumstances of the case, have occurred.

That a shrunken and collapsed state of the tissues is not necessarily due to loss of fluids, is a matter of common observation. In hernia, or internal strangulation of the intestine, it may occur in as marked a degree as in Cholera itself, and, on the contrary, very large effusions may take place from the intestinal membrane both in Choleraic diarrhœa, and from artificial means, without the patient falling into this condition.

The College received evidence of the following kind, in answer to a query bearing on this subject.

Mr. French of Marlborough Street says:—

"I have repeatedly seen cases in which the evacuations appeared to be wholly insufficient to account for the fatal collapse." (Followed by the recital of a case.)

Dr. Shapter of Exeter says:—

"These cases were numerous: the following are examples in which collapse and death were preceded by scarcely any amount of vomiting, purging, or sweating.

"J. W., male, æt. 50, left London on the 20th August, having at that time a yeasty diarrhœa. He travelled for three days, and on the 23rd arrived in Exeter. He immediately fell into collapse. The vomiting and purging were scanty, the whole scarcely amounting to two pints. He died in 21 hours.

"A. J., male, æt. 61, left London on the 8th September, on the 9th attended to his professional avocations, on the 10th at 2 A.M. fell into collapse. The discharges were but scanty. By noon he was insensible, at 5 P.M. died.

"J. B., male, æt. 40, strong and healthy, had comparatively speaking, neither purging nor vomiting. He died 12 hours after collapse set in.

"J. D. W., male, æt. 58, vomited the food he had taken a few hours before, was but slightly purged, gradually passed into collapse, and died 41 hours after the first and only vomiting. This case was characterised by an absence of all active symptoms, having neither cramps, vomiting, copious purging, nor sweating. He early became lethargic, and so continued till death."

Mr. Millar of Emsworth says :—

"Many of my cases of diarrhœa have sustained a greater loss of the fluids of the body than those which fell victims to the incurable collapse so peculiar to Cholera."

Dr. Williams and Mr. Hickes of Gloucester say :—

"We have seen about six cases where the fatal collapse bore no relation to the severity of the diarrhœa or vomiting. Some of these patients were warm and perspiring to the end, and sunk after vomiting and purging had ceased."

Mr. Horton of Hammersmith says :—

"On the 12th August, a female, æt. 42, was attacked with symptoms of Cholera at 1 P.M. The diarrhœa was soon checked, and the sickness ceased ; the sweats were not very profuse. She rapidly fell into collapse and died in 13 hours. I have attended other similar cases."

Dr. Beadle of Tewkesbury says :—

"Miss D——, æt. 33, was seized with purging but not severe. In half an hour cramps came on, and rapid failure of the pulse. In spite of stimulants, &c., she was in fatal collapse in 4 hours. A male, æt. 30, died under my care in 3 hours after slight diarrhœa."

Dr. Peacock, in his report of the children from the Asylum at Tooting, admitted into the Royal Free Hospital, says :—

"In one of the most rapidly fatal cases no diarrhœa was present after the occurrence of the urgent symptoms. The child was seized with vomiting during the night, and almost immediately became collapsed. In another case two evacuations, one very copious, and the other scanty, occurred in quick succession, and the patient then rapidly sunk into fatal collapse. In two other fatal cases, the collapse seems to have ensued upon two or three more or less copious evacuations."

Dr. George Burrows, after stating that he had never seen a case either during the epidemic of 1832-33 or 1848-49, in which the discharges were quite out of proportion to the symptoms of prostration, says:—

"The case of most rapid collapse which I witnessed during the present epidemic, was in a male, æt. 29. This young man stated, that an hour before his admission, he felt himself quite well; he was suddenly seized with profuse diarrhœa, vomiting and cramps, which - symptoms continuing, he died in 18 hours."

Dr. Basham says:—

"Several cases have come under my observation, in which the fatal collapse has borne no relation to the amount or duration of the previous serous discharges. The master of a vessel lying opposite the Horseferry at Millbank, went into the city at eight o'clock in the morning, and returned at 10, complaining of not being well. He went and lay down in his berth. At 12 he was brought to the hospital in a state of complete collapse. There was no vomiting and he had had but one serous evacuation. He died at eight o'clock the same evening.

"Whilst discharging the duties at the Millbank Prison for my friend Dr. Baly, two cases occurred amongst the convicts, illustrating this inquiry. They had been but eight days in the prison, and were reported to have gone to bed quite well. One complained of being taken suddenly ill with prostration and looseness at 2 A.M. The other with the like symptoms at 4 A.M. Both were passed to the Infirmary at the hours mentioned, I saw them at 11 A.M. They were both livid and cold and pulseless. There was no vomiting or purging, but most urgent cramps. Both died before sunset. I could repeat several similar instances."

Dr. Burchell of Kingsland says:—

"I have several times observed perfect collapse fully established after only two serous evacuations, and from that time the discharges have ceased."

Dr. Gordon Bailey says:—

" I can bear testimony to the fact, but, from want of time, was unable to note the particulars of cases."

Together with these replies were many others of a negative kind, stating that in all the cases observed, the severity of the symptoms was in proportion to the amount and rapidity of the discharges.

There is in most of the above evidence a want of precision, inseparable, in a great degree, from the nature of the case, it being scarcely possible to estimate accurately the amount of fluid lost. The frequency of the evacuations is obviously no test whatever, for the amount passed at any one time may be out of all proportion greater than at another; and, moreover, it is to be borne in mind that, during severe collapse there was often a continued draining of fluid from the body without any effort at evacuation; and after death it was not uncommon to find the cavity of the small intestines distended with effusion.

Notwithstanding the incompleteness of the data, we conclude that, although, in a large number of instances, the intensity of the symptoms is in a general way proportionate to the amount of the effusion, yet that this will only in part explain the attendant collapse which often appears to be in no inconsiderable degree due to the adynamic state of the ganglionic nervous system, induced either primarily by the poison or secondarily by the lesions of the affected mucous surface. A further elucidation of this subject is yet a desideratum.

PATHOLOGY OF THE STAGE OF REACTION.

The Cholera poison is comparable to those deleterious agents whose action on the body is transient, what after-phenomena there are being due to the accidents of the primary operation.

The normal issue of the disease is to a uniform and complete restoration of the several functions without any degree of reaction which can be considered morbid.

Such a result is not unfrequent, even where the previous symptoms have been severe. "I have seen," says Mr. Grainger *, "a man stand at his door on Wednesday, who on Monday was in perfect collapse;" and his observation accords with the experience of others.

When the powers of life are feeble or greatly reduced by the violence of the disease, reaction is often imperfect and protracted, and there is a tedious fluctuation between collapse and recovery. The pulse returns to the wrist, but the circulation remains embarrassed, the warmth of the skin is partial, and often attended with sweating. The urinary secretion is suppressed, and there is a tendency to coma. After a longer or shorter struggle death may ensue or the several functions be slowly re-established as in the more normal cases. The pathological conditions are here those of the cold stage, except that in general the lesions in the gastro-intestinal membrane are less marked.

A third issue of Cholera is into the so-called consecutive fever, which has been divided into different forms according to the prominence of particular symptoms. Such divisions are but of little practical value, as their boundaries are not constant, and they mislead by fixing the attention exclusively upon one organ, where, from the circumstances of the case, the whole system is more or less deranged.

Amongst the more important lesions are those of the kidneys. Not only are these organs, in the first stage, occasionally subject to the cholera-process, but, from the complexity of their circulation, the state of the blood, and the depressed nervous power of the ganglionic system, they slowly recover their function, and, from the persistent congestion, the secreting structures undergo changes similar to those found in acute albuminuria from other causes. In addition to the evidence on this subject given in another part of this report, we may add the following from Dr. Gairdner †, who says, "The kidneys appeared in many cases to have undergone morbid changes; the cortical sub-

* Report on the Epidemic Cholera of 1848–49.
† Monthly Journal of Medical Science, 1849.

stance being pale and turgid, and the tubuli uriniferi gorged with im-
perfectly-developed epithelium, which was mostly loaded to an unusual
extent with oleo-albuminous granules."

The urinary secretion was correspondingly affected, being either
entirely suppressed or small in quantity, and of low specific gravity.

As to the frequency of albumen in the urine after the cold stage of
Cholera, there is a universal accordance amongst different observers
both in this country and on the Continent. In more than 40 cases
observed on board the *Dreadnought*[*], in every instance but one, the
urine first passed was albuminous. Of 67 cases in which the urine
was examined by Dr. Begbie at the Cholera Hospital in Edinburgh[†],
the results were noted as follows : —

Decidedly coagulable	.	16 cases.
Highly coagulable . . .	.	17 „
Slightly or very slightly coagulable	.	20 ,
Not coagulable	.	14 ,

Reinhardt and Leubuscher found the urine coagulable in most of
their cases, and Hamernik[‡] attributes the principal pathological
phenomena of the typhoid state to disorder of the kidneys; he terms
it " reaction with uræmic phenomena."

When albumen was present, a microscopical examination of the
urine discovered the desquamated epithelium of the uriniferous tubules,
and at different times all the varieties of fibrinous casts met with in
Bright's disease, and frequently blood corpuscles.

Eighteen specimens of urine were analysed by Dr. Begbie, in order
to determine the amount of urea present in them. In eight the
quantity was too small to admit of being estimated, and in the other
ten below the normal proportions. These observations would have
been complete had the whole amount of urine passed in 24 hours
been noted, but we may conclude, from the general history of such
cases, that it was below the average.

Dr. Letheby[§] also made two analyses of urine passed after protracted suppression. The first specimen was passed on the fourth
day from the accession of severe symptoms; the second on the fifth.
In both the amount of urea was deficient, and neither contained
albumen. The extractives were in great excess in both. The results

* Lancet, June 9, 1849.
† Month. Journ. Med. Science, 1849.
‡ Die Cholera Epidemica, p. 235.
§ Medical Gazette, 1848, p. 1011.

were as follows, the standard of healthy urine being given for comparison :—

	Health.	Cholera. No. 1.	Cholera. No. 2.
Specific gravity	1015	1018·2	1017
Reaction . . .	Acid.	Very acid.	Very alkaline.
Albumen . . .	——	Not present.	Not present.
Solids in 1000 grains .	35	38	26·2
100 grains of solid matter yield :—			
Urea	42·03	12·35	8·41
Uric acid .	1·57	·62	1·85
Extractives . .	38·15	82·59	76·8
Alkaline sulphates .	10·35	1·70	6·84
„ phosphates .	5·94	1·90	3·93
Phosphate of lime and magnesia . . .	1·66	·80	2·17
	99·7	99·96	100·

Whilst attention is drawn to these derangements of the urine, we cannot leave out of consideration the state of the blood and the disturbances of the general circulation from the previous collapse, conditions which would greatly favour the retention of the urinary excreta in the system.

The following comparison between the symptoms of ordinary uræmia and of the typhoid stage of Cholera will serve to exhibit their identity. Those which characterise the Cholera typhoid we have set down from the excellent treatise of Reinhardt and Leubuscher on Cholera in 1849, and those depending upon ordinary uræmia are described mostly in the words of Dr. Addison's paper of 1839 [*]; thus avoiding the influence of any hypothesis as to the relation here insisted upon.

CHOLERA TYPHOID.

[1] Dull pain in the head.
[2] Dimness of sight—double vision.
[3] Giddiness — drowsiness — [4] slight wandering of intellect.
[5] Spasms, tonic or clonic, of an epileptic form.
[6] Pupil normal.
[7] No paralysis.
[8] Pulse various, commonly quickened or normal, sometimes below the average.

ORDINARY URÆMIA.

[4] " Dulness of intellect—sluggishness of manner. [5] Drowsiness proceeding to coma, and more or less stertor, with or without [5] convulsions." These symptoms being " very frequently preceded by giddiness, [2] dimness of sight, and [1] pain in the head." There is [8] " a quiet pulse, a contracted, or undilated, or [6] obedient pupil, and the [7] absence of paralysis."

* Guy's Hospital Reports, 1839.

CHOLERA TYPHOID.	ORDINARY URÆMIA.
9 Temperature of the skin at the beginning slightly raised; in further course normal, with extremities cool.	9 Temperature of skin natural.
10 Tongue moist and furred, and, later in the disease, dry and brown.	10 Tongue at first natural, afterwards dry and brown.
11 Vomiting, which ceased when the cerebral symptoms became more intense. Evacuations feculent—their consistence various.	11 Vomiting an early symptom, coming when the brain becomes oppressed.
12 Frequent excitement and irregular rhythm of the respiratory movements with stertor.	12 Respiration frequently with stertor. Rhythm irregular and quickened.
13 Urine suppressed or small in quantity, albuminous.	14 Urine albuminous.

The lesions of the kidneys in Cholera did not lead to permanent changes of structure. In the severest cases, if the patients recovered, the urine generally became normal in eight or ten days, and, where reaction was otherwise uncomplicated, within one or two, or not unfrequently, only the first urine passed contained albumen. These varieties depended upon the intensity and duration of the previous collapse. Hamernik * mentions a case where Bright's dropsy followed upon Cholera four weeks after the attack, and a similar case came to our knowledge during the past epidemic, but Bright's disease is so common, from other causes, that these were probably mere coincidences, and are not to be attributed to the lesions set up during the Cholera attack.

The communications received by the College show that the symptoms of the consecutive fever were most frequently referrable to the defects in the urinary secretion.

Dr. Roupell directed attention to the renal disorders in the first epidemic, and now adds :—

"The confusion and disturbance of the cerebral circulation, in the absence of any organic lesions, may be referred to an abnormal state of the blood, and is apt to terminate fatally unless the urine and bile be abundantly secreted."

Dr. Rae, Royal Naval Hospital, Plymouth, says :—

"The symptoms resembled typhus, the sensorium was much affected."

Dr. Gwynne Bird, Swansea, says :—

"The symptoms were those of adynamic fever."

* Op. Cit., p. 238.

Dr. Williams and Mr. Hickes of Gloucester say :—

"Cerebral congestion appeared to be the most prominent pathological condition."

Dr. Plomley of Maidstone says :—

"In 43 deaths amongst the hop-pickers at East Farleigh in Kent,
only 16 died in collapse, and 27 during the stage of reaction. The
chief cause of this mortality appeared to be the suspended action of
the kidneys, the recovery being very rapid in those cases where the
urinary secretion was restored. The symptoms were of a typhoid
character, with stupor and delirium, complicated in many cases with
pneumonia. During the first days of recovery, both in adults of
both sexes and children, it was not unusual to have retention of
urine requiring the use of the catheter. Of the 27 cases fatal during
reaction, 18 died with total suppression of urine, complicated in 7
with pneumonia; 3 died after the secretion had been partially restored, in all 3 there was pneumonia; 2 died with incessant vomiting two or three days after the cessation of the diarrhœa, the urine
being partially restored; 1 died with dysentery aftenthe secretion of
urine was quite normal; 3 died with gastro-enteric symptoms, the
urine being in 2 completely restored and partially in the other."

Dr. George Burrows says :—

"The pathological conditions observed by me in the consecutive
fever are—1st, congestion of the encephalon with typhoid symptoms;
2nd, pain at the epigastrium with hiccup and an irritable state of the
stomach; 3rd, the appearance of a rubeoloid exanthema."

Dr. Dickinson of Liverpool says :—

"The pathological conditions were principally those of congestion
of the brain and kidneys, as evidenced by the injection of the conjunctiva, the stupor, and coma, &c., and by the suppression of urine."

Dr. Basham says :—

"The pathological conditions of the consecutive fever have appeared to me to consist essentially in inflammatory congestion of the
intestinal mucous membrane and congestion of the kidneys. There
is stupor, drowsiness, headache, and other cerebral symptoms, and
the patients mostly die comatose."

of simple fever, lasting for about a week, and in 2 the form was 'gastro-enteric,' there being extreme tenderness over the stomach, with vomiting and a red, dry tongue. The recovery in these two cases was retarded by one or two relapses, with gastric irritability."

Dr. Moore of Tunbridge Wells says:—

"In the single case which occurred to me, the symptoms were those of a bilious remittent fever."

Mr. Paul of Bermondsey says:—

"Secondary diarrhœa was, in my experience, a very unmanageable complication, several cases dying under it; the other state, which frequently occurred, resembled typhus. The temperature of the skin was, however, generally normal or rather cooler, the pulse regular, brain oppressed."

Dr. Barlow says:—

"Generally there was suppression of urine for two or three days after the severe collapse, and when it was passed it was albuminous. The accompanying symptoms were vomiting of a green bilious fluid, listlessness, or stupor, or coma. The pulse sharp, with a slight back stroke, but very compressible. A miliary eruption was common."

Dr. Moore of Edinburgh says:—

"I have had 15 cases of consecutive fever, and in all the cerebral symptoms were the most prominent."

Dr. Shapter of Exeter says:—

"The face was generally flushed. Skin of a dusky hue. Pulse small and frequent. Tongue dry, frequent vomiting as in sea-sickness. Pain in the head, restlessness, and an expression of unconsciousness, but still the patient could be roused. The urine was of a brownish colour. The dejections dark, bilious, and fœtid."

In many of the communications received, it is stated that, after the urine was secreted, there was occasionally an inability to void it, attended with neuralgic pains about the bladder; we find the same circumstance referred to by authors.

The cerebral and thoracic complications of Cholera typhoid are obviously dependent upon the retention of the urinary excretious in the blood, and do not present any special relation to the Cholera poison itself. The pneumonia was generally limited to the posterior and inferior parts of the lungs. Its characters were commonly those of hypostatic engorgement with œdema, or reddish grey consolidation with diffused puriform infiltration. The symptoms, both on account of the cerebral oppression which co-existed, and the character of the lesion itself, were generally obscure.

In those parts of the intestinal tract where, during the cold stage, the hyperæmia and other changes were most marked, there was not unfrequently during reaction persistent congestion, and inflammation of the mucous membrane, with diphtheritic exudation. In such cases the consecutive fever had the characters of gastro-enterite, or, where the large intestine was much affected, of dysentery. As these conditions were generally complicated with uræmia, it was difficult to distinguish whether the gastric irritation which accompanied them arose from this source or depended upon the state of the mucous membrane itself.

, The pathological indications of the diphtheritic exudations appear to be of the most general kind, since such effusions occur upon mucous surfaces wherever there is long-continued congestion, and the plastic powers of the part are depressed. They are in no way peculiar to Cholera. Their presence indicates in this, as in other diseases, an adynamic condition of the system.

Frequency of consecutive fever. We have no exact data whereby to determine the frequency of "consecutive fever." Some practitioners rarely met with it, though, according to others, it was of frequent occurrence. There is some reason to believe that this difference may have depended in part, although not to the extent generally supposed, upon the medicines administered during collapse.

Frequency of mortality from consecutive fever. The mortality in this stage may in some degree be determined by a table in the Registrar-General's report, recording the duration of fatal cases at different ages. When death took place within 48 hours, we may conclude that it resulted from the primary effects of the disease. The cause of death during the third and fourth days is more difficult to appreciate, but from the general history of cases having that duration, it is probable that most of the deaths in this period depended upon an imperfect reaction, and belonged rather to the stage of collapse than to that of consecutive fever. After the fourth day the effects of the secondary lesions would become obvious, and the deaths then occurring might be referred to them. The only fallacy in the numbers included in this period depends upon the time at which the disease is supposed to have begun. In general the commencement is dated from the onset of severe symptoms, but sometimes from the first occurrence of diarrhœa; therefore, by assuming that all the cases fatal after the fourth day were complicated with consecutive fever, we obtain too high an average of its mortality, and hence we may conclude, that it was less than that indicated below. To avoid, as far as possible, this source of error, the deaths between 25 and 45 years of age have been taken, this being the time of life at which the course of the disease is most regular. Of 16,901 cases, the results were as follows :—

Died during first 24 hours	9,150 ⎱	Period of collapse.
„ „ 2nd day .	4,435 ⎰	
	13,585	
Died during 3rd day	966 ⎱	Period of imperfect
„ „ 4th „ .	656 ⎰	reaction.
	1,622	
Died during 5th day . . .	438	
„ „ 6th „ . . .	302	
„ „ 7th „ . . .	367	
„ „ 8th „ . . .	119	
„ „ 9th „	102	Period of "consecutive
„ „ 10th „ . . .	188	fever."
„ „ 14th „	128	
„ „ 21st „ . . .	32	
Upwards	18	
	1,694	

Therefore, nine-tenths of the deaths took place in collapse or during imperfect reaction, and not more than one-tenth in the consecutive fever, this being probably above the average.

Cholera exanthem.

Dr. B. G. Babington [*] was the first in this country to call attention to the occurrence of an exanthem in the "consecutive fever" of Cholera, and his description has, in most particulars, been confirmed by later observers.

"This eruption," he says, "I have found to make its appearance in protracted cases of Cholera when the disorder has assumed that typhoid character which is marked by extreme debility, drowsiness not amounting to stupor, injected conjunctiva, and general indications of cerebral congestion.

"After this state has existed several days, some red spots are observed about the wrists and hands, and the face becomes tumid as on the approach of erysipelas. If this occur in the evening, on the

[*] Medical Gazette, 1832, p. 578.

following morning the arms, the forehead up to the roots of the hair, and the face generally, will be covered with large elevated patches of a bright red colour, more vivid than measles, and more defined than scarlatina, much resembling nettle-rash, especially in the circumstance of their disappearance on pressure and instant recurrence when that pressure is removed. They vary in hue at different times, being occasionally purplish, especially on the hands; and again resuming their bright tint without any apparent cause. On the second day the efflorescence is found over the whole trunk, and the sensation produced by it is not that of tingling and heat alone, but of intense itching. To allay this the patient scratches himself incessantly, until he has removed the cuticle in numerous places over his body and extremities, leaving patches of encrusted blood and subsequent scabs wherever this abrasion has taken place. The eruption is very well marked about the third and fourth days; the outline around the edges of each patch being then more distinct than before, and bearing a greater contrast to the central portion. It declines about the sixth day, and terminates by a general desquamation of the cuticle. In this respect, as well as in its definite duration, it is needless to remark, that it differs altogether from nettle-rash."

Before discussing the pathology of this eruption, it may not be uninteresting to compare the account given of it by Dr. Babington in 1832, with that of those excellent observers Reinhardt and Leubuscher in 1849 [*], especially as the observations were made in two epidemics, and the patients had been under different treatment during the primary symptoms.

These writers continue thus:—

"We observed this, in many instances very characteristic rash, in 15 cases. It appeared without any observable change in the general condition of the patient; without restlessness, heat, quickening of the pulse, or other symptoms generally attendant upon the development of an acute cutaneous eruption. In many cases, particularly in young and strong subjects, a diffused redness of the skin preceded the exanthem. It was particularly marked on the hands and face, where it was occasionally so bright, and attended with so much swelling, as to have the appearance of erysipelas. After 12 or 24 hours the swelling decreased, and the redness was more partial. In some places it gradually lessened and disappeared altogether, whilst it continued unchanged in others. At this time there appeared over the hands and arms numerous large, irregular, and for the most part indistinctly defined, red patches. Where the diffused redness

[*] Op. Cit., p. 470.

and swelling were absent, the exanthem appeared first in the form of large, irregular, undefined erythematous patches. Sooner or later these became gradually concentrated into the exanthem. The skin was then covered with small round defined spots, from the size of a pin's head to a linseed, more or less bright in colour, and not elevated above the skin. This gradual development of the exanthem could be best seen on the hands and feet, on the other parts of the body it was not generally preceded by any diffused redness. The exanthematous spots subsequently increased in size, and when near together became confluent and produced a roseolous appearance. In some cases the eruption remained in this condition but increasing for 24 or 36 hours, and then after two or three days became pale and disappeared altogether with a fine branny exfoliation of the skin. This abortion of the exanthem, if it may be so called, occurred in 3 out of 15 cases; in these it was limited to the extremities, and principally affected the joints. The exanthem generally, however, underwent a further development, the spots became raised, and at the same time increased in circumference, forming an eruption like measles. By a further increase in size, and a greater elevation of the skin, wheals like urticaria were formed as large as a lentil or a silver penny. This similarity to urticaria was in some instances greater from the wheals being in part paler in the centre than at the periphery. As the exanthem advanced, these wheals enlarged, at the same time their centres generally became depressed, and the edge was more raised above the skin. They either remained distinct or were more or less confluent, as about the joints, elbows, shoulders, and knees. In this stage the exanthem lasted from one to two days, sometimes from three to five, before it underwent any particular change. It afterwards became pale, gradually sunk to the level of the skin and formed yellowish or reddish yellow, indistinctly-defined patches, which faded, and were followed by exfoliation of the cuticle. For the most part, this was in small branny scales, but in two instances, where the rash was extensive, the cuticle, especially on the hands and feet, separated, as after scarlet fever, in large membranous laminæ."

That this exanthem is not of frequent occurrence, and when it happens but of subordinate pathological importance, we may conclude from the fact, that in the communications received by the College, it was spoken of in only a few instances, and then somewhat incidentally. It appears to be nearly allied to *urticaria febrilis*, nor do we think the objection that it differs from this affection in having a more or less definite duration and terminates by desquamation, a valid one, since the same occurs in urticaria febrilis, which, according to Willan, lasts seven or eight days, and terminates by slight exfoliations of the cuticle.

In its abortive forms, where it did not become developed in wheals, the eruption had not unfrequently the characters of *erythema papulatum.*

It was independent of any form of treatment which had been employed in the preceding stage of the disease, and occurred sometimes in mild cases where the patient had been kept to cold water or other simple diluents, as well as in the severe forms where stimuli had been freely administered. Although it is not ascertained what were the proximate conditions which determined its appearance, yet, since similar eruptions are known to be intimately dependent upon disorders of the gastro-intestinal mucous membrane, and these are, after an attack of Cholera, frequent, we cannot but refer it in a general way to such a source, admitting, as we must in ordinary urticaria and erythema, that the individual peculiarities which determine its presence are not obvious.

Other appearances occasionally occur during reaction, such as petechiæ in the lower extremities, erysipelas of the face and furuncles.

Predisposing causes of Cholera. Whatever may be the nature of the Cholera poison, it requires no definite predisposing conditions in the system to enable it to produce its effects. It was fatal at all ages, nearly equally to both sexes, and neither the weakness of infancy, the vigour of manhood, nor the decrepitude of age, was a safeguard against its inroads.

Age. The total number of deaths in England in 1849, from Cholera and diarrhœa together, was, with a few exceptions, in which the age was not named, and 20 persons over 95 years not included, 72,110, as follows :—

DEATHS from CHOLERA and DIARRHŒA from Birth to 95 Years. 1849 *.

Age.	Sex.	Cholera.	Diarrhœa.	Total.
		Deaths.		
Under 5......	Males	3,866	6,393	19,381
	Females ...	3,470	5,652	
„ 10......	Males	2,458	292	5,404
	Females ...	2,358	296	
„ 15......	Males	1,349	109	2,785
	Females ...	1,217	110	
„ 25......	Males	2,578	188	5,561
	Females ...	2,573	222	
„ 35......	Males	3,837	232	8,666
	Females ...	4,303	294	
„ 45......	Males	3,712	259	8,364
	Females ...	4,068	325	
„ 55......	Males	3,417	333	7,468
	Females ...	3,387	331	
„ 65......	Males	2,605	506	6,530
	Females ...	2,909	510	
„ 75......	Males	1,610	679	5,016
	Females ...	1,954	773	
„ 85......	Males	576	521	2,525
	Females ...	827	601	
„ 95......	Males	710	119	410
	Females ..	97	124	
	*	53,241	18,869	72,110

By dividing the whole term of life into periods, we obtain the following results :—

Infancy and childhood (under 5 years)			19,381
Youth .	(5–15	„)	8,189
Adult age	(15–45	„)	22,591
Middle age	(45–65	„)	13,998
Old age	(65–95	„)	7,951

These numbers give the absolute mortality at the different periods of life, but, in order to obtain a correct idea of the influence of age, it is necessary to compare them with the number of persons living at

* Registrar-General's Report on the Mortality of Cholera, 1848–49.

these periods, by which the mortality per cent. is determined to be as follows:—

DIAGRAM I.

*Mortality from the Epidemic of 1849 per cent. of Persons living at different Ages **

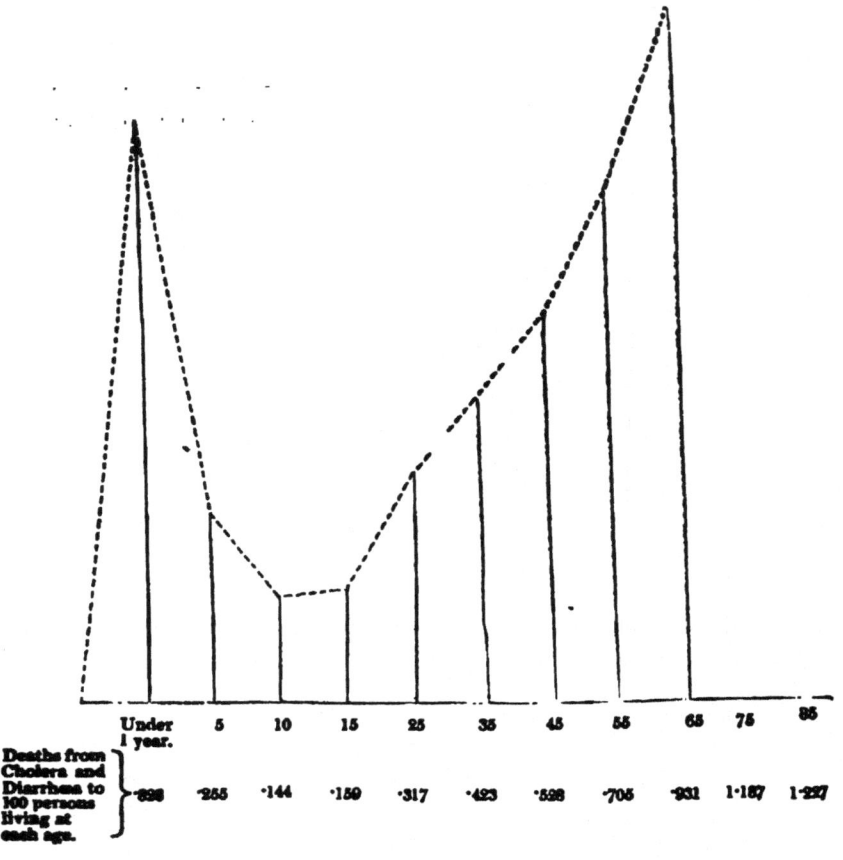

	Under 1 year.	5	10	15	25	35	45	55	65	75	85
Deaths from Cholera and Diarrhœa to 100 persons living at each age.	·896	·255	·144	·159	·317	·423	·596	·705	·931	1·157	1·227

Such a calculation shows that the epidemic was, in proportion to the number of persons living, most fatal to infants and persons over 55 ; that the mortality was lowest from 5 to 15 ; and that from the latter age upwards, it rose by an almost regular gradation, being among infants nearly six times greater than among children of 10 years,

* Op. Citat., p. xlii.

at 15 remaining nearly the same as at 10, when it was at the lowest point, and at 35 increasing to three times, and at 55 to five times beyond this.

The epidemic was especially fatal in early life and old age, in accordance with the tendency to fatal disease at those periods, the mean mortality per cent. from all causes at different ages when Cholera does not prevail, being as follows :—

Deaths from all causes to 100 persons living at each age (1838—1844).

Under 1 year.	5	10	15	25	35	45	55	65	75	85
6·554	·918	·526	·819	·988	1·245	1·662	2·961	6·249	18·797	28·599

By a diagram (Diag. 2), similar to the former, it is readily seen that the curve indicating the mortality from Cholera rises as the curve for general disease rises, it falls with it, and subsequently rises by almost the same gradations.

DIAGRAM II.

Annual Mortality from all Causes (1838–44) per cent. of Persons living at different Ages.

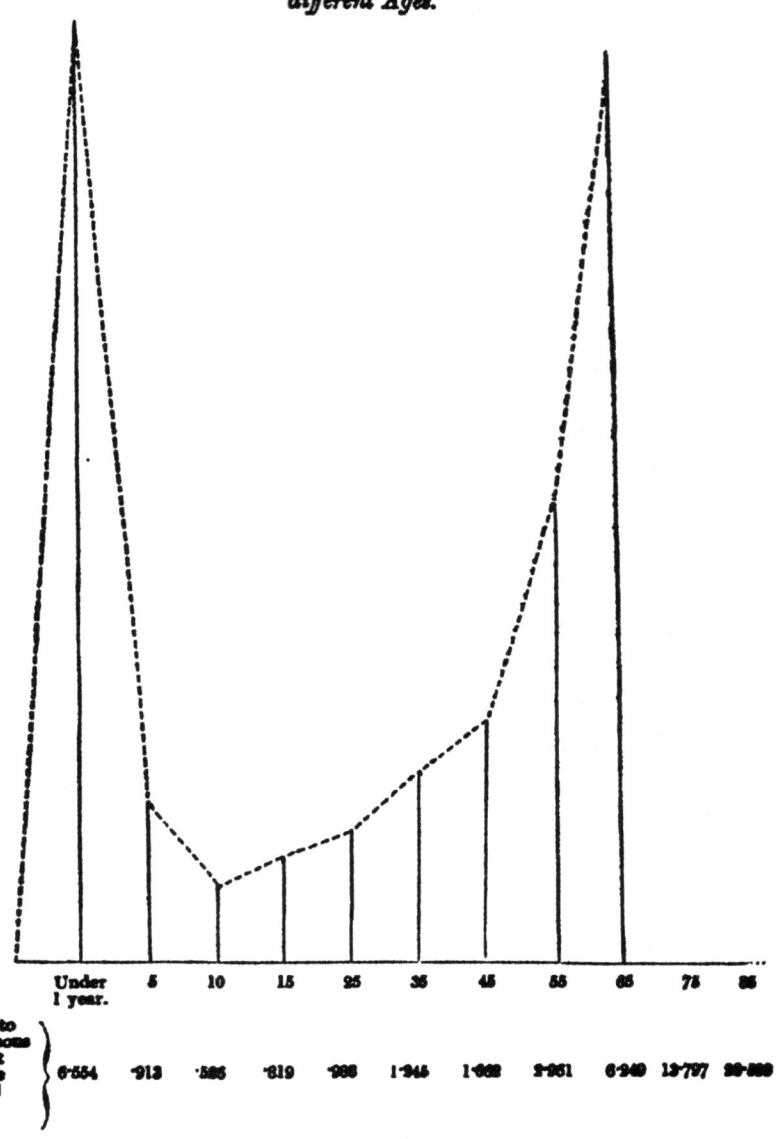

	Under 1 year.	5	10	15	25	35	45	55	65	75	85

tenths to 10 persons ving at each age um all ages, 38-44.

6·554   ·913   ·585   ·819   ·988   1·245   1·682   2·951   6·249   13·797   29·880

There are, however, some points of contrast in these two curves deserving consideration. Although the epidemic was very fatal to infants and aged persons, it was less so in proportion to the mean percentage of mortality at these ages than it was during the vigorous periods of life. This is shown by placing the two series of numbers together, and noting what fraction of the whole mean mortality Cholera reached at the different periods as follows:—

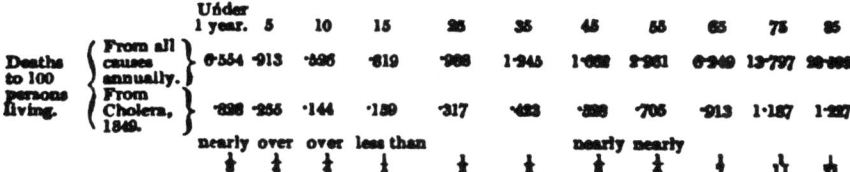

	Under 1 year.	5	10	15	25	35	45	55	65	75	85
Deaths to 100 persons living. { From all causes annually. }	6·554	·913	·596	·819	·966	1·245	1·662	2·961	6·249	13·797	20·699
{ From Cholera, 1849. }	·896	·255	·144	·159	·317	·422	·559	·705	·913	1·187	1·227
	nearly $\frac{1}{7}$	over $\frac{1}{4}$	over $\frac{1}{4}$	less than $\frac{1}{5}$	$\frac{1}{3}$	$\frac{1}{3}$	nearly $\frac{1}{3}$	nearly $\frac{1}{4}$	$\frac{1}{7}$	$\frac{1}{11}$	$\frac{1}{16}$

At 5 and 10 years the mortality from the epidemic was as high as ¼, and from 25 to 45, as high as ⅓ of the whole mean mortality per cent., whilst in infants under a year, it was not ⅐, and in aged persons not more than 1⁄11 or 1⁄13. These facts appear to prove that general constitutional tendency to disease had but a subordinate influence as a predisposing cause, for although, as we have said, the absolute number of deaths in infancy and old age was high, yet in proportion to the mean mortality at those periods it was low compared with that in youth and middle age. It may, therefore, be concluded that, although the delicacy of infancy and the infirmity of age were, as in other diseases, predisposing conditions, yet that the Cholera poison was independent of them and asserted its power over the vigour of the constitution in the highest ratio to the mean of all other causes at that period of life least prone to disease. This is made apparent by placing together the two former curves as in Diag. 3.

DIAGRAM III.

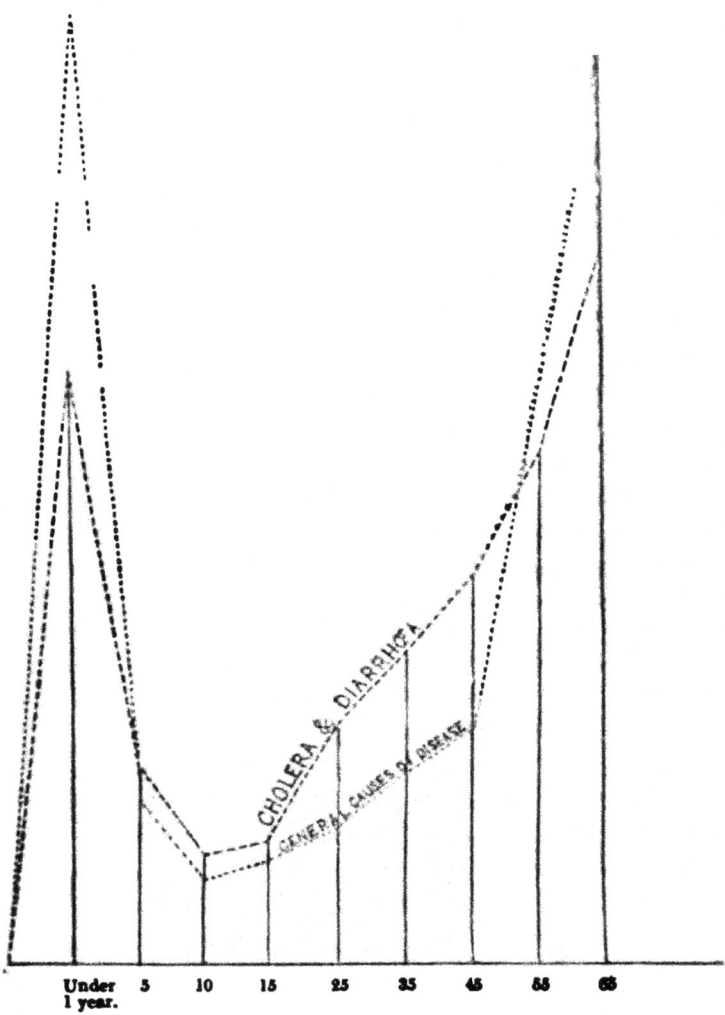

| | Under 1 year. | 5 | 10 | 15 | 25 | 35 | 45 | 55 | 65 |

It is here seen that the curve indicating the mortality from Cholera at different ages cuts that for general disease at 5 years, and continues above it until 55, when it again dips below it. In the above calculations, the cases of epidemic diarrhœa are included with those of Cholera, as they are probably effects of the same cause, varying only in degree.

Age had much influence in determining the *character* of the phenomena. Under a year the proportion of fatal cases of diarrhœa to those denominated, from their severity, Cholera, was high, nearly as 5 of the former to 3 of the latter. From 5 years to 45, this was reversed, there being, as a mean, but 1 of diarrhœa to 10·5 of Cholera ; over 55, as the debility of age increased, the proportion gradually changed again, being, at 55, 1 of diarrhœa to 5 of Cholera ; at 65, 1 to 2·5 ; at 75, 3 of diarrhœa to 4 of Cholera ; and at 85, 14 of diarrhœa to 9 of Cholera. Cases of diarrhœa were, therefore, more frequent, or, in other words, the effects of the epidemic were less intense, at those ages when the vital powers are most feeble. The accompanying diagrams (Diag. 4 and 5), showing the curves for Cholera and diarrhœa,

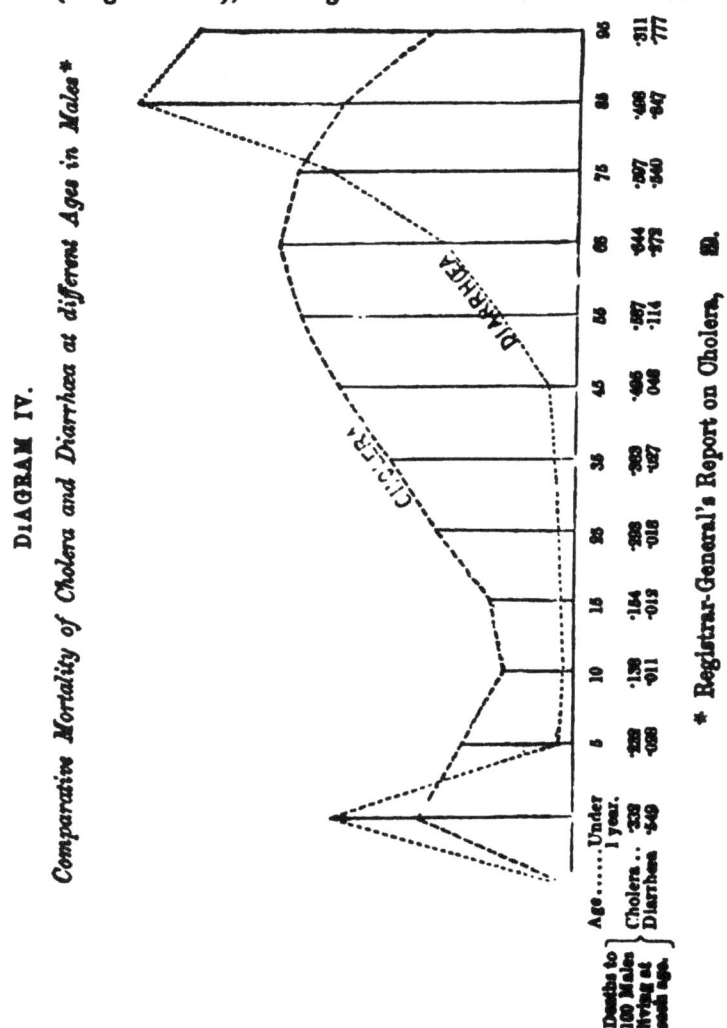

DIAGRAM IV.

Comparative Mortality of Cholera and Diarrhœa at different Ages in Males *

* Registrar-General's Report on Cholera, p.

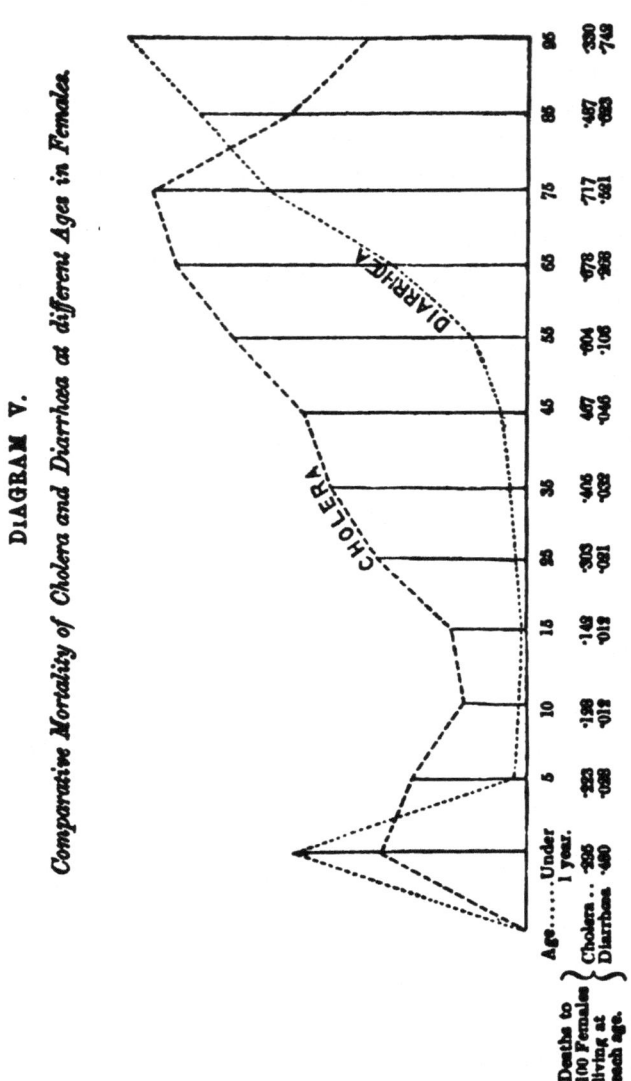

DIAGRAM V.

Comparative Mortality of Cholera and Diarrhœa at different Ages in Females.

Age......	Under 1 year.	5	10	15	25	35	45	55	65	75	85	95
Cholera ..	·935	·323	·198	·148	·303	·406	·467	·504	·678	·717	·467	·330
Diarrhœa	·480	·088	·012	·012	·091	·032	·046	·108	·268	·081	·033	·743

Deaths to 100 Females living at each age.

present the same contrasts, and cut each other at nearly the same periods of life as those indicating the specific effect of the epidemic taken as a whole, and the mean effect of other morbific causes: from which we draw the conclusion, that when the epidemic poison affects the system already predisposed to disease, the phenomena will be less intense, death occurring in the stage of diarrhœa; but when, on the other hand, the predisposition is less, the resistance in the constitution will favour the development of the more characteristic phenomena.

Of 200 patients whose condition was noted by Briquet and Mignot[*]—

77 were strong and of good constitution.
57 of moderate strength and constitution.
56 were either feeble or much emaciated or cachectic.

" It results, "they add, " from these facts that the majority of our patients were of good, or of moderately good constitution, and that in common life weakness alone was not a very evident predisposing cause of Cholera."

Sex.   " The deaths from Cholera were 26,108 males, and 27,185 females ; and from diarrhœa, 9637 males, and 9250 females. The population of England and Wales returned at the census without revision was on March 31, 1851, males 8,762,588 females 9,160,180. And correcting for increase of population, the mortality from Cholera at all ages in 1849, was :—

Males, 1 in 331.
Females, 1 in 333.

The mortality was thus a shade less among females than it was among males ; but the difference is much less than it is from all other fatal diseases in ordinary years ; where the total deaths among males is invariably greater than the deaths among females. Thus, in the year 1848, the deaths of males from all causes amounted to 202,949, of females to 196,851. And in the severe years 1838-44, the annual rate of mortality among males was 2·270, females 2·104." In many districts there was a discrepancy in the results from that indicated above ; the proportion of females to males being reversed. In the Middlesex districts of London 3388 males and 3612 females died of Cholera ; in the Surrey districts the discrepancy was much greater, 2814 males and 3509 females. In Liverpool, Manchester, and the adjacent districts, the deaths of females also exceeded the deaths of males, being in Liverpool 1895 males and 2278 females. In Tynemouth and South Shields, Sunderland, Chester-le-Street, as well as in several other places, the deaths of females were in excess. In Newcastle-upon-Tyne, they were nearly equal. On the other hand, the proportion of males was in some places greatly in excess of the average. In Gloucester, Stroud, and Tewkesbury,

* Op. Cit., p. 21.

the number of males that died of the epidemic exceeded the females in the proportion of 133 to 96. At Madeley and Shrewsbury 10 males and 71 females died. Also in Stoke-upon Trent, Wolverhampton, West Bromwich, and Dudley, the deaths of males considerably exceeded the deaths of females *.

Similar variations occurred, also, at certain periods of the epidemic. Mr. Farr has drawn attention to the fact, that at the beginning of the epidemic the deaths of males exceeded the deaths of females very considerably, but the reverse obtained when the mortality was at a high rate. Thus in the months of October, November, and December, 1848, the beginning of the first outbreak, the numbers were, males 612, females 493, or 100 to 80; but in the following quarter, ending March, 1849, the deaths of males amounted to 250, of females to 266, or as 100 to 106; at the age of 25 and upwards, the excess of deaths among females being considerable. Again, in June, at the commencement of the *great outbreak*, the males furnished the most numerous victims; but at the close of July, when the intensity of the epidemic was greater, the females died in greater numbers than males, and this proportion continued to the end. In the week the mortality was highest the deaths were 895 males and 1131 females, or 100 to 126. These fluctuations obviously depended in some instances upon accident, in others, probably, upon the relative numbers of the two sexes, and their occupations. They illustrate the uncertainty of deductions from too restricted data.

It has been often stated that pregnancy is a predisposing condition to a fatal attack of the epidemic. Such an opinion is in some degree supported by the mortality at the child-bearing period. Thus from 25 to 45, the average mortality per cent. was among females ·424, among males ·420, the reverse of the general average. Too much weight must not, however, be laid upon this fact, since from 55 to 75, the mortality among females maintains a still higher average, being ·964 per cent., and only ·918 for males.

Predisposing influence of disease.

It is generally assumed that the weak and cachectic are peculiarly liable to Cholera. This has been shown not to be strictly so, and here we have to add that the existence of other disease did not obviously predispose to an attack. Chronic lesions were rarely found in the bodies of those who died of Cholera. Gairdner† says, in his experience they were

* Registrar-General's Report, p. 40.
† Edinburgh Monthly Journal, 1849.

very rare.   In 89 cases examined by him, the liver presented traces of chronic lesion but once, the kidneys only four times, in only two of which was the disease progressive.   The intestines were in all uniformly free.   The cases we have tabulated give nearly a similar result.   The general absence of chronic and other lesions is also noted by Schmidt.

The following table gives the number of physicians' patients attacked with Cholera whilst under treatment for various diseases, in five of the larger metropolitan hospitals, from the 1st of June to the 1st of November, 1849, the period during which the epidemic chiefly prevailed.

The average duration of their stay in the hospital was from four to six weeks.

Physicians' patients under treatment from June 1st to Nov. 1st, 1849.		Attacked with Cholera.	Labouring under
Bartholomew's	934	None.	
St. Thomas's	998	6	1 Bright's disease. 1 Convalescent from rheumatism and endocarditis. 1 Chronic rheumatism without constitutional affection. 3 Not noted.
Guy's	913	3	1 Acute rheumatism. 1 Pleurisy. 1 Malignant disease of lumbar glands.
St. George's	640	1	Ascites.
Middlesex	474	1 (suspected only).	Indigestion.

Without inferring that those who laboured under previous disease enjoyed an immunity from an attack of the epidemic, it would appear that they were not in any marked degree predisposed to it.   Yet Hamernik * states that Cholera supervenes more frequently upon other diseases than is usual with other epidemics, but gives no numerical proof of this.

Briquet and Mignot found that amongst the Cholera patients brought to La Charité, a little less than half were in good health before the attack, less than a fourth were delicate, and a third were subject to different affections, of which they give the following analysis:—

Fifteen of them, all females, had for a long time been troubled with dyspepsia and pains in the stomach.   One laboured under gas-

* Die Cholera Epidemica, p. 46.

tralgia resulting from a former attack in 1832. Thirteen had enteric affections, chronic disorder of the colon, or habitual diarrhœa for one or two months. Three had gastro-enteritis. The remainder were 4 cases of hysteria, 2 of phthisis, 1 of chronic bronchitis, and 2 of epilepsy. In 4 the attack occurred at the onset of acute pneumonia, and in one of typhus fever.

" The character of the pre-disposition," they add, " is obvious, since we find that of 45 cases there were, including the 2 of phthisis, 33, and including the 4 of hysteria with pain more or less acute at the epigastrium, 37 suffering under morbid conditions (probably in-flammatory) of a part or whole of the alimentary canal."

These facts appear to us too vague and limited for any certain con-clusions to be drawn from them.

Influence of habits, &c.   It is difficult to estimate separately the various noxious influences which in large cities are naturally associated with intemperance. This vice soon entails all those conditions which not only impair the vigour of the body, but favour the dissemination, and probably the generation, of the Cholera poison. But notwithstanding this, there is sufficient evidence that not only habitual drunkenness in itself, but also the immediate effects of an occasional carouse, induced a predisposition to an attack. In the communications received by the College from various practitioners these facts are frequently alluded to, in some instances the illustra-tions are striking. Thus Dr. Plomley of Maidstone states, that the first 9 cases of Cholera in that town were in persons of intemperate habits. In the private practice of Dr. Wright of Wakefield, of 7 adults who had Cholera, 3 were of intemperate habits; of 8 cases which came under the care of Mr. Millar, of Emsworth, 4 were or had been of intemperate habits. Others bear the same testimony, but state their experience without numerical details. Mr. Grainger, in his report, says, " Abundant evidence was afforded during the late epide-mic, that habitual drunkards were highly predisposed to Cholera, and of them a large number perished."

The depression of the nervous system and the derangement of the digestive organs following immediately upon occasional intoxication had apparently a marked predisposing influence. In the Registrar-General's report *, it is shown that there were certain days in the week on which the deaths from Cholera were far above the average. These

---

* Page xlix.

fatal days were Monday, Tuesday, Wednesday, and Saturday. "In the whole country Tuesday was the most, Friday the least fatal day of the week. The disparity was greater in London, where 2194 persons died on Mondays, 2136 on Tuesdays, and only 1927 on Thursdays, and 1824 on Fridays;" making a difference of 370 between the highest and the lowest day, or rather more than a sixth of the whole average, as shown in the following table of the number of deaths on the several days of the week in the whole epidemic.

Number of fatal Cases on the several Days of the Week.

	Mondays.	Tuesdays.	Wednesdays.	Thursdays.	Fridays.	Saturdays.	Sundays.	Average.
All England and Wales......	7693	7826	7621	7607	7167	7769	7610	7614
London	2194	2136	1978	1927	1824	2067	2011	2020
Other parts of England and Wales......................	5499	5690	5643	5680	5343	5702	5599	5594
All England and Wales......	+79	+212	+7	−7	−447	+155	−4	
London	+174	+116	−42	−93	−196	+47	−9	
Other parts of England and Wales......................	−95	+96	+49	+86	−251	+108	+5	

"In reading the table it must be recollected that the days given are the days on which the deaths occurred, and that half the deaths happen in the 24 hours after the attack. The weekly wages are generally paid on the Saturdays, and the Mondays in London and other cities are days in which a certain proportion of the population indulge in intoxicating drinks. The Fridays are days of comparative abstinence."

If we confine our observation to London, where the influence of intemperance would probably be greatest, it will be seen that the mortality formed a more or less regular wave from Saturday to Monday and Tuesday, when it reached its highest point, and then subsided through Wednesday, Thursday, and Friday. Similar facts are alluded to by several practitioners who favoured us with their experience, and that without any knowledge of the data given above.

"Many more cases," writes Mr. Michael of Swansea, "occurred on Sunday nights and Monday mornings than at any other period of the week; this I believe to be attributed to the prevailing habit of intoxication on Saturday nights."

"Occasional excesses," says Mr. Grainger, "led to a vast number of attacks; thus at Hamburgh it was observed that there was among the sailors in that great port a regular accession of Cholera every Monday and Tuesday, owing to the men going ashore and getting drunk on the preceding Sunday. In London also several medical men informed me they had noticed the same thing; excess either in drinking or eating, particularly if improper food was used, such as pork, cabbage, &c., being followed by attacks, which thus became more frequent on Sunday night and Monday."

Occupation. Apart from elevation and the other sanitary conditions of the locality in which the occupation is carried on and the general habits of those employed, but little can be said of the predisposing or preventive influence of occupation. Whatever appears to have depended upon it may probably be referred to other concomitant conditions.

Dr. Guy classified under their different professions and occupations 4312 males of the age of 15 years and upwards, who died of Cholera in London during the last epidemic 1848–49*, and by comparing the numbers with the probable number of persons occupied in the several divisions, he obtained the ratio of mortality for each, so far as it could be arrived at by such limited and rather uncertain data. It appears from this inquiry that Cholera was least fatal to persons occupied in the learned professions, not excepting general practitioners in medicine. It was in an equally low ratio to undertakers. Footmen and other men-servants appear to have been highly favoured, probably from the part of the town in which they are principally employed, and the great care they take of themselves, being, perhaps, less exposed to fatigue, either bodily or mentally, than any other class; hence we are not surprised that whilst amongst physicians, surgeons, and general practitioners of medicine, the mortality was 1 to 265, amongst footmen and other men-servants it was but 1 to 1572. Amongst tradesmen there are too many discrepancies to admit of any general deductions. Amongst common labourers the mortality was high, especially to ballast-heavers, coal-porters, and scavengers.

No occupation appears to exempt those employed in it from an attack. Pfaff, in his pamphlet on the Berlin epidemic, quotes the testimony of Bergson of Warsaw, that manufacturers of tobacco and cigar-makers were altogether free from the disease, and adds, in

* Weekly Report of the Registrar-General, Dec. 22, 1849.

confirmation of this, that among 250 workmen and 609 helpers so employed in Berlin, only three fell sick during the winter epidemic, and but one died in the summer; yet we learn from Dr. Guy's table, that six fatal cases occurred to tobacconists in London, which is in the ratio of ˙1 to 75, and from inquiry we have learned that those employed in this calling suffered like other persons from the milder effects of the epidemic.

The immunity of Jews in this metropolis was better ascertained, and according to good authority, depended upon their attention to hygiène. Their houses are cleansed annually, and are not over-crowded. They are as a class sober, and in their diet scrupulous. There is no extreme destitution among them, the wealthy classes relieving those in distress. Their Sabbath is rigidly observed as a day of rest.

> " Wealth," says Mr. Farr*, "appears to influence the mortality from Cholera. It represents food, lodging, clothing, cleanliness, medical advice in sickness to a certain extent, as large masses of people supply themselves with these necessaries in proportion to their means. If the 19 wealthiest districts of London are compared with the 19 poorest districts, the mortality from Cholera is found to be inversely as the wealth measured by the value of house-room."

But, he further adds, elevation considerably interferes with these results, so that in lower elevations the reverse occurs; for if

> " The 10 districts, not differing greatly in elevation, but all lying on an average under 10 feet, are arranged in the order of wealth, the singular result is obtained that the five poorest districts experienced the least average loss from Cholera."

After enumerating other particulars, showing that at higher elevations wealth did bring some slight exemptions, he adds :—

> " Under these circumstances I find it difficult to establish any definite relation between the various degrees of wealth and the mortality of Cholera, further than that, in districts of some elevation, wealth does exert a certain influence on the mortality both of Cholera and of ordinary causes."

Supposed identity of Sporadic and Epidemic Cholera.
The occasional occurrence in European countries, in the autumn, of cases of sporadic Cholera, presenting the symptoms and general character of the epidemic form, and the insensible gradations by which such cases are connected with the bilious diarrhœa

Registrar-General's Report on Cholera, p. lxvi.

prevalent at that season, have given rise to the opinion that the epidemic or Asiatic Cholera is only the ordinary endemic disease increased in intensity by a greater prevalence of the causes which originate it to a more limited extent in other years.

In a consideration of this subject it is necessary to premise that a general correspondence in symptoms and a similarity of morbid products do not prove identity of pathological conditions, and that, in determining how far a disease is specific, we must include the whole clinical history.

Epidemic Cholera has principally prevailed in this country in the autumn months, the period of the year to which the sporadic form is chiefly limited. This fact, however, proves no necessary connection between the two diseases, since other epidemic pestilences with which this country has been visited have prevailed at the same season. The sweating sickness made its first appearance in the early part of August, 1485; it was at its height in London about the middle of September, and declined during October. The second visitation was in the summer of 1506; and the third time, it broke out in London in July, 1517, reaching its height in about six weeks. At the 2nd of May, 1528, it began again to appear; and in July, August, and September of the year following, "brought a scene of horror upon all the nations of Northern Europe scarcely equalled in any other epidemic."[*] In its fifth visitation it broke out in London on the 6th of July, and lasted until the end of September; having begun to show itself on the banks of the Severn about the middle of April of that year.

The influence of the autumnal season upon the prevalence of epidemics is not limited to Cholera and the sweating sickness, for the plagues of the 17th century[†] prevailed at the same season. In 1603 the plague was at its height at the beginning of September. In 1625, when it visited us a second time, it was within a week of the same period of the year that the greatest number of deaths took place; and in the Great Plague of 1665 the deaths rapidly rose in number from the end of July till the end of September; the disease maintaining its intensity from that time to the beginning of October, when it as rapidly declined.

We may conclude, therefore, that the influence of season upon the

[*] Hecker's Epidemics, &c., p. 238.

[†] See Map of the Plagues of London, Registrar-General's Report on Cholera.

spread of Cholera, as upon other epidemics, is a general one, and depends rather upon temperature and other concomitant conditions in and out of the body, than upon any intimate relation between the Cholera poison and the causes of common autumnal diarrhœa, whether in its milder form or as sporadic Cholera.

Sporadic Cholera is limited in its severe form to infants and aged or debilitated persons, whilst the epidemic, on the contrary, manifests its greatest intensity when the powers of life are most vigorous.

The mortality from sporadic Cholera and allied intestinal affections follows the general law of mortality; whilst the epidemic, as we have shown in another place, was disproport'onately fatal in youth and middle age. We have endeavoured to illustrate this in the following table; taking the deaths from English Cholera, diarrhœa, and dysentery at different ages in London, in 1847, and comparing them with a similar number of fatal cases of epidemic Cholera in the year 1849.

Thus, 2400 cases of epidemic Cholera would be distributed over the different periods of life as follows :—

Under 5 years	10	15	25	35	45	55	65	75	85
646	180	93	185	287	278	249	217	167	84

On the other hand, if we take a similar number of sporadic cases of diarrhœa, dysentery, and Cholera, there will be a different distribution as follows :—

	Age—Under .	5 years	10	15	25	35	45	55	65	75	85
In London in 1847.*	Diarrhœa . .	1475	5	11	26	31	32	52	118	165	59
	Dysentery . .	123	3	6	19	25	26	28	41	26	9
	Sporadic Cholera .	59	3	2	6	7	7	5	8	14	6
		1657	11	19	51	63	55	85	167	205	74

By comparing two curves, so arranged as to express the distribution of the two sets of cases over the different periods, the contrast in respect of age is at once made apparent :—

* Tenth Annual Report of the Registrar-General, Abstracts of 1847, pp. 304, 305.

DIAGRAM VI.

Curve (A) of English Cholera, Diarrhœa, and Dysentery, at different Ages in London in 1847, compared with the curve (B) of the same number of Cases of Epidemic Cholera in 1849.

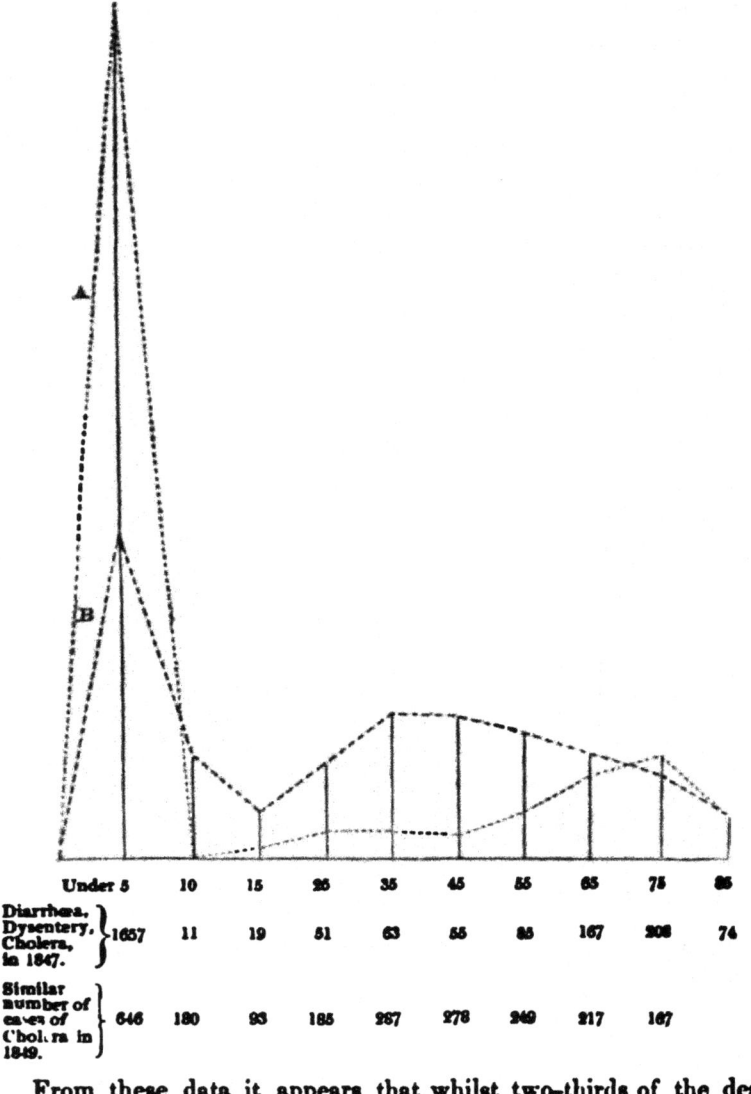

	Under 5	10	15	25	35	45	55	65	75	85
Diarrhœa, Dysentery, Cholera, in 1847.	1657	11	19	51	63	55	85	167	208	74
Similar number of cases of Cholera in 1849.	646	180	93	185	287	278	249	217	167	

From these data it appears that whilst two-thirds of the deaths from English Cholera, &c., occurred under 5 years, only one-fourth

M 2

of a similar number would have occurred within the same period from the epidemic. Again, between the ages of 5 and 55 the deaths from the sporadic form, &c., were but one-ninth of the whole; whilst from the epidemic, at the same period of life, they would have amounted to one-half. Nothing can be more striking than the contrast between the two curves in the diagram from 15 to 55, nor more indicative of a difference in the morbific agents whose results are thus compared.

The poison of epidemic Cholera, though in general very acute in its operation, did not, so far as we know, observe any law as to the *time* in which it produced its effects, and in this respect accorded with the ordinary sporadic disease; but still, on taking an average of a large number of cases, there was a wide difference

Of 39,468 cases of epidemic Cholera, in which the time of death from the commencement of the acute or characteristic symptoms was registered, 20,684, or more than one-half, were fatal within 18 hours; the average duration of all cases being 2·08 days, whilst the sporadic or summer Cholera has a duration of 5 days;[*] although Sydenham says, " Ægrum in viginti quatuor horarum spatio interimit."

This difference becomes more obvious when we select those ages at which the two diseases occurred in their most marked form. Thus of 8567 fatal cases of epidemic Cholera in children under 5 years, only 1745, or about one-fifth, terminated in 24 hours; whilst in 8281 fatal cases in adults between the ages of 20 and 35, when the symptoms are most characteristic, as many as 4449, or more than one-half, terminated in that time. The reverse of this occurs in sporadic Cholera, which is most acute in infants, and most prolonged in adults.

Our knowledge of the morbid anatomy of sporadic or English Cholera is too defective to enable us to institute a strict comparison on this head between it and the epidemic form; nevertheless, the above facts are sufficient to show that there is an essential difference between the two diseases.

* Registrar-General's Report on Cholera, page 120 and xiv.

REPORT

ON

THE TREATMENT OF CHOLERA.

Treatment of the period of invasion. IT is well ascertained that in the largest proportion of cases, at least in European countries, the poison of Cholera produces its first effects on the system *gradually*, as indicated by diarrhœa, varying in duration from a few hours to several days before intense symptoms supervene. This period may be called the period of invasion.

The numerous communications received by the College establish the importance of recognising this stage at its commencement, and render it highly probable that the morbid effects may then be often successfully combated.

The popular theory that the discharges are an effort of nature to throw off a *materies morbi*, is not only unsupported by any known facts of the disease, but, when applied to practice, is found to increase the violence of the symptoms.

At present no antidote or specific medicine is known to neutralise the cause of Cholera, or with certainty to arrest its early effects; but the subjoined quotations, from the communications received, show that the diarrhœa was, in a large number of cases, arrested by various combinations of such remedies as generally suppress discharges from the intestines, and prevent the exhaustion of nervous energy.

Opium was an almost constant ingredient, and was given in conjunction with astringents, aromatics, and diffusible stimuli.

A recumbent position is proved by experience, and also from the nature of the case, to be a most important measure. It prevents exhaustion, favours the circulation, and lessens the frequency of the evacuations. It is highly probable that cases, which otherwise resisted the action of medicines, would have readily yielded had the horizontal position in a warm bed been strictly enforced.

Enemata were not, as might have been anticipated, of much service, since the small intestine and duodenum are the principal source of the effusion.

The indications for treatment in this stage are formed entirely from the mucous membrane itself, independently of any hypothetical derangement of the liver. This organ does not appear to be in any way the cause of the symptoms; the diminution of bile in the evacuations, as they become more and more fluid, being an effect rather than a cause of the disease.

The character of the fluid thrown out—the attendant symptoms—the absence of pain—the passiveness of the evacuations, and their occasional retention to a large amount in the intestine, indicate a depression of all the energies of the affected surface.

The amount of success obtained by early treatment is not yet determined; there is a general opinion that it was very great, but this must be received with some limitation, as the facts upon which it is founded are not unequivocal. By far the larger number of cases of diarrhœa would probably never have passed beyond this stage if no medicines had been administered; and, on the contrary, in many instances the symptoms were uninfluenced by any treatment, and fatal collapse came on in spite of every effort to prevent it.

Notwithstanding this uncertainty, the general results of preventive measures were apparently very favourable, as shown by the small proportion of cases which passed into the severer forms of the disease subsequently to early treatment.

Although this is sufficient to establish the great practical importance of house-to-house visitation amongst the poor, the results at present obtained indicate a degree of success which an exact scrutiny of the circumstances does not permit us to infer.

This system was not brought into operation in the metropolis until the first week in September, 1849, the period at which the mortality had reached its acmé, the disease having already, on the 7th of September, numbered 13,520 victims. We cannot therefore think with Mr. Grainger* that the uniform success which attended the preventive system in all parts of London was independent of the natural decline of the epidemic.

* Report on the Epidemic Cholera, 1848–49, p. 151.

Epidemics cease at last, as fire does, from the want of combustible materials; and on this point we may quote from the communication made to the College by Dr. Burrows:—

"According to my experience," he says, "the facility with which the serous diarrhœa may be checked depends mainly upon the period of the epidemic when the treatment is adopted. Those remedies which are powerless in the height of the epidemic in any locality, will prove efficacious towards its decline. Thus, cases of serous diarrhœa, with symptoms of exhaustion short of collapse, appeared, in spite of unremitting attention, to be quite uncontrollable in the month of July; whilst cases of equal urgency at the time of admission, in the month of September, were controlled with a facility which often quite astonished me when I reflected upon my want of success at an earlier period of the epidemic."

On comparing the curve indicating the decline of the epidemic in the whole country in the autumn of 1849, with that for London in particular at the same time (see the Maps in the Registrar-General's Report), there is the closest coincidence between them; from which we may conclude that the causes in operation were the same in both, and hence we cannot attribute the diminution of the mortality in the latter, in any great degree, to the interference of preventive treatment.

The following are the results of the house-to-house visitation in the metropolis, from September 1 (4?) to October 27, 1849:—

Cases of Diarrhœa discovered.	Cases approaching Cholera discovered.	Cases which passed into Cholera after treatment.
43,737	978	52

The town of Dumfries is referred to in Dr. Sutherland's* report as having afforded a striking instance of the advantages of a house-to-house visitation, but the same objection obtains as before. It was not until the 10th of December, 1848, that the system was begun, and not until the 13th that it was in efficient operation, when 250 persons had already died in a population of 10,000. On referring to the Table accompanying the Report, it appears that the mortality had reached its highest point nearly a week earlier than the above date, and was already declining when the preventive system was instituted.

* Report on the Epidemic Cholera, 1848–49, p. 63.

In the case of Glasgow the same objection does not apply, as the visitation system was commenced at an earlier period of the epidemic and so efficiently carried out that, in the words of the Report,

"Whether we consider the extent of the machinery employed, or the zeal with which it was sustained, or the expense cheerfully incurred, no provision more munificent was ever made for the relief of a great public calamity than that carried out by the humane and enlightened citizens of Glasgow."

We are therefore greatly interested in learning the result. The epidemic began on the 11th of November, 1848, and by the 26th of December there had been 214 fatal cases. The house-to-house visitation was instituted " in the city parishes about the 26th or 27th of December, and in the barony parishes a day or two later." Notwithstanding this the mortality steadily increased for a fortnight, and maintained a high rate for nearly a month, and even then declined but very slowly; the deaths after the house-to-house visitation was begun being 898, and in the whole epidemic 1112.

Dr. Sutherland, however, concludes that a very marked effect was produced upon the comparative mortality of the disease even in this instance. He compares the percentage of deaths with the percentage of recoveries, as deduced from the whole number attacked at different periods of the epidemic, and finds that after the preventive system was in operation the ratio of deaths to those attacked was greatly diminished. But as the latter series is somewhat arbitrary, and would of necessity be more numerous when every case was recorded, the conclusions thus drawn do not inform us so certainly of the value of the remedies employed, as does the absolute rate of mortality.

The following are the general results of the preventive measures employed for the city and barony parishes of Glasgow :—

Parishes.	Premonitory Cases.				Cholera.	
	Applicants at Dispensaries.	Diarrhœa Cases discovered.	Rice-water Purging Cases discovered.	Total Premonitory Cases treated.	Premonitory Cases passed into Cholera.	Cholera Cases.
City . .	3066	2736	473	6,215	15	1331
Barony .	3113	3255	506	6,874	12	1003
Total .	6119	5991	979	13,089	27	2334

A large amount of evidence bearing upon this subject is further contained in the reports by Mr. Grainger and Dr. Sutherland, which, after all the abatements in it, arising from the sources of fallacy indicated above, is yet sufficient to place the preventive system in the first position of importance as a measure for counteracting the development of the disease into its severer forms. It cannot be a matter of doubt that the earlier the disease is encountered, the greater, in an infinitely high ratio, are the advantages under which medicines are employed to counteract it. This statement is confirmed by the communications received by the College, from which the following are selected, without any reference to the means advocated or the success obtained, so as to show the results of treatment in various localities and under different conditions of practice.

Dr. White, Winchester:—

"When called to a case of purging and vomiting, with cramps and cold extremities, but with the pulse tolerably perceptible at the wrist, I gave from one to two grains of solid opium, which almost invariably stopped the vomiting and the cramps, and generally the purging also. I followed this up in about a quarter of an hour by the administration of the following draught:—Sp^t. ammon. comp., 3j; Tr. camph. c., 3j; Tr. nucis vomicæ, ꯮iij; ex Mist. camph. I always insisted upon the patient going to bed, and generally placed a large mustard poultice over the stomach. This treatment was highly satisfactory; for I cannot call to mind one single case which did not speedily rally and recover, when seen before the pulse had much failed."

Dr. Shearman, of Rotherham:—

"I found alum, aromatic confection with opium, catechu, acetate of lead and opium, and small doses of calomel, generally check the serous diarrhœa."

Dr. Brown, Sunderland:—

"It accords with my experience, that Cholera, in the stage of serous diarrhœa, may with certainty be checked; and I would add, that powerful astringents, combined with opium, are the means which I have found most effectual in attaining this object. The tendency to depression must be counteracted by external warmth as well as by repose in bed, to which the patient should be confined until the diarrhœa is completely subdued. Of all astringents I have found the acetate of lead the most generally efficacious, conjoined with opium."

Dr. Peacock, H. M. Dockyard, Chatham :—

"The serous diarrhœa could not with certainty be checked; but in the majority of cases I have found the common chalk mixture, with aromatic confection and tincture of catechu, answer well; and, in obstinate cases, the acetate of lead and opium, in the form of pill."

Mr. Painter, Westminster :—

"I think not invariably, but, I believe, in the great number of cases, serous diarrhœa, if taken at the commencement, may be checked. In both fæculent and serous diarrhœa, I gave either chalk mixture, with compound chalk powder, or decoction of logwood and chalk. If the case was severe without symptoms of collapse, opium was added; it was omitted if symptoms of collapse supervened. Acetate of lead and opium was extensively used when there was no depression."

Dr. Williams, Gloucester :—

"I have found chalk mixture, combined with astringents, opium, capsicum, and other warm aromatics, of great utility, and sometimes acetate of lead and opium, or quinine with or without opium, and combined occasionally with creosote."

Dr. Beadle, Tewkesbury :—

"A compound of opium and camphor was found effectually to control diarrhœa."

Dr. Barlow :—

"According to my experience watery diarrhœa could generally, though not certainly, be checked. The most effectual means, and one which I have never dispensed with, was opium. I have most frequently given it in combination with calomel, often a grain of each every hour, or sometimes the first dose was two grains. I generally found it well borne until signs of impending collapse set in. Vegetable astringents, as hæmatoxylon, kino, catechu, were also valuable adjuncts; and chalk was useful when the tongue was clean. The recumbent position was indispensable."

Dr. Borland, Surrey Dispensary :—

"The number of cases admitted under my care at the Surrey Dispensary during the epidemic was unusually large; the majority of these were cured by mist. cretæ, tr. catechu, and opium."

Mr. Bainbridge, St. Martin's Lane :—

"It accords with my experience that serous diarrhœa can, almost without an exception, be checked, provided the depression is not great. The most valuable remedial agent was opium."

This gentleman states that he had under his care 1454 cases of simple diarrhœa, and 190 cases of diarrhœa with cramps and rice-water dejections; and adds, that only two passed into Cholera after treatment. One of these was aged 67, and one aged 65, both delicate persons.

Dr. Fincham :—

"Several scores of cases of diarrhœa fell under my care at the Western Dispensary whilst the epidemic was raging; many of these had thin, colourless, and profuse evacuations, but I never had any difficulty in checking the flux. The chief means employed were equal quantities of the compound chalk mixture, and infusion of catechu, with tincture of opium administered in frequency according to the urgency of the case."

Sir Duncan McArthur, Deal :—

"In reference to treatment, I found in the premonitory diarrhœa opiates and aromatic confection of great benefit."

Dr. Shapter, Exeter :—

"The most effectual means for arresting the diarrhœa were aromatics and opium, followed by mercurials."

Dr. Oke, Southampton :—

"My own experience of the epidemic has been limited, when compared with the experience of those who had charge of parochial districts; but I can support their testimony by stating that the treatment of the serous diarrhœa with calomel and opium or morphia was attended with success in every case that came under my care."

Mr. Mallett, Bolton :—

"With regard to treatment, I found calomel and opium, in frequently-repeated doses, the only remedy on which I could confidently rely, and was much gratified by the result in those cases in which there was no prostration."

Mr. Allen, Oxford :—

"Serous diarrhœa can be checked, but not with facility or certainty. I found calomel and opium the best remedy, but consider confinement to a warm bed an important part of the treatment."

Dr. Lang, Heavitree, near Exeter :—

"I found the best preventive treatment for adults in the earliest stage to be the pulv. cretæ comp. c. opio, with a grain of calomel, repeated after every loose motion. It appears from the experience of the last few weeks, as well as from a multitude of cases similarly treated during the previous visitation, that the full development of the disease can thus be almost always prevented."

Dr. Peacock, on the epidemic amongst the Tooting children :—

"When the children from Tooting were first received into the Free Hospital, a careful inquiry was instituted once or twice daily to ascertain whether any of them laboured under diarrhœa or other premonitory symptom, and if so, powders were given, composed of pulv. Doveri and hydr. c. cretâ, and afterwards the compound chalk powder, with opium, in a carminative mixture every three or four hours, until the affection was arrested. When with the diarrhœa there was any sickness, or the slightest tendency to collapse, the child was placed in bed, and wrapped in warm blankets, and after the powder a mixture was given, containing compound sulphuric ether, aromatic spirit of ammonia, or brandy and laudanum. Under this course of treatment the attack subsided in all but two instances without going into marked collapse."

Dr. Johnstone, Birmingham :—

"I, as well as other physicians of our medical institutions, have seen a great many severe cases of diarrhœa, though by early attention most of the patients have recovered. Of 3186 cases of bowel complaint which have occurred among the out-patients of the General Hospital during the last month (September, 1849), in many of which there were cramps, only 22 were fatal, and these were all in children. Small doses of calomel and opium were of more service than any other remedy. Astringents alone were of little use."

Dr. Davie, Plymouth :—

"A great number of persons have come under my care suffering from diarrhœa, which has been controlled by the common form of astringents in general use. The most decided and immediate good was derived from one-grain doses of the acetate of lead with one-quarter of a grain of opium every hour."

Dr. Plomley, Maidstone :—

"My experience has proved that Cholera, in the stage of serous diarrhœa, may with facility be checked, if treated early, and provided it was preceded by fæculent diarrhœa of one, two, or more days' duration. If the premonitory diarrhœa should pass into the serous form within a few hours, the difficulty of subduing it becomes much greater. The most effectual means for arresting the discharges were either the acetate of lead or alum, alone or combined with small quantities of opium."

Dr. Young, Plymouth :—

"When diarrhœa was the prominent symptom, acetate of lead, combined with opium, was useful. When the premonitory symptoms were slight, opium alone, or combined with ammonia and aromatics, was sufficient."

Mr. Field, Margate :—

"Some few cases resisted the employment of calomel and opium, and passed into the second stage, when the purging invariably yielded to eight-grain doses of the acetate of lead."

Dr. Davies, Hertford :—

"I am sorry to be obliged to state (but I do so most positively) that my experience does not accord with the assurances constantly published that there is no difficulty in checking the diarrhœa premonitory of Cholera. When it is characteristic of the epidemic I have been so unfortunate as to meet with very ill success. The discharges will continue for days, in spite of the remedies said to be always successful in checking them. In the majority of instances diarrhœa terminates favourably, as it probably would if left to itself; but in a few cases the disease progresses into the stage of collapse, in spite of all the remedies yet employed."

Dr. Strange, Bridgenorth :—

"In answer to the inquiry I must say decidedly, No! the most fatal cases of Cholera having been those which were seen early, and against the increasing symptoms of which nothing seemed to avail."

Mr. French, Great Marlborough Street :—

"I have not found that Cholera, in the stage of serous diarrhœa, can with certainty be stopped."

Mr. Michael, Swansea :—

"Serous diarrhœa has not proved in every case easily manageable. It has at one period been amenable to one class of remedies, which, at another, have been laid aside as useless. In spite of every modification of the treatment, I have known many cases uninfluenced by any."

Treatment of impending and complete collapse.

The total disappearance of the epidemic from the metropolis and other parts of the country soon after the date of the letter issued by the Committee requesting the co-operation of the profession in making a systematic trial of such plans of treatment as seemed best adapted to counteract the conditions of impending and complete collapse, prevented the suggestions contained in it from being carried into effect.

390 communications on this subject were, however, received from different practitioners. In by far the larger number the general results of treatment are given unsupported by any detail of cases; a defect almost unavoidable in general practice during the height of an epidemic.

A small part only of the information thus conveyed to the College can be made the basis of any certain conclusions, since in general no uniform plan of treatment was steadily employed throughout, but, as the symptoms persisted and became more urgent, various combinations of means were in turn employed, and often for so short a time, or so imperfectly, or under such unfavourable states of the constitution for their operation, as that when recovery took place it was impossible to say to which of them it was due, if, indeed, to any.

Numerical results in the treatment of Cholera are most fallacious. Without a scrupulous regard to the state of the patient at the commencement and at different stages of the treatment, and a note of the period of the epidemic when the observation is made, almost any conclusion may seem to be established.

There is but little hope that any specific remedy will be found to counteract the severer effects of the disease, and it is certain that none having in any way pretensions to such distinction are as yet known.

In the fully-developed stage, medicines administered internally must be of small power. The pathological condition of the gastro-intestinal membrane is such that absorption is then almost, if not quite, suspended, and medicines when retained in the stomach form but an inert accumulation.

The theory of their occasionally acting by sympathy must be regarded as a relic of a therapeutic superstition long since exploded, and, untenable in any condition of the system, is especially so in the collapse of Cholera.

On this division of our subject we can do little more than point out, according to the evidence before us, what forms of treatment seem to have been of some service, or useless, or injurious; and by thus clearing the ground, prepare the way for better directed efforts.

An enumeration of all the means proposed for the treatment of this stage would be useless; it is, therefore, only upon the principal of them that we shall make any report.

Use of
Calomel.

Calomel stands foremost, from having in this country been more fully tested than any other remedy. The theory of the disease which has chiefly led to its employment is not supported by anatomical facts. The absence of bile from the evacuations appears to be merely a subordinate result. Calomel can be administered only on empirical grounds, and its value must be determined by the results so obtained ; for there appears to be no argument in favour of its exhibition either from analogy or pathology.

The results in 365 cases treated by this remedy in small and frequent doses were as follows :—

Results of Cases treated by Calomel in small and frequently-repeated doses.

	Deaths.	Recoveries.
Mr. Bainbridge	3	0
Dr. Basham	3	3
Dr. Blackall . .	31	39*
Dr. R. Chambers	22	18
Dr. Davies (Hertford) .	9	1
Mr. Dabbs (Unité Convict Ship)	18	12
Mr. Eccles (Plymouth)	12	27
Dr. Fearnside	5	5
Cases in St. George's, reported by Dr. Barclay	5	3
Dr. Hill (Peckham Asylum) . .	12	0
Dr. McIntyre	5	7
Mr. Livett .	8	1
Mr. Michael (Swansea) . .	2	1
Dr. McWilliam	12	4
Melville Hospital, Chatham	5	1
Mr. Merry (Hemel Hempstead)	12	40†
Dr. Shearman (Rotherham) .	0	2
Dr. Shapter (Exeter) . .	5	6
Mr. Statter (Wakefield) . .	11	8
Dr. Reid (St. Giles's Infirmary) .	7	0
	187	178

* Fifteen were not in collapse, and 14 in only slight collapse, when the treatment was begun.

† From the report it is doubtful whether many of these cases were in collapse.

This list might be extended by including cases treated with variable doses at irregular intervals, but the result will not thereby be much affected :—

	Deaths.	Recoveries.
Dr. Hawkins (Middlesex Hospital) .	20	17
Tooting Pauper Asylum (Mr. Kite) .	80	61
	100	78

Dr. Ayre forwarded to the College a detail of his theoretical views upon the use of calomel, and with his letter a printed report, from which we extract the following :—

"In the Table will be seen the number of patients and the results of the treatment employed for them; and it is with no inconsiderable degree of just pride, and with yet greater thankfulness, that I bring them under your notice. Of the cases here given, it is to be understood that those of Cholera were in full collapse when they came under treatment, and those in the premonitory stage were entering into that state; whilst of the diarrhœa cases the patients were in that threatening condition which almost constantly precedes and leads into (?) the full disease.

Cases of diarrhœa attended by six house visitors .	1430	
Cases of diarrhœa attended by six district visitors	606	
Cases of diarrhœa attended at dispensaries .	868	
Cases of Cholera in full collapse . . .	725	
Cases of impending collapse .	138	
		3764
Deaths from diarrhœa	6	
Deaths from Cholera . .	365	
		371
Recoveries		3393

Such are the numbers of the patients whom we had under treatment, and such are the results of it."

Extracts from private letters to Dr. Ayre, and from public journals, accompanied the above report, and were all expressive of great confidence in the curative powers of calomel in Cholera.

The numbers here given do not sustain this favourable opinion. The deaths were 365 out of 725 unequivocal cases.

Under various and opposite plans, the recoveries, even in severe cases, averaged from 45 to 55 per cent., according to the period of the epidemic; they should therefore exceed the highest of these numbers before they can be adduced in proof of the value of any particular method of treatment.

In general no appreciable effects followed the administration of calomel, even after a large amount in small and frequently-repeated doses had been administered. For the most part it was quickly evacuated by vomiting or purging, or, when retained for a longer period, was afterwards passed from the bowels unchanged. Salivation but very rarely occurred, and then only in the milder cases.

We conclude that calomel was inert when administered in collapse; that the cases of recovery following its employment at this period were due to the natural course of the disease, as they did not surpass the ordinary average obtained when the treatment consisted in the use of cold water only.

The following quotations are arranged so as to show the balance of general evidence on this point; those which are in favour of the calomel treatment are placed first.

Dr. Oke, Southampton :—

"The Cholera broke out with fearful violence in 'Charlotte Place,' an assemblage of houses on a high situation to the N.E. of the town, and detached from it. The population of this place was estimated at 600, of whom 40 died of the epidemic. Two gentlemen volunteered their gratuitous services to the pauper patients. They decided on adopting a modification of Dr. Ayre's plan, giving two grains of calomel every ten minutes to adults, and somewhat less to children, but without any opium whatever, except when it was demanded by severe cramps.

"In order to insure its regular administration, nurses were employed to give the doses when the medical attendants could not remain with the sufferers. The result was most satisfactory; the vomiting and purging were soon controlled, and by persisting in the treatment the alvine discharges became of a dark green colour, which was considered as prognosticating a favourable termination. As soon as this change was effected, the calomel was given less and less frequently till the disease was subdued.

"Under this treatment, children in whatever stage, whether of diarrhœa or collapse, generally recovered; and it is calculated that *a third part* of the adults in a state of collapse were saved by the same."

Mr. Robert Merry, Hemel Hempstead :—

"I have much pleasure in bearing testimony to the value of Dr.

N

Ayre's plan of calomel with morphia every quarter of an hour (with mustard epithems), over every other plan of treatment I have tried. Out of 52 cases of decided Asiatic Cholera, I believe 40 have been saved by this treatment."

Dr. Shearman, Rotherham :—

"This year I have had in my own practice only two cases of true Cholera, both boys of about eight years, living in the midst of an ill-drained, unventilated, and filthy neighbourhood. They both recovered under very small and frequently-repeated doses of calomel, with very little laudanum, with the addition of the following solution for common drink :—

> Chloride of sodium, gr. 175;
> Chloride of potassium, gr. 17½;
> Tartrate of soda, gr. 40;
> Tribasic phosphate of soda, gr. 122½;
> Sulphate of soda, gr. 17¼;
> Water, a gallon.

"I quite agree with Dr. Ayre that his plan of treatment is the most successful."

Dr. Dick, Bedford :—

"The diarrhœa was treated by ordinary astringents; but the more severe kind attendant upon Cholera was best met by five-grain doses of calomel given in quick succession ; and on collapse appearing, the calomel was increased to a single half-drachm dose, followed by smaller ones of five grains every hour."

Dr. Dick gives no particulars of his success with this plan ; but of the 69 cases under his care, 35 died, the treatment being various.

Mr. Allen, Oxford :—

"Dr. Ayre's plan was tried, but abandoned, because by disturbing the patient so often, the restlessness and exhaustion were increased, and no compensating benefit ensued; but larger doses of calomel at first, followed by smaller ones at intervals of half an hour or an hour, were substituted with advantage."

Dr. R. Chambers :—

"In the collapse of Cholera I have chiefly relied upon calomel (gr. v. at first, and gr. ii. every half hour afterwards) with cold water. I witnessed 18 recoveries in 30 cases."

Dr. Robert Semple, Islington :—

"I have tried all the plans enumerated in the circulars sent to me, and found them to fail, except in some instances the calomel treatment."

Mr. Shillitoe, of Hitchin, after recommending "small and repeated doses of calomel," adds :—

"I am doubtful whether any kind of treatment is of use in the stage of collapse."

Mr. Joseph Taylor, Fever Hospital, Liverpool :—

"The diarrhœa, when unchecked, gradually assumed the serous character, the stools becoming thinner, and devoid of colour, and passed with rapidity. In this stage calomel in small doses, frequently repeated, appeared the most efficacious remedy. In very few instances did it produce salivation, and then only in the mildest cases. One person took 1160 grains, another 500, without any ill effect whatever."

Mr. Henry Perry, Stonehouse :—

"I carried out, in numerous cases, to the fullest extent the plan advised by Dr. Ayre, and unquestionably with marked success; but finding from large experience that the laudanum narcotized my patients, I gave it only in occasional doses, and exhibited the calomel alone in a mixture of tragacanth and mucilage. I attribute my success in several instances to this method of treatment. In candour, however, I must state that when collapse was fairly set in, calomel exhibited in any degree too often led to no good result, and the disease continued its course unchecked to the end."

Mr. J. H. Roberts, Finchley Road :—

"In my hand the calomel plan has succeeded in 8 out of 11 cases of collapse, more or less severe. I considered 3 of those who recovered moribund when I first saw them."

Mr. Roberts gives the report of only one case, a female, who was under impending collapse when first seen ; two grains of calomel were given every ten minutes, with ether and chloroform to allay the cramps, but she never rallied, and died the same day.

Dr. Shapter, Exeter :—

"Mercury in small and repeated doses is less fatal than a treatment conducted without mercury."

Mr. Statter, Wakefield :—

"I have had the exclusive treatment of 19 cases of Cholera (11 deaths and 8 recoveries), and have been called in to several others ;

in all calomel was more or less administered, but I must confess that my faith in its efficacy has considerably diminished. I have tried Dr. Ayre's plan in several of them, and it has failed."

Mr. Mallett, Bolton :—

"I tried calomel in small and frequent doses; I gave it in large doses, but all in vain."

Dr. Wood, Winchester :—

"Calomel in small and repeated doses I have employed without satisfactory results, nor have I seen the advantage of calomel with opium."

Dr. Strange, Bridgenorth :—

"Calomel in large doses was not successful. At first most of us began its use, but after the first few cases I abandoned it, as it appeared to lower the resisting powers of the system, without having any marked effect on the disease. Salivation occurred but in a few cases, when it did (in two or three) recovery resulted. In one case when I used large doses (ten grains every four hours) profuse salivation followed, but the collapse returned three times, and the patient was with difficulty saved."

Mr. Hovell, Clapton :—

"Calomel, in small and frequent doses, was partially tried, with no good results."

Mr. Bainbridge, St. Martin's Lane :—

"I have tried the plan recommended by Dr. Ayre in three cases; it did not appear to do the least good: they all died."

Dr. David Lewis, Finsbury :—

"Calomel, in my experience, both in large and small doses, was totally useless."

Dr. Davies, Hertford :—

"Mr. Woodhouse, the Union medical officer of the town, was much prepossessed in favour of calomel in small doses frequently repeated. Ten cases, varying but little in their symptoms, and watched by myself, were successively treated with calomel alone, according to the mode already described (2½ grains every quarter of an hour), and 9 out of the 10 died; some at the end of 12 or 15 hours, and others after the expiration of several days. Hence the treatment, by calomel only, was abandoned. The single case of recovery was mild from the beginning. Of 33 cases treated with calomel, either alone or in combination with opium, camphor, and other ingredients, 24 died and 9 recovered."

Dr. Parkes :—

" I did not feel myself at liberty to try the effect of large doses of calomel, since I had satisfied myself that they were hurtful, but I gave Dr. Ayre's plan a trial in several cases. In one or two the method was carried out literally (calomel in two-grain doses every five minutes) ; in others it was not used so rigorously, yet sufficiently so to enable me to form an opinion as to its efficacy. I saw no striking benefit from its use, and I may mention that I tried a similar plan (viz. two grains of calomel every ten minutes) in 1843, in India, without finding it of any use."

Dr. Rayner, of Stockport : —

" I found that in the cases treated on Dr. Ayre's plan, the stage of collapse was more prolonged than in those treated by opium, but that under both plans of treatment death eventually took place."

Dr. A. W. Barclay, Report from St. George's Hospital :—

" In 8 cases, calomel was repeated at intervals of from 5 to 15 minutes, in small doses, with or without a larger previous dose ; 5 died, and 3 recovered. Of those which recovered, 2 were comparatively mild cases, and were never completely collapsed, the other was pulseless upwards of 4 hours."

Mr. Dabbs, surgeon of the *Unité*, convict ship, gives a list of 30 cases treated with calomel, conjoined, according to the urgency of the symptoms, with salines and occasionally with stimuli, the use of the warm bath and sinapisms. They were males, between the ages of 20 and 35 ; 12 are stated to have been in feeble health and labouring under some disease : 7 of these recovered. Of the whole 30 cases there were 18 deaths and 12 recoveries. The frequency of consecutive fever is not noted.

Dr. Fearnside, of Preston, gives the details of 10 cases treated by calomel in small doses, a large quantity of the medicine being given in all the cases. There were 5 deaths and 5 recoveries. Of those that recovered, 2 were very mild cases; in one of these salivation occurred. No obvious effects of the treatment were observed in the others. The ages were 2, 4, 9, 18, 36, 36, 63, 67, 76.

Mr. Kite gives an outline of 235 cases of Cholera occurring amongst the children in the pauper asylum at Tooting; males, 122 ; females, 113 ;—187 passed into a state of collapse with the following results :—

		Collapsed.	Recovered,	Died.
3 years and under	5	21	4	17
5 „ „	10	84	31	53
10 „ „	15	82	44	38
		187	79	108

Of these, 141 were treated by calomel (doses and frequency not given); stimuli, as ammonia and brandy, were occasionally administered; and sinapisms and the warm bath used. The deaths were 80, the recoveries 61.

Of the deaths, 61 died in collapse, 19 with fever and prostration.

Of the recoveries, 44 were without fever, 17 after fever and long-continued prostration.

Dr. J. Reid, St. Giles's Infirmary:—

" Dr. Ayre's plan was tried in 7 cases in succession in the infirmary, but as all died quickly the plan was not persevered in."

Melville Hospital, Chatham:—

5 cases are carefully detailed. In 3 a fair trial was made of the value of calomel and opium for arresting the premonitory diarrhœa, but the treatment was ineffectual. In 4 of the cases the plan recommended by Dr. Ayre was precisely followed; in the fifth, the calomel was given in larger doses. 4 died in the stage of collapse, and 1 on the ninth day, in consecutive fever.

Mr. Livett, of Wells, gives a table of 9 cases "treated with calomel in small and frequent doses, combined with a small proportion of opium." All the patients died but one, a boy of 14 years.

The patients were in a state of collapse when first seen. One was in the eighth month of pregnancy, and gave birth to a dead child on the second day. The case that recovered was pulseless for 24 hours.

Six of the patients were males, and three females. The ages were respectively 14, 28, 28, 28, 35, 36, 40, 60, 80. Death occurred in collapse, except in two cases.

Dr. Blackall sends an abstract of 101 cases treated by calomel. In 31, the tartarized antimony formed part of the treatment, with, in some cases, bleeding or leeches.

Of the 70 cases treated by calomel alone, the following are the details. They were males:—

Ages.

From 15 to 20 . . .	16
„ 20 „ 40 . . .	49
„ 40 „ 50 . . .	3
., 50 „ 60 . . .	2
	70

Results :—

	Recovered.	Died.
15 were not in collapse when the treatment was commenced	14	1
14 were in slight collapse . . .	12	2
23 in marked, but moderate, collapse .	11	12
18 in extreme collapse	2	16
	39	31

In 39 cases calomel was given in doses of 5 grs. every half-hour.

In 10	„	„	5 „	quarter of an hour
In 14			20 „	half-hour.
In 3			5 „	hour.
In 1			10 „	half-hour.
In 2			5 „	2 hours.
In 1	„	„	30 „	3 hours.

There is no mention of obvious effects, immediate or remote.

Of the 39 recoveries, 17 had consecutive fever; of the 31 deaths, 7 had consecutive fever.

In 14 of the worst cases a salt-and-water emetic was given. In 11 venæsection was used; in 2 the hot-air bath; some took saline draughts, containing chlorate of potash.

In 27 other cases, *stimulants* were given with the calomel. They were males.

Ages.

From 10 to 15 . . .	5
„ 15 „ 20 . . .	2
„ 20 „ 40 . . .	13
„ 40 „ 50 . . .	2
Over 50	-
	27

Results :—

	Recovered.	Died.
2 not in collapse when the treatment was commenced	0	2
5 in slight collapse	1	4
4 in moderate collapse	1	3
16 in extreme collapse .	8	16

8 took calomel, 5 grains every half-hour.
9　　　„　　　5　　　„　　　quarter of an hour.
1　　　„　　　5　　　„　　　hour.
2　　　„　　　20　　　„　　　half-hour.

Others uncertain.

16 died without passing into consecutive fever; 9 had consecutive fever ending in coma.

Dr. Shapter makes a return of 11 cases treated by mercury in small doses; of these, 6 recovered and 5 died. 6 had secondary fever, of which 2 recovered and 4 died.

Dr. Hawkins returns 37 cases treated with calomel in the Middlesex Hospital. The dose was, in most of the cases, gr. ii. every half-hour. In some the intervals were longer or the doses larger, according to the urgency of the symptoms. The deaths were 20, the recoveries 17. In addition to the employment of calomel, a salt-and-water emetic was given when the patients were first admitted, and the vomiting was encouraged by copious draughts of warm fluids. With a few exceptions, they were all placed in a hip bath of 104° Fahr. for ten minutes, and with marked relief to the spasms. The hot-air bath produced a distressing oppression of the breathing, and was therefore discontinued.

Salines were given with the calomel, and occasionally stimuli, as ammonia and brandy.

Dr. James Hill, Peckham House Lunatic Asylum:—

"In 2 cases I employed calomel and opium in small doses frequently repeated, as recommended so highly by Dr. Ayre, of Hull, and most faithfully carried out his plan to the letter. Both cases, however, proved fatal, as likewise did all of those (and they were several) treated in a similar manner during the prevalence of the epidemic in November last. As the epidemic did not leave us for a month after this, and the balance of evidence was much in favour of Dr. Ayre's plan, I resolved on giving it a further trial, notwithstanding its previous ill success in my hands. I accordingly adopted it in 10 other cases, and most attentively carried out his recommendations in every point, but with the same fatal results; so that out of 12 cases treated on this plan I was so unfortunate as not to save one."

Dr. McIntyre, of the Western General Dispensary, records 12 cases, 4 females and 8 males, all but 2 being between the ages of 30 and 40. The deaths were 5, recoveries 7.

The treatment consisted in small and frequent doses of calomel, with occasional stimuli and salines, according to the urgency of the symptoms. 4 of the cases which recovered were mild. Salivation occurred in one of these.

Dr. McWilliam :—

"Thus much I can say for calomel, when it was given before collapse, so as to be taken into the system, the bilious tinge given to the stools and the discharge of urine were coincident events. Until there was sure evidence of mercurialization upon the general system I have seen no benefit from its use."

Of 16 cases treated principally with calomel by Dr. McWilliam, 12 died.

Treatment by calomel, opium, and stimulants. This is termed the "rational method" of treatment, and was intended to combine those remedies which seemed best fitted to fulfil the supposed indications of this stage. The calomel was given to restore the functions of the liver, and as an alterative of the morbid action in the gastro-intestinal mucous membrane ;—the opium to allay irritation and arrest the discharges ;—and the stimuli to counteract the depression of the nervous system. Experience did not confirm the theory: the results were unfavourable, and not altogether so indifferent as when calomel was exhibited by itself.

Although opium and diffusible stimuli, brandy, camphor, and ammonia were useful at an early stage of the disease, as collapse set in, they not only failed to produce any favourable result, but often aggravated the symptoms.

It seems well ascertained that opium in large doses was at this period injurious; by increasing the cerebral oppression and embarrassing the system during reaction. It was probably less and less applicable as the disease advanced to its characteristic development.

Stimuli, especially the various preparations of alcohol, did not act as restoratives in collapse, but often increased the irritability of the stomach, and added to the sense of oppression at the præcordia.

The expectations excited by the early success apparently obtained by the use of chloroform, were not realised in its subsequent employment. It not unfrequently allayed the vomiting and cramps, but did not in any degree arrest the course of the disease.

The perchloride of carbon in 5 or 10 grain doses, and a solution of camphor in chloroform, acted as powerful stimuli, but the results did not indicate that they possessed any especial therapeutic value. Although they produced symptoms of reaction, this apparent improvement was generally, in severe cases, but transient, and their continued use seemed to exhaust the little remaining power, rather than to restore the patient.

21 cases were treated by calomel, opium, and stimulants, in St. Bartholomew's, by Dr. George Burrows, from July 19th to 25th, 1849—12 males, and 9 females.

Ages.

Under 20	.	.	.	.	.	.	.	6
20 to 40	.	.	.	.	.	.	.	12
Over 40 .	.	.	.	.	.	.	.	3

	Deaths.	Recoveries.
3 not collapsed	0	3
3 slight collapse .	0	3
11 marked collapse	7	
4 extreme collapse	4	0

The dose of the medicines was calomel five grains, opium one grain, every two or four hours; the first dose being sometimes double. All the patients had a warm bath. According to the urgency of the symptoms, ammonia, brandy, wine and chloroform were given, and they were also allowed to take freely cold water and ice. Sinapisms to the epigastrium.

The results were as follows: 5 died within 24 hours, the shortest time of the treatment being $9\frac{1}{2}$ hours; and 6 in from 3 to 5 days; 10 recovered; Dr. Burrows adds :—

" During this period of the epidemic the remedies employed seemed to have little or no influence ; the patients were neither salivated by the mercury, nor narcotized by the opium."

In contrast to the above, Dr. Burrows gives 14 cases treated from September 20th to 25th—7 males and 7 females.

Ages.

Under 20	.	.	.	.	.	.	.	3
20 to 40	.	.	.	.	.	.	.	9
Over 40 .	.	.	.	.	.	.	.	2

	Deaths.	Recoveries.
4 not collapsed	0	
2 slight collapse	0	2
8 marked collapse, but symptoms not extreme }	2	6

The treatment was that employed in July. Dr. Burrows says:—

"In July the mercury and opium produced no effect on the symptoms, whilst in September, the same remedies appeared to give relief, and in several cases quickly produced their respective specific effects on the system."

16 cases (9 males, 7 females) were treated by Dr. Basham with calomel and opium, brandy, ammonia, chloroform, sinapisms, and the warm bath. In some cases, enemata of acetate of lead were used.

Ages.
Under 20 5
20 to 40 7
Over 40 4

The recoveries were 2, deaths 14. 11 of the cases were in marked collapse when the treatment was commenced; in the other 5 diarrhœa was urgent, with symptoms of depression. 8 of the deaths took place in collapse, with symptoms of coma; 6 died in consecutive fever. The two cases of recovery had mild consecutive fever. Except in one instance, where slight reaction followed the application of the wet sheet, no obvious effects resulted from the means employed.

Dr. Shapter, Exeter, gives the results of 68 cases treated with calomel and opium, 41 recovered, and 27 died; 24 had consecutive fever, of which 18 recovered, and 6 died. He adds:—

"This combination appears to avert death more successfully than mercury by itself; nevertheless, those cases which recover, whether from incipient or complete collapse, are, if the use of the opium be long persevered in, more likely to pass into consecutive fever than if no opium be given."

Drs. Dunn and Milner, Wakefield Prison.—In the prison at Wakefield, in January, 1849, 27 cases of Cholera occurred. They were all males.

Ages.
18 to 35 20
35 to 50 6
70 1

The deaths were 16, recoveries 11. In 16 cases diarrhœa preceded the symptoms of collapse, and the discharges were in 11 of these characterised as bilious. The whole 27 cases had symptoms of collapse, viz. cramps, feeble or imperceptible pulse, cold dusky surface, &c. They were treated in the following manner:—

"As soon as a patient was received into the hospital, he was placed in a hot bath of 105° for five or ten minutes. Mustard poultices were applied large enough to cover the greater part of the front of the chest and abdomen, and frictions were used, with turpentine liniment, to the back and limbs. Calomel and opium were given in small and repeated doses, and also ammonia and brandy, effervescing salines and cold water, as freely as the patients desired."

Dr. Hawkins reports 21 cases treated with calomel (two to three grains) and opium (half a grain to one grain) every half hour or hour, according to the urgency of the symptoms. Brandy, chloroform, camphor, and effervescing salines, were also prescribed, and external stimulants and the hot-air bath used. 17 were in marked collapse, and 4 in the incipient stage, when the treatment was commenced; 15 died, and 6 recovered. Most of the deaths took place in collapse.

Mr. Clarke, Hackney:—

"The plan which I have pursued with the greatest success has been to give calomel (gr. iii.) with opium (gr. ss.) every ten minutes, quarter of an hour, or half hour. Out of 20 cases I have saved at least one in three."

Dr. Dickinson and Dr. Burgess, Liverpool Fever Infirmary:—

"These remedies (calomel and opium) combined have been the most successful in our hands previous to the state of collapse, in which we have found opium decidedly injurious. The dose usually given to adult males was two grains of calomel with half a grain of opium every half hour. Opium in large doses alone we have found in all cases prejudicial, in the severe cases manifestly hastening on coma and death, and in the milder cases producing or aggravating the consecutive fever. We are so fully convinced of these facts from ample experience, that we dare no longer prescribe it by itself."

Dr. McIntyre, Western General Dispensary, gives 3 cases treated by opium, stimulants, and astringents, with external warmth and frictions—2 females, æt. 29 and 56, and a boy; all died, two in collapse, and one in consecutive fever.

"The irritable condition of the stomach was not in the least controlled in two of the cases, nor any of the symptoms alleviated."

Dr. Rayner, of Stockport, reports 11 cases; 5 males, 6 females, aged respectively 3, 28, 30, 42, 49, 54, 54, 62, 65, 71, —. 3 of the cases were in collapse when first seen. In 1, the severe purging was arrested and collapse prevented. The treatment was opium in large doses, with brandy, ammonia, &c. In 2 mild cases, calomel was given with the opium. There were 8 deaths, and 3 recoveries. One died comatose, one in consecutive fever, and 6 in collapse. The 3 recoveries are stated to have been in mild cases. Dr. Rayner remarks:—

" I think in the cases treated with opium, the stage of collapse was certainly shortened by the death of the patient, for in those to whom it was not administered, though death eventually took place, the state of collapse was prolonged."

Dr. Hawkins gives a list of 7 patients—2 males and 5 females— treated by opium, astringents, capsicum, ether, and effervescing salines; 4 recovered, and 3 died.

Dr. Beadle, Tewkesbury:—

" There is great tolerance of opium in the stage of serous diarrhœa, and one or two large doses at an early stage of the disease I have seen attended with benefit, but if administered at too late a stage I consider it highly injurious, producing narcotism, and rendering the subsequent fever more severe and complicated."

Dr. Dick, Bedford:—

" Opium we had every reason to suppose was injurious."

Dr. Basham:—

" Opium in large doses I believe to be injurious."

Dr. Strange, Bridgenorth:—

" Opium was not much used by me, but in the practice of others I saw that the result was decidedly injurious. The coldness of the surface and the clammy sweats of collapse seemed to be increased, and death hastened by it."

Dr. Shapter, Exeter:—

" Stimulants are useful in the premonitory disease and earlier stages of collapse, but their use is more doubtful after collapse is fully established. These remedies were notably employed in 40 cases: of these 21 died, and 19 recovered, and as many of these recoveries were not the severer cases, the adoption of this treatment generally cannot be considered advantageous. The cases varied somewhat in their tolerance of this class of remedies, but few were anxious for them, whilst by far a larger proportion expressed a repugnance to them.

" Camphor appeared to exert, in many cases, the greatest and most prompt benefit, giving direct comfort to the stomach. Combined with hydrocyanic acid it tended greatly to relieve the epigastric and painful vomiting, retraction of the præcordia, and cramps."

Dr. Blackall reports 28 cases, males.

Ages.							
Under 20							. 10
20 to 40	.		.		.		. 11
Over 40	.	.	.		.	.	. 7

				Deaths.	Recoveries.
2 not collapsed	.	.	.	0	2
6 slight collapse	.	.	.	1	5
7 marked collapse	.			6	1
13 severe collapse	.	.	.	12	1

The treatment was brandy and laudanum in 5 cases: camphor, chloroform, and ammonia in 10 cases; chloroform and brandy in 7 cases; oil of turpentine in 3 cases; camphor alone 3 cases. There were 9 recoveries, and 19 deaths; 6 recovered without consecutive fever; 3 after consecutive fever; 7 died in consecutive fever; 11 in collapse, and 1 not recorded.

Dr. McWilliam gives an account of 8 cases treated by stimuli and tonics. They were males, from 25 to 45 years of age; 4 recovered, and 4 died.

Dr. Barclay's report of cases in St. George's Hospital:—

"Stimulants were administered in large quantity in 5 cases—3 of these recovered. They were administered in moderate quantity in 15 cases; of these 4 recovered. They were altogether withheld in 4 cases; of these 2 recovered. In no case in which the collapse was complete, did stimulants restore the circulation: in one or two instances, they seemed to produce a transient effect in rallying the powers of life, but they produced no permanent good effect."

Dr. Wood, Winchester:—

"Against large doses of opium I am decided, as well as against alcohol."

Dr. Raynor, Stockport:—

"In some of the early cases of the epidemic, I administered brandy and camphor, but soon discontinued them. I do not believe that large doses of stimulants are attended with benefit in the stage of collapse, but that they rather tend to depress the heart's action."

Mr. Mallett, Bolton:—

"I tried the stimulating plan with warm fomentations of mustard, &c., but all in vain."

Mr. Burchell, Kingsland :—

"Stimulants appeared quite useless."

Dr. Strange, Bridgenorth :—

"Stimulants generally, whether brandy, ammonia, ether, camphor, or aromatics, were given by me in some cases, and freely by some other practitioners. In the more advanced cases they appeared to do harm, especially when the pulse was flagging, and the surface cold."

Dr. Paul, Bermondsey :—

"An extensive experience in the use of stimulants both in 1832–33, and in 1848–49, has entirely convinced me of their worse than uselessness. I have not known a case in which that practice has been mainly depended on do well. In 1832, the first appearance of the disease, 7 cases occurred in the immediate vicinity of the mill-streams in this neighbourhood; 6 were treated with opium, and the free use of stimulants; they all died. The seventh drank freely of cold water, and recovered."

Dr. White, Winchester :—

"I watched the treatment by stimulants alone which was pursued in several cases by one of the surgeons here, and I tried that mode of treatment in the first 5 cases which occurred to myself, and it appeared to me to be more than ordinarily unsuccessful. Brandy gin, ether, and ammonia, each appeared to aggravate the sickness. I saw them injected per anum, I believe with injurious effects."

Dr. Borland, Newington :—

"I have tried all kinds of stimulants without the slightest benefit."

Dr. R. Semple :—

"In 1832, I had, in conjunction with another surgeon, charge of a Cholera Hospital, and found brandy, even in pint draughts, quite useless."

Dr. Lang, Heavitree :—

"Ether, ammonia, brandy and opium all aggravate the disease, and augment its virulence." "Musk is quite useless." "Camphor doubtful."

Dr. Theophilus Thompson :—

"I have seen a few cases in which reaction from a state of collapse appeared to be promoted by administering six drachms of the spirits of turpentine, and afterwards repeating small doses at inter-

vals of a quarter of an hour, but in other instances I did not observe any effect from the remedy."

Dr. Dickinson, Liverpool :—

    " In the first stage, when the evacuations have been profuse, and
the prostration proportionate, we have found ammonia and alcoholic
liquids in moderate doses serviceable, but they appear to exert a
decidedly injurious effect on the consecutive fever."

Dr. Davies, Hertford (first report), gives the particulars of a
case in which chloroform was administered by inhalation.

    " The patient was a monthly nurse, æt. 62 ; the treatment for the
first 8 hours consisted in frequent doses of opium and catechu.
The inhalation began about 15 hours after the seizure. The patient
fell asleep in a few seconds, and continued to sleep almost constantly
for two hours. The inhalation was repeated four times at intervals
with the like effect, relieving the cramps, and giving general ease,
but it did not retard the course of the disease in the least degree."

He adds :—

    " In 22 cases, as severe symptoms came on, the chief remedy was
chloroform administered internally in doses of from seven to ten
minims every hour, half hour, or quarter of an hour, according to
the severity of the symptoms, but of these 22, 8 terminated fatally,
and 14 recovered."

Dr. Davies (second report) :—

    " Out of 9 cases of Cholera, and 13 of the worst cases of diarrhœa,
occurring in my own practice, and treated with chloroform, one
died. All these were in the better ranks of life. In some of them,
the warm salt-water bath was used as an auxiliary, and the diet
consisted of nothing but cold milk and water, with some carbonate
of soda ad libitum. The fatal case was that of a drunkard, who
probably did not take the remedy.

    " These cases varied in degree of severity, from sickness and diar-
rhœa, and some amount of collapse, to sickness, diarrhœa, severe
cramps, and great collapse, with almost clear watery evacuations
passing away involuntarily.

    " Of 14 cases of Cholera treated by my friend, Mr. Towers, Me-
dical Resident of the infirmary, many of them under my observation, one died. The fatal case was that of a woman, æt. 63, in a
state of great destitution."

Dr. Davies (third report) :—

    " It will probably be remembered by the Committee, that in my
second report, I expressed a very favourable opinion of chloroform
in this deadly malady. I considered I had strong grounds for so

doing, after observing the large proportion of cases which recovered under its administration. From the history of this last visitation in the county prison, however, the fact turns out, that, under some uncertain circumstances, the use of chloroform will not prevent the proportion of deaths being considerable. I have reason to believe that it was, from over anxiety, given in too frequent doses in some cases, and that it thus rather added to the coma, which is one of the characteristics of the malady.

" At the commencement of the outbreak, the doses were repeated every hour, or every two hours, and it is to be noted, that the first 7 cases recovered. As the cases multiplied, the remedy was given every half hour, and in some instances, every quarter of an hour; the result was, that the next 6 cases died. Whether these cases had anything in them inherently more fatal, it is difficult to tell; the symptoms at first were about equal, and the differences did not show themselves until towards the end. There was next a recovery of 7 cases in succession; in these the remedy was administered less frequently, but subsequently 2 deaths occurred under the less frequent administration.

" The chloroform was administered also by inhalation in some of the more severe cases of cramps, with the effect of affording relief in every instance. The inhalation was not carried so far as to produce perfect insensibility.

" Although I am still of opinion that chloroform, properly regulated, is the remedy, of all others hitherto tried, to be depended upon, yet it cannot be considered as a ' specific' for Cholera. In one of my fatal cases the chloroform mixture had been taken for two or three days, about every four hours, during the stage of diarrhœa, yet the patient sank rapidly into collapse, and died in two days."

Dr. Davies' subsequent statement:—

" I found that no reliance could be placed on chloroform alone. It is true the cramps and pain were greatly relieved by it if the inhalation was carried so far as to produce insensibility, but the course of the disease did not seem to be at all impeded."

Mr. Vines, Reading:—

" Chloroform was tried, but its effects were evanescent."

Mr. Butcher, of Ware, in a letter to Dr. Davies, speaks in high terms of the value of chloroform for arresting the early symptoms of Cholera, viz. vomiting and cramps. It does not seem to have been successful in rallying patients under impending collapse, nor in arresting the onward course of the disease. 4 cases of urgent Cholera were treated by Mr. Butcher with stimulants, the warm bath, and chloroform ; 2 died and 2 recovered.

The Commissioners in Lunacy forwarded to the College the copy of a letter from Dr. Hill, of the Peckham Lunatic Asylum, giving his experience of the use of chloroform.   Dr. Hill says :—

> " We have had in all 17 cases.
>
> Deaths 5
> Recoveries 8
> Under treatment 4
>
> 17"

The first 3 fatal cases were not treated with chloroform.   The following are the details of the first case so treated :—

> " A fourth case occurred in which the vomiting was incessant, and the cramps excruciating, the purging severe, the skin cold, clammy, and blue, and the patient apparently sinking from collapse.   Chloroform had the effect of tranquillizing the nervous system, and of checking the vomiting and spasms, and of restoring the animal heat.   The patient was kept gently under its influence for upwards of 24 hours ; whenever it was suspended, or the patient began to recover consciousness, the distressing symptoms immediately returned. In the intervals small quantities of brandy and water were administered, with arrow-root and milk for nourishment. This case is now convalescent.   9 other cases have been treated in this manner, all of which have recovered, or are now convalescent."

No mention is made of the other 4.

As the intensity of the symptoms in the several cases was not noted, a letter was addressed to Dr. Hill, inquiring if his further experience corresponded with the favourable report here given, to which the following reply was received :

> " In the epidemic of 1849, I must candidly admit I did not find the treatment of Cholera by means of the chloroform inhalation nearly so efficacious as in the previous year. The type of the disease was of a more virulent character both in this establishment and in the neighbourhood, and but a small proportion (little more than one-fourth) were saved."

Dr. A. W. Barclay's report from St. George's :—

> " Chloroform was administered in combination with camphor in 3 cases, 2 of which proved fatal ; in 1 it was employed in the premonitory stage every half hour, for several hours, and was

abandoned only when decided symptoms of Cholera occurred. It was also administered at the close of another fatal case, without apparent benefit."

Mr. Perry, Stonehouse:

" At the outset of my practice, when I found my patient suffering horribly from cramps, I prescribed 5 minims of chloroform combined with tincture of opium, lavender, and camphor every half hour. This draught was rejected from the stomach so soon as swallowed, and when repeated was attended with the same result, until at length I lost all confidence in its use."

Dr. Blackall :—

" 7, cases were treated with chloroform, of these, one was in articulo mortis, and therefore not to be considered. 4 in collapse, 3 died, 1 recovered ; 2 in approaching collapse, both recovered.

Use of cold water and ice.

The obvious requirements of the system, and the urgent thirst, were sufficient indications for the use of diluents, and the experience of the profession appears to be uniformly in favour of permitting patients to gratify their appetite for them. Cold water was generally preferred, and good results were often observed when it was taken freely in repeated and copious draughts, although it excited vomiting. In smaller quantities, and iced, it was refreshing to the system, and allayed the irritability of the stomach.

Ice was generally grateful to patients in impending or approaching collapse, and probably acted favourably upon the mucous membrane, and served to arrest the discharges.

Dr. Arnott * proposed to push the therapeutic action of cold further, by administering a mixture of ice and salt in large quantities. 2 patients submitted by him to such a treatment recovered. There is no further experience respecting it.

Reinhardt and Leubuscher† write as follows :—

" The principal result of therapeutical experience during the present epidemic is, in our opinion, the general introduction of the use of ice and cold water.

" Ice relieves the burning feeling of thirst, and in many cases favours reaction more than the most powerful stimuli.

" In the typhoid state we have in some cases continued the use of

* Med. Gazette, 1849, p. 375.
† Archiv. für Path. Anat., &c., 2 Band, p. 516.

iced water in place of all medicines. It appears to be the only rational means adapted to the anatomico-pathological condition of the intestinal mucous membrane, as opposed to warm fluids, which only increase the irritation. It is also that which gives the greatest relief to the patient."

This encomium on the use of cold water is in accordance with the unanimous expression of opinion in the communications made to the College, and is confirmed by other reports. Thus Dr. C. J. Müller, in his pamphlet on the Cholera in Riga, says :—

" All observers here agree in the praise of ice and iced water."

And in the report on Cholera in the Obuschowschen Hospital in Petersburgh, it is stated that—

" Warm drinks were avoided, as they increased the discharges and did not revive the patients. Ice and iced water were certainly most serviceable ; they refreshed the system without oppressing the stomach."

The desire for cold drinks was not, however, universal. In the severest cases the patients lay in a state of apathy without expressing any want, and when urged to drink, did so with indifference.

Salines.   Salines of low specific gravity were sometimes given instead of common water, the intention being to restore to the blood a fluid similar to that lost in the early stages of the disease.

We have no evidence that they possessed any influence over the local morbid action in the mucous membrane. It was not until this surface had in part recovered its function of absorption, that any good resulted from their employment.

When given at an early period and in a more concentrated form, they appeared to favour the discharges.

Dr. Burton, of Walsall, reports 20 cases, treated mostly by salines, 15 males and 5 females.

Ages.
7 years	1
20 to 40	11
40 to 50	3
60 to 80	4
Unknown	1

9 of the cases were in the promonitory stage, 4 in approaching collapse, and 7 in collapse, when the treatment was commenced. The saline given was :—

"Sodæ sesquicarb. Ɖj; sodæ chlorid. Ʒj; potass. chlorid. gr. viij; aquæ Oʃ; and occasionally the sulphate of magnesia largely diluted."

In 5 cases, reaction seems to have been accelerated by the use of the wet sheet. There were 6 recoveries, and 14 deaths. Of the recoveries 3 were mild cases, the symptoms of collapse never having been severe, one had consecutive fever. Of the deaths, 11 took place in collapse, and 3 in consecutive fever.·

Thirty-seven cases treated by mercurials and salines in the Middlesex Hospital are reported by Dr. Hawkins; of these 17 recovered, and 20 died. Of several it is stated, that secondary fever ensued, but as, in many cases, there is no note, the proportion in which it occurred to the whole is not known.

Mr. E. E. Hooper, Haggerstone:—

"At the first outbreak of the disease in Haggerstone in July last, I watched 6 cases treated by the parish officer, Mr. Burchell, under Dr. Stevens' saline plan; no good effect was perceptible. The evacuations were increased, not the slightest attempt at rallying seemed to be made, and they all quickly died. I had previously felt great reliance on this method, as well from believing in the theory, as from the success reported to have resulted therefrom during the outbreak of the Cholera in 1832."

Dr. Haycraft, Greenwich:—

"The modification of the saline plan of Dr. Stevens, as recommended by Dr. Marsden, was fairly tried by us and failed."

Dr. Beadle, Tewkesbury:—

"So far as I used the saline treatment of Dr. Stevens, I could not put any faith in it."

Dr. Parkes gives a report of 13 cases treated on the saline plan; sodii chloridi Ʒss, sodæ tart. gr. xij, sodæ phosphat. grs. viij. aquæ Oj. Specif. grav. 1008. Salines were also occasionally given in an effervescing state. There were 6 recoveries and 7 deaths. The treatment produced no obvious effect upon the symptoms. The vomiting and purging continued unabated. In 6 cases there was secondary fever, in 3 it was mild, and ended in recovery.

Of the 6 cases that recovered, it is remarked that 3 were mild. In addition to the above 13 cases, 4 others are also reported, in which—

"Salines were prescribed and persevered in, until no reasonable hope of recovery remained, after which recourse was had to injections into the veins. They all ended fatally."

Dr. Basham :—

" The saline plan recommended by Dr. Stevens has been attended with such apparently favourable results, that I shall continue to employ it until more numerous failures convince me of its inefficacy. 4 cases out of 5, in which it was employed by me, recovered."

Emetics.   Emetics were sometimes given at the onset of the disease, with the intention of cutting short the morbid action, by distributing the blood to the surface, and relieving the congestion of the intestinal mucous membrane.

They were given in collapse in the hope of bringing about reaction.

And they were given for the purpose of superseding the irritability of the stomach set up by the disease.

It is probable that, when administered early, they were occasionally of service ; but the results appear to have been too uncertain to admit of their forming any part of a routine system of treatment.

In collapse, they were not generally admissible ; for, although they occasionally produced symptoms of reaction, this effect was but of short duration, and was followed by increased exhaustion ; at least, such was the more common sequence ; in rare instances, the improvement, thus begun, continued.

When emetics, given with the third intention, were effectual in lessening the irritability of the stomach, it is still doubtful how far such a result was curative.

The amount of evidence in the communications received is too small to admit of any definite conclusion as to the conditions under which these remedies are applicable ; but the general deduction is, that in the early stages they were sometimes of use, and in collapse the effects were equivocal. .

Dr. Haycraft :—

" Emetics failed to produce any benefit."

Dr. Basham :

" Emetics have been employed in 2 cases only ; reaction speedily followed their administration ; but both cases fell back again into collapse, and died."

Dr. Barclay, Report of Cases in St. George's Hospital :—

" Emetics were employed in 11 cases with the view of rousing the system generally, and with apparent success. 3, in a state of imperfect collapse, recovered. They were given with probable benefit in a fourth case, in the stage of complete collapse; and with no permanent benefit in the other 7 cases, all of which were fatal. The emetic was, in 8 cases, mustard, or mustard and salt, and in 3, sulphate of zinc."

Dr. Rae, Royal Naval Hospital, Plymouth:—

"I have used emetics with, I think, injurious effects."

Dr. Rayner, Stockport:—

"All the cases of Cholera under my care, which were not in collapse, were treated by mustard emetics, and one or two large doses of opium: I was satisfied with the result. The vomiting and cramps were much relieved; and, in many cases, a strong desire for drink was manifested. In my own case, nothing arrested the purging before an emetic was given. Of 39 cases with profuse watery evacuations and cramps, and in impending collapse, thus treated, there were 6 deaths."

Sir Duncan McArthur:—

"In the premonitory diarrhœa, opiates and aromatic confection were of great benefit; but when it assumed the Cholera form, ipecacuanha, as an emetic, was more useful than other means; the patients, at the same time, being allowed to drink as much barley-water, or cold water, as their thirst demanded."

Dr. Roupell:—

"Emetics will rouse the system, even in the stage of collapse; but their chief advantage is in the earlier period, when collapse is threatened. Their immediate effect is often to arrest the diarrhœa, and, secondarily, to check the vomiting."

Dr. Hawkins:—

"During the earlier stage, emetics have appeared to me beneficial. A signal instance of their value, even in the advanced period, occurred in the case of a male patient, aged 30; he was perfectly blue and pulseless, with great restlessness and dyspnœa. Death seemed impending. With the forlorn hope of relieving the oppression complained of at the epigastrium, I directed a salt-and-water emetic to be given, which, as soon as it operated, gave great relief, and from that time the patient began steadily to recover."

Report on Cholera in the Obuschowschen Hospital, St. Petersburgh:—

"In the second stage, we have never seen emetics act as stimulants; but, on the contrary, they seemed to hasten dissolution

Given at the onset of the disease, they sometimes arrested its further course; but they oftener failed."

Reinhardt and Leubuscher * :—

"Emetics frequently relieved the sense of oppression complained of by the patient, and the muscular effort of vomiting, in many cases, produced reaction; we cannot, therefore, determine unconditionally to reject those remedies, although we are willing to confess, that their universal adoption, as by us at the beginning, is not to be recommended."

Bleeding. Bleeding was employed in the premonitory stage of Cholera, for the purpose of arresting the discharges by relieving the congestion of the intestinal mucous membrane. This practice was not much resorted to in the last epidemic; and the communications to the College contain but little mention of it. The early reports in its favour, by Annesley and other writers on the disease as it occurs in India, have not been confirmed by further observation; and hence, except in rare and exceptional cases, it is not usually had recourse to in the premonitory stage, or at the onset of the more severe symptoms. Its general inadmissibility is to be inferred from its almost entire disuse in the last epidemic.

Dr. Brown of Sunderland says :—

"I employed bleeding eighteen years ago, because I was then inexperienced in the disease, and the practice came recommended from India; but I soon abandoned it, from finding its effects invariably pernicious."

The uncertain course of the disease, in its early stages, makes it difficult to estimate the value of any remedy employed at this period, unless the observations are numerous; and hence, the contradictory statements, respecting almost every means which has been employed in Cholera, bleeding being no exception. In contradiction of the above opinion, expressed by Dr. Brown, who had a large experience in the epidemic, is the following from Dr. Strange of Bridgenorth, who writes as follows :—

"Bleeding was employed by myself and two other practitioners; and we all concur in the great benefit derived from it, especially when the patient was seen early. In many cases of approaching collapse, when coldness of the tongue and general surface, small pulse, cramps, and serous discharges, were present, all these symptoms yielded to prompt bleeding, from 8 to 16 ounces, followed by

* Page 520.

the immediate exhibition of iron and quinine. Employed at a later period, it had no good effect; on the contrary, in 2 cases it appeared to increase the symptoms of collapse, and to hasten the fatal issue."

Dr. C. J. Müller* says:—

"During the first epidemic, 1830–31, bleeding was vaunted as the principal means for rescuing the patient in the premonitory stage; but in the present epidemic, its use has been questioned by most observers, and its value generally denied. When the pulse begins to fail, and the skin to become cool, and there is vomiting, serous dejections, and cramps, bleeding is injurious, by increasing the depression. It was employed in 4 cases, whilst the pulse was still marked at the wrist, though feebly; increased collapse immediately followed in all the cases, and none recovered. Similar results were obtained in the General Hospital. In plethoric subjects, if the disease was mild, the loss of blood seemed to do good; yet, it must be added, that similar cases did equally well without it. In 10 cases, which, on admission, were cold, blue, and pulseless, vomiting and purging continuing, from 8 to 12 ounces of blood were with difficulty obtained; in only 3 were the effects obvious by increased restlessness, oppressed respiration, and increased blueness of the surface. Of 23 other cases, in only 8 was there a favourable change. Sometimes the patient felt himself better for a short time; but more frequently (and this was very remarkable in 5 cases), immediately after the bleeding, there was increased debility and collapse, quickly terminating in death. In the Nicolai Hospital, bleeding was employed in 6 cases; only once was the result favourable, the patient being in the first stage; in the other 5, death followed very quickly with coma. .... From all that has been recorded, and from the experience of the author, blood-letting, in the advanced period of the second stage (commencing collapse), is injurious, and at the beginning, is useless, or at least doubtful."

Dr. Zeroni†, in his report, writes as follows:—

"We found by experience that both mild and severe cases might recover under simple regimen. The chief effort of art being to prevent collapse, or, when it occurred, to lessen the oppression of the brain in the stage of reaction, it was determined to try the value of blood-letting."

The details of 9 cases accompany the report. The results were as follows:—

* Report on Cholera in Riga.
† Report on the Treatment of Cholera in Mannheim.

"Male, æt. 44.   Impending collapse ; no cramps : bled to 8 ounces.
                  Death.
Female, æt. 22.   Impending collapse : bled to 8 ounces. Death.
Male, æt. 55.   Premonitory stage : bled to 8 ounces ; gradual
                  development of the disease. Death.
Male, æt. 56.   In collapse : bled to 10 ounces. Death.
Female, æt. 22.   In collapse : bled to 7 ounces. Death.
Male, æt. 34.   Pulse weak and frequent : bled to 6 ounces, and
                  24 leeches to the epigastrium. Death.
Female, æt. 40.   In collapse : bled to 4 or 5 ounces. Death.
Male, æt. 58.   Impending collapse : bled to 4 ounces ; blood
                  black. Death.
Female, æt. 25.   Impending collapse ; cramps : bled to 4 ounces ;
                  cupping to epigastrium. Recovered."

The quantity of blood obtained was, in many of these cases,
obviously too small to influence the course of the disease in any
degree. The conclusions of the writer are as follows:—

"The result was altogether unfavourable. After the bleeding,
the blueness of the surface changed to a grayish tint, the features
were more collapsed, the tendency to coma was more marked, the
pulse, which was previously to be felt at the wrist, became indistinct, the symptoms of prostration seemed at once to come on to a
more marked degree, and the patient was rapidly brought to the
last stage."

In a report on the epidemic in Petersburgh*, it is stated :—

"Venæsection is admissible only in particular cases, and under
rare conditions. When the vomiting and purging are urgent,
blood-letting is injurious by producing exhaustion and preventing
reaction."

Mr. Bell† gives a table of cases treated by bleeding in the Castle
Hospital in Edinburgh, in 1832. He is an advocate of this practice
in every case of Cholera with symptoms of asphyxia ; but the results
obtained by him are not such as to recommend it. The table contains—

       44 cases in the first stage, of these 7 died,
        6 „   verging on collapse . . all died,
        9 „   in collapse . . . . . 7 died.

The quantity of blood drawn in the first set of cases varied from

* Report from the Obuschowschen Hospital.
† Edinburgh Medical and Surgical Journal, 1849.

12 to 30 ounces. Of the 6 cases verging on collapse, in 4, 12 ounces, in 1, 24 ounces, and in 1, 8 ounces, were taken. In the 9 cases in collapse, from 5 to 20 ounces were taken. Sinapisms, stimuli, calomel and opium, and Dover's powder, were also used, as well as those measures, general and local, which arrest the discharges and restore heat, &c. The mortality in the first stage was as high as 16 per cent.; and of the remainder, 13 out of 15, or 86 per cent.

These scattered facts correspond with common experience, and lead to the conclusion that, in the premonitory and early stages, bleeding is in general to be avoided. In the stage of collapse, it is for the most part impossible to remove an amount of blood sufficiently rapidly to produce any obvious effects. A few cases, however, are contained in the communications received, and similar ones occurred in the practice of most who were occupied with the disease, in which the abstraction of a few ounces of blood relieved the cramps and sense of oppression complained of at the precordia, and was followed by favourable symptoms of reaction.

The following case, reported by Dr. Havcraft of Greenwich, is remarkable :—

"In one severe case (a male æt. 27), which ended fatally in ten hours, and which, from the beginning, was marked by great prostration and extreme oppression at the epigastrium, we tried cupping. The blood, contrary to expectation, flowed freely to the extent of 8 ounces, and the patient expressed himself strongly and thankfully, as much relieved ; but within five minutes, he fell back and died. Before the cupping, the voice was husky ; but immediately afterwards its tone was clear and distinct."

In the consecutive fever, local depletion seems more directly to be indicated ; nevertheless, experience shows that its employment requires much caution. Leeching the temples, or cupping the back of the neck, were sometimes of service in obviating the cerebral congestion of this period ; but, if carried to any great extent, were injurious by exhausting the patient. Dr. C. J. Müller* reports that, of 69 cases in the typhoid stage, treated by general and local depletion, 48 died. In only 2 did the treatment produce any improvement, the results for the most part being negative or unfavourable. In the experience of others, leeches to the temples sometimes re-

* Op. Citat.

lieved the coma, and the patients were so much benefited as
their recovery from their application.

In a note subjoined to the report from the Obusche
Hospital, it is stated that blood-letting, in the stage of
requires much discretion, though well-marked signs of pn
may exist. Of 18 cases of pneumonia in the consecutive
6, treated by bleeding, died; of 12 not bled, 5 died and
vered.

Leeches were applied, with occasional advantage, to the
trium in the consecutive fever, when there was tenderness, v
and hiccup. Occasionally, under these circumstances, local
tion by cupping was employed with good effect.

The general inference, from all we have observed of the
and collected from the experience of others, is, that larg
of blood, in the consecutive fever, are injurious; but that occi
good results follow its local abstraction according to the indi
the symptoms.

Empirical treat- Quinine, strychnia, arsenic, sesquichloride
ment. Specific   nitrate of silver, nitrous acid, chlorine water,
remedies.   sulphuric acid, bichloride of mercury, charco
                 &c.

The failure of those methods of treatment, which, from bei
upon some supposed indications of the disease, may be called
led naturally to the employment of almost every active mec
the materia medica.

It is notorious that the results have been discouraging,
standing the bold assertions to the contrary. The communi
made to the College contain no data for determining the
nor is anything deserving the name of evidence in favour
value of these means, to be gathered from the numerous jour
published treatises in this country and on the Continent. Thi
our report must, therefore, be defective, although an unlimited
of time and labour has been bestowed upon a perusal and con
of the statements brought before us.

The suggestions contained in the letter issued by the Comn
the 6th of September, 1849, and which, from the rapid subsi
the epidemic, could not then be put in practice, may be
here :—

    " It is not to be expected that the doubts and discrepa
isting will be finally settled by the evidence which any in

member of the profession may adduce ; but the Committee have a confident hope that valuable and conclusive results, in regard to at least some of the disputed points, might be obtained by collecting and comparing the observations of hospital physicians, and the many other members of the College.

"Such a method of inquiry appears to be especially applicable, and indeed indispensable, in any endeavour to estimate the relative values of the various modes of treating Cholera, respecting which the evidence is so conflicting.

"It seems desirable that every member of the College who has the necessary opportunity, should submit one or more remedies to a *systematic trial* in a *series of cases*."

The therapeutic history of Cholera leads us to guard the above suggestions, by expressing our conviction that for empirical inquiry to be pursued to a good end, the most favourable opportunities are required for noting the state of the patient at the commencement, and different stages of the treatment, by which alone discrepancies in the results can be reconciled.

Again, the employment, without definite scope, of one remedy after another, with the vague hope of at last finding a specific, is to be deprecated, not only because it can lead to no good result, but because it deprives the patient of that assistance which established experience affords.

The state of the patient in the collapse of Cholera is so unfavourable to the absorption of medicines, that even if we knew the remedy in itself most appropriate, we could not anticipate great results from its administration by the mouth at this period. Every consideration of this formidable malady urges upon us the paramount importance of obviating the causes which give rise to it, and of arresting the symptoms at the onset.

External means; heat. The application of heat to the surface has been largely tried. The hot bath, alone, or with mustard or salt, &c., the vapour bath and the hot-air bath, have been principally employed. It appears to be the uniform experience of the profession, that in collapse these means are but of little value.

When the depression of the circulation is great, and the surface cold and clammy, although heat may be imparted to the body, it rarely excites reaction in the system itself; on the contrary, it is oppressive to the patient and increases the exhaustion. These means are better adapted to an earlier stage of the disease, or when it is less

severe, and whilst the pulse indicates a moderate degree of power.
Under such circumstances the hot bath and the vapour bath are grateful to the patient ; they allay cramps, and if continued for a short time, may serve, with other means, to arrest the symptoms ; they are, however, in general only palliative.

For the purpose of producing perspiration, external heat is not required. In the worst cases the sweating is profuse, and without any favourable influence over the course of the disease.

It is not found by experience, that the degree of reaction, which may be sometimes excited by such means, and by internal stimuli, is of any permanent advantage, nor was this to be anticipated from a consideration of the conditions of the system in the collapse of Cholera. The state of the blood, and the extreme depression of the nervous power, necessarily render abortive such attempts at restoring the circulation. The whole tendency of the evidence yet acquired from the treatment of this stage, is towards a more restricted use of powerful excitants of the kind alluded to.

Cold affusion.   On the Continent, in the former*, and in the last† epidemic, cold affusion was highly spoken of as a means of producing reaction. The patient was placed in a warm hip-bath, and cold water poured or thrown over the head, back, and chest. This was done quickly, and the patient then placed between warm blankets. If the first application was followed by any improvement, the operation was repeated every three or four hours. The results appear to have been, on the whole, more satisfactory than from the hot bath.

"Wet sheet."   The "wet-sheet envelope" was more commonly used in this country. The effects varied according to the state of the patient ; in the milder cases it favoured reaction, but when the disease was severe, it was useless or injurious. The sweating caused by it added to the exhaustion, and had no influence in arresting the intestinal discharges. In none of the cases, which were many, in which we saw it tried, did it produce any good effect.

Dr. Roupell :—

    " I have used the wet sheet without any permanent good."

* Extracts from Casper's work, "On the Application of Cold in Cholera," translated by Dr. George Burrows, Med. Gazette, 1833.

† Archiv. für Path. Anat., Band 2, p. 518.

Dr. Paul, Bermondsey :—

"In the Bermondsey Workhouse, many cases (their exact number I cannot say) were treated with charcoal, soda water, and the wet sheet, stimulants and nourishment ; but, so far as I could observe, without any favourable result."

Dr. Burchell, Kingsland :—

"I found the wet sheet answer in producing reaction, but in the instances in which I tried it, the patients died even more rapidly than under other modes of treatment."

Mr. Painter, Westminster :

"Next I tried the 'wet sheet,' and was much pleased with it as a means of bringing about reaction. I gave at the same time calomel and brandy. The time required for the effect of the sheet was from half an hour to two hours. I have great faith in its use, and believe it saved many lives in this district ; nevertheless I am free to confess I have not the confidence in it that I had at one time."

Dr. Borland, Newington :—

"I have seen the wet sheet applied, and iced water given to drink, but without any good effect resulting, but rather otherwise."

Dr. Burton, Walsall :—

"Out of 20 cases, in which the chief treatment was the administration of salines and the free use of cold water, and, except in the infirm, the wet-sheet envelope, the deaths were 14. The wet sheet produced reaction."

Dr. Basham :—

"The wet sheet, as a means of bringing on reaction, certainly holds out inducements for its employment. In all the cases in which it was tried by me, reaction followed its application. In some cases this was but slight, in others more permanent."

Mr. Tebay, Westminster :—

"I have found the wet sheet a valuable means for bringing on reaction, when properly applied ; if long continued it appears to produce exhaust'on by the profuse perspiration and warmth it occasions."

Dr. Haycraft, Greenwich :—

"The application of the wet sheet, and afterwards packing the patient in blankets, was tried in several cases during collapse ; it induced reaction, and relieved the cramps and vomiting, but neither prolonged life, nor seemed in any way efficacious as a means of cure."

Dr. Dickinson and Dr. Burgess, Fever Hospital, Liverpool :—

> "The cold sheet was used in collapse. It appeared to restore to a certain extent the functions of the skin, causing warmth of surface, and augmenting the force of the pulse at the wrist; but the effects were not permanent."

Dr. White, Winchester :—

> "I have seen the wet sheet, and superimposed blankets and bedding, tried by others. In one case only did the patient recover."

Reinhardt and Leubuscher *:—

> "We have frequently employed the cold envelope. The patient was closely wrapped in cloths, wrung out of ice-cold water ; and so soon as sweating came on, the same process was repeated. This treatment was soon abandoned. It certainly proved that it was not difficult to produce sweating in the asphyctic stage of Cholera, for the patients perspired most freely, nevertheless the other symptoms continued to progress."

Stimulating epithems.   In the milder cases, stimulating epithems of mustard or turpentine were of some use in relieving local symptoms, and for obviating the nervous depression. Frictions, chloroform liniments, and warm fomentations allayed the cramps.

In the severer cases these means were quite ineffective, even the flame of alcohol producing but little more reaction in the skin than it would have done on the dead body. This powerful stimulant was, indeed, tried by Casper, by placing linen, dipped in spirits of wine, on the epigastrium, and igniting it for a few seconds. "At most it produced only a redness around the edges of the linen, and in many cases not the slightest traces of its application remained."

Oxygen and galvanism.   A few cases are reported in which oxygen was inhaled in the stage of collapse with asphyxia, at the same time galvanism was employed to stimulate the respiratory function. The effects upon the circulation and respiration were such as might have been anticipated. The heart's action was, for the time, increased, and there were slight symptoms of general reaction, but no permanently-favourable influence was exercised, by these means, upon the course of the disease in the majority of the cases.

Dr. Burton, of Walsall, gives the particulars of 5 cases of Cholera,

---

* Op. citat., p. 519.

occurring in the year 1832, which, in the stage of collapse, were treated by galvanism. The action of the heart was excited, but the effect was not permanent. All the cases died.

Mr. Allen, Oxford:—

"Galvanism, by shocks from a coil, was tried in three instances, but too late. In a patient in extreme collapse, a girl, aged 21, one wire was applied to the posterior cervical region, and the other to the epigastrium. Powerful inspirations, with great expansion of the chest, followed by an expiratory shout, was the result. The leaden hue of the features was changed to a ruddier tint, which lasted for a few minutes each time the stimulus was applied; but the blueness soon returned, and the patient died."

Dr. A. W. Barclay, Report from St. George's:—

"In two fatal cases galvanic electricity was applied to the region of the heart, and in one of them oxygen diluted with about an equal bulk of atmospheric air was inhaled, on several occasions, without perceptible benefit."

Dr. Oke, Southampton:—

"Galvanism and electricity have been fairly tried in the state of partial and complete collapse by Mr. A. Mordaunt of this town, who is practically acquainted with their therapeutic use. In one or two instances electricity seemed in some measure to increase the temperature of the skin, but no further benefit was observed from these means."

Dr. Roupell:—

"Galvanism was tried in one of my cases; it produced excitement, which appeared afterwards injurious."

Dr. Peacock:—

"In one of the cases (of the Tooting children) in collapse, the most decided benefit followed the employment of galvanism. The patient, a little girl 8 years of age, who had been seized 8 hours before, was apparently rapidly sinking; she lay with her eyes closed, insensible to what was passing around her, the respiration was very feeble, the pulse could not be felt at the wrist, and a thermometer placed under the tongue indicated a temperature of 88°. Slight shocks were passed at short intervals from the sides of the neck to the epigastrium, with the view of stimulating the diaphragm, and also occasionally from side to side across the lower part of the chest, and through the region of the heart. The application was continued from ten minutes to a quarter of an hour, and the effect of the remedy was most satisfactory. The child immediately opened her eyes, and complained of pain, the respiration became fuller, the pulse was again perceptible at the wrists and the thermometer indicated a temperature of 92° under the tongue. The improvement thus manifested was maintained, and after six days' illness and slight febrile reaction, the child entirely recovered. The beneficial effects of galvanism in this instance induced us to employ it in the case of one of the nurses, a female, æt. 20 years, who was attacked with Cholera in the institution and sunk into the state of collapse. In her case, however, though she was roused by the stimulus, no very marked benefit resulted."

Dr. Nicholson, Deputy Inspector General of Army Hospitals, reports to the Committee the particulars of five cases treated by oxygen and the electro-galvanic battery under the superintendence of Mr. C. Nettleton, of Torquay. In the report it is stated, that the cases were not thus treated until they had been in a state of collapse for some hours, and had been given up by the ordinary medical attendant. They were 2 males and 3 females. 2 recovered, aged 8 and 16. 3 died, aged 7, 43, 59.

" The immediate effects of the galvanic stimulus and of the oxygen inhaled were, a return of the pulse to the wrist and a greater freedom of respiration."

Messrs. Dunn and Milner, in their report upon Cholera in the Wakefield Prison, state that in one case oxygen gas was inhaled without any beneficial result.

Mr. Allen, Oxford :—

" Oxygen gas was administered in four instances. A mouth-piece, having an inspiratory and an expiratory valve, was attached to a mackintosh bag containing 4 gallons of pure oxygen. After about six inspirations the countenance slightly improved, but no permanent benefit ensued."

Saline injections into the veins. — This method of treatment was not much investigated during the last epidemic. The results were, as in 1832–33, generally unfavourable. Its value, however, cannot be determined by statistics collected from various sources. The operation in all its details is a delicate one, and requires not only a careful discrimination of the cases to which it is applicable, but also an exact attention to the physical characters and composition of the fluid to be injected, and other collateral circumstances. Until these points receive greater elucidation the results obtained are form no sound basis for an opinion respecting its merits. Saline injections appear to be especially indicated where the loss of fluid has been very great, and where, consequently, the physical condition of the blood in itself opposes an important obstacle to recovery. A more careful diagnosis on this head is yet required, for it must be admitted that the intensity of the symptoms is often in no inconsiderable degree greater than can be accounted for by the amount of the effusion. Under such circumstances we cannot anticipate good results from their employment. Again, the period of the stage of collapse, to which the operation is adapted, requires a nicer discrimination. Hitherto it has not generally been had recourse to until the patient has been in extreme collapse for several hours. It may be suggested whether, by further observation of such cases, an earlier period might not be determined upon.

In reference to the operation itself, the points to be considered are, the *composition, physical properties*, and *quantity*, of the fluid to be injected, the *rapidity* with which it should be thrown into the system, and the necessity for repeating the operation.

The end aimed at is, the supplying to the blood an amount of fluid having some relation to the quantity lost, and possessing as nearly as possible the same physical and chemical properties.

An accurate determination of the amount to be employed at one injection is difficult. This must be arrived at by a consideration of the previous history of the case, and by the effects produced. In general, too great anxiety has been manifested to witness immediate and striking results, and some have probably fallen victims to a large amount of fluid suddenly thrown into an enfeebled circulatory system, whereby the lungs and brain have become seriously embarrassed. In an adult, probably not more than from 40 to 60 ounces should be injected without intermission. The operation may be repeated after a longer or shorter interval, according to the necessities of the case; and this is, for the most part, to be preferred to throwing in double the quantity at once. Cases have terminated successfully where such an amount of injection has been repeated five or six times. Our physiological knowledge of the constitution of the blood shows the importance of the saline fluid being slowly mixed with it, otherwise a serious injury may be inflicted upon its organic constitution. From the data afforded by successful cases we may conclude that about 2 to 3 ounces per minute may be set down as the mean rate.

The temperature requires further investigation; that of the blood has been generally taken as a standard.   Dr. Latta at first proposed 112° Fahr., he subsequently reduced it to 105°, and in his later operations to 98°; in Dr. Macintosh's experiments it varied from 106° to 120° (!); in Dr. Little's it was 110°.

A temperature higher than that of the blood in its normal condition has been chosen in order to obviate the depression of the animal heat which occurs in collapse, and in itself to serve as a stimulus.   Dr. Little's cases, of which 3 out of 4 in severe collapse were successful, at least prove that 110° is not injurious; but whether this or a lower degree is to be preferred, is not determined.

The specific gravity and composition of the fluid to be injected would readily be known were it possible to collect and analyse all that is effused, but a difficulty arises from the unequal constitution of the "rice-water" dejections at different stages of the disease.

During the earlier period, when the discharges are profuse, the proportion of water to the salines is greater, and the soluble salts are in a higher ratio to the organic matters than they are as the disease advances into prolonged collapse.   Analyses of the evacuations at different periods are, therefore, necessary in a series of cases, in order to arrive at an accurate mean of the salines thrown out.   Taking the data before us (page 26) we find that seven analyses give 8 parts of soluble salts per 1000 [*].   On comparing these results with the amount of soluble salts in the liquor sanguinis, we find a very close correspondence between the two fluids; in the liquor sanguinis the soluble salts, as determined from Schmidt's analyses (page 47), being 9 parts per 1000 of water.

---

[*] Mr. Herapath (Medical Gazette, 1849, p. 841) gives two analyses of the evacuations, in which the numbers closely coincide with the above. In the first, the ash obtained from the dried matters of 1000 grains of the fluid, contained

Carbonate of Potash	. . .	0·6507
„ Soda	. . .	2·5960
Sulphate of Soda	. . .	0·8795
Phosphate of Soda (3 Na O PO⁵)	.	0·0260
Chloride of Sodium	. . .	3·6334

Soluble salts.

                                            ——— 7·7856
Earthy Phosphates and Carbonates, &c. 2·1400

                                            9·9256

We may therefore conclude that this is near the proportion in which they should enter into the fluid to be injected. 8 parts per 1000 would give a spec. grav. of 1005.

The fluid employed by Dr. Latta was 1003·5; that by Dr. Macintosh 1002·5; and that by Dr. Little 1003·75.

The apprehension that a fluid so low in spec. grav. as 1005 would injure the red corpuscles by too ready an endosmosis into them, is unfounded under the circumstances in which such a fluid is transfused into the veins in Cholera. When this operation is indicated, the blood is much increased in density by the loss of the water and soluble salts of the liquor sanguinis. The albuminates, which in health are to the soluble salts in the ratio of 10 to 1, are after the loss of fluids in collapse as 20 to 1 (see page 45). If, therefore, a fluid constituted like that effused, but *less in quantity*, be injected, no danger of over-dilation is incurred, nor will the normal balance of endosmosis of the corpuscles be disturbed, for the fluid slowly introduced will by union with the albuminates be brought up to or above the normal standard of the liquor sanguinis*.

In the second analysis the results were:—

Carbonate of Potash	. . .	0·2923	⎞
„ Soda	. . .	2·8068	⎟
Sulphate of Soda .	. .	1·0492	⎬ Soluble salts.
Phosphate of Soda	. . .	traces	⎟
Chloride of Sodium	.	3·6194	⎠

$$\overline{}\ 7·7677$$

Earthy Phosphates and Carbonates, &c. 0·3721

$$\overline{}$$
$$8·1398$$

"It ought," says Mr. Herapath, "to be mentioned, that although only two analyses of these fœcal evacuations have been recorded here, at least two dozen specimens of them have been examined more or less minutely, and all with very nearly similar results."

* In the Lancet, October 1st, 1853, Dr. Rees advises the injection of a saline fluid of the sp. grav. of the serum, 1030, at 60°, his reasons being, that a lower density would endanger the integrity of the corpuscles from too free an endosmosis into them; a danger, he adds, increased in Cholera, owing to their contents being concentrated by the drain of fluid which has occurred. After a consideration of his statements, we see no reason to modify the conclusions given in the report. A fluid owing its density to salines only, has a different action on the blood corpuscles from one, like the serum, whose density is principally due to albumen. Again, an

The constitution of the fluid to be employed cannot be strictly determined until we have a larger series of analyses of the Cholera evacuations, including the whole fluid thrown out. There is some reason to believe that the soluble salts of the liquor sanguinis are not effused equally, the exosmosis of the alkaline salts (see page 27) being in a higher ratio than that of the neutral chlorides, and of the salts of soda in a higher ratio than of those of potash (page 47). Until, however, this is established by further investigation, it may be safer to take the analysis of the blood in health as a standard for our artificial mixtures.

The following table, from data by Schmidt, gives the composition and proportion of the salts in 1000 parts *of the water* of the liquor sanguinis.

Soluble salts in 1000 *parts* of the water *of the Liquor Sanguinis, in health.*

Chloride of Sodium	5·72
„ Potassium	·627
Phosphate of Soda	·367
Sulphate of Soda	·176
Carbonate of Soda	2·13
	9·02

From this it will be seen that in Cholera the water transudes in a rather higher ratio than the salts it holds in solution.

From the above table we deduce the following formula for the constitution of the salt to be used:—

Approximative constitution of the salt to be used for injection into the veins in Cholera.

Chloride of Sodium	60 parts by weight.
„ Potassium	6 „
Phosphate of Soda	3
Carbonate of Soda	20 „

By dissolving 140 grains of this salt in 40 fluid ounces of distilled water, and filtering, we obtain a fluid having a decidedly saline taste,

artificial fluid having 50 parts of salines for 1000, instead of 8 or 9, which is the amount in the liq. sanguinis, could hardly, with safety, permeate our tissues, at least its innocuousness requires to be tested by actual experiment.

a faintly alkaline reaction, and nearly approximative in its constitution to the fluid effused, minus the organic substances. These are small in amount, and their loss has apparently no important influence on the constitution of the blood.

Medicated venous injections.

The arrest of the function of absorption in the stage of collapse, and the consequent inertness of all medicines administered by the stomach at this period, naturally led to the suggestion of injecting them into the veins. From the discovery of the circulation to the present time various experiments of this kind have been instituted by different observers, which prove that medicinal substances can thus with safety be employed. The trials which have been made in this way in Cholera are too few to admit of any deduction from them. In the former epidemic, laudanum, camphor, quinine, &c., were used unsuccessfully. In some cases in University College, under the care of Dr. Parkes in 1849, quinine was again tried at the suggestion of Mr. Marshall, but without good effect. These failures do not, however, decide the question of the utility of such measures, since the operation was not performed until the patients were *in extremis.*

The addition of a small quantity of alcohol to the saline injections, which was made by Dr. Little in 1832, was repeated by him in his cases during the last epidemic, and with success. In one, a male æt. 22, 250 ounces of saline fluid was injected at four times, each pint containing two drachms of alcohol. "This patient," he says, "therefore, received into his veins, in the course of a few hours, a quantity of alcohol equal to that contained in six ounces of brandy."* The recovery was complete. This subject certainly deserves a more extended inquiry.

Treatment of imperfect reaction.

Of those who resist the fatal influence of the Cholera poison in the stage of collapse, a large number yet fall victims to its protracted effects.

After hopes of recovery have been excited by a partial restoration of the functions to their normal condition, the favourable prognosis we may have formed is disappointed by a failure in the system to maintain its upward tendency, or by a recurrence of the more characteristic phenomena of the cold stage. Probably half the cases fatal after the first 48 hours of severe symptoms belong to this category.

We may, therefore, infer that much care is required during the

* Hunterian Oration, 1852.

early period of reaction, since circumstances, in themselves apparently trifling, may at this time determine the issue.

The indications for treatment are the same as in the cold stage, but although our remedies are applied under somewhat more favourable circumstances for their operation, the therapeutic effects hitherto obtained are uncertain.

A strict observance of the horizontal position, moderate external warmth, stimulating applications to the extremities, region of the heart, or epigastrium, and the administration internally of diffusible stimuli in small quantities, with the free use of ice, cold water, and other diluents, appear to constitute the principal part of the treatment as far as it is yet determined.

The cerebral oppression and delirium of this period are probably due to exhaustion and the asphyotic condition of the capillary circulation, the blood being imperfectly aërated and deficient in water. The state of the brain which gives rise to these symptoms is to be distinguished from that which occurs at a later stage from retention of the urinary excretions. It is not benefited by local or general depletion, but is slowly removed as the circulation is re-established.

Although the analysis of the so-called consecutive fever is not complete, enough has been done to shew that it is resolvable into a series of secondary lesions varying in character and intensity. It does not, therefore, admit of one form of treatment, but requires an adaptation of remedies to the several exigencies of the system. The fruitless search after specifics which occupies the mind in the preceding stages of the disease is now tacitly given up, and we are content to be guided by the pathological indications, as in other diseases.

Treatment of "consecutive fever;" uræmia.

But whilst our attention is directed to the local and more visible complications, it must not be forgotten that they are the effects of an agent which has remarkably depressed the whole of the vital powers, and, consequently, rendered necessary, modifications in the activity of the measures otherwise adapted to their removal.

The most important indication for treatment is the depuration of the blood from the urinary excretions. The conditions following collapse are favourable to their retention, viz., the blood is of high specific gravity, the circulation is embarrassed, and lesions of the kidneys are frequent.

It is well known that uræmia may be developed even with healthy

excreting organs, if there be a want of fluid in the blood.   The
phenomena preceding death from thirst are from this cause, and the
same results follow whenever absorption of fluid is long prevented
by irritability of the stomach ; in Cholera, therefore, such a condition
cannot be overlooked.

The affection of the kidneys appears to be somewhat similar
to that following scarlatina, but the inflammatory action is less
marked.   For the most part the derangement is rather con-
gestive than inflammatory, and these organs regain their normal condition as the general circulation is restored.   In severer cases, the
evidence of nephritis, from the character of the exudations found
in the urine, is more distinct.

These considerations show that the treatment must include such
means as allay irritability of the stomach and promote absorption,
restore the circulation, and remove the lesions of the kidneys.   Of
these may be enumerated the use of ice and cold water, effervescing
draughts or weak solutions of the alkaline salts, the warm bath,
emollient enemata, dry cupping to the loins, and counter-irritation
over the stomach.

Stimuli are sometimes necessary for the purpose of counteracting
the nervous depression, but their employment, whilst the system is
poisoned with urea, obviously requires careful regulation.

Stimulating diuretics, as cantharides, squilla, turpentine, &c., are
not adapted to the great majority of the cases.   The spontaneous occurrence of profuse diuresis, when the intestinal mucous membrane
recovers its functions, shows that the matters to be excreted are,
in themselves, sufficient to stimulate the kidneys, if the conditions
favourable to their action be present.

Occasional doses of mercurials, followed by laxatives, were found
to be useful, probably by quickening the circulation through the liver
and promoting absorption, as well as by depurating the blood, but
their use was necessarily limited, whilst the excretive function of
the kidneys was defective.

The cerebral and thoracic complications were treated as in the
ordinary uræmia of Bright's disease.

The following quotations give the general tenour of the replies
received in answer to a query respecting the means found most
serviceable in re-exciting the functions of the kidneys after the stage
of collapse was passed.

Dr. Miller, Western General Dispensary :—

"In bad cases of consecutive fever I have invariably failed to restore the functions of the kidneys, although blood-letting, blistering, and salines have been employed. In less severe cases, where calomel had been given, the suppression was less marked, but the secretion was preceded by hæmorrhage. In some instances the kidneys have almost suddenly recovered their function."

Mr. W. F. Horton, Hammersmith :—

"Probably through my rather liberal use of mercury, I have not had much difficulty on this point."

Mr. Snape, Bolton-le-Moors :—

"The most successful means which I have found for re-exciting the kidneys after the stage of collapse, are small doses of calomel repeated every two hours."

Dr. Shapter, Exeter :—

"Effervescing salines and mild purgatives, with the free use of cold water and demulcent drinks."

Dr. Barlow :—

"As long as the sickness remains unchecked, there is but little hope of urine being secreted in any quantity. For fulfilling this first indication I found a little calcined magnesia in water most serviceable. When the sickness began to subside, 5 grains of the chlorate of potash in half an ounce of water appeared to act as a diuretic. A most important measure, however, was the introduction of the catheter as soon as there was reason to suspect that even a few ounces of urine might be in the bladder, for the drawing off of a small quantity was generally followed by a more copious secretion. The restoration of the functions of the kidneys was not necessarily followed by recovery; several patients under my care became suddenly comatose after the urine had been freely secreted for some days. As long as the dusky colour of the skin indicated capillary obstruction, the danger was urgent."

Dr. Beadle, Tewkesbury :—

"Under the use of mild salines, with Hydr. č cretâ and Pulv. antimonialis, the secretion of urine returned with returning strength."

Dr. Shearman, Rotherham :—

"The application of leeches or cupping to the region of the kidneys, the warm bath, and diaphoretic salines."

Dr. Haycraft, Greenwich :—

"The calomel given in the stage of collapse generally favoured the secretion of urine ; this, and the carbonate of soda, or other salines, with beef-tea ad libitum, were chiefly trusted to."

Dr. George Burrows :—

"The means I have employed for re-exciting the functions of the kidneys have been frictions over the loins, with liniment. camph. co. ð R̄. lytt., occasionally cupping, the warm hip-bath, and the internal use of salines combined with more stimulating diuretics. The catheter was sometimes introduced and urine drawn off, although its presence was not suspected."

Dr. Williams, Gloucester :—

"I have tried various remedies, yet cannot say that any were particularly successful."

Dr. Strange, Bridgenorth :—

"The means for restoring the action of the kidneys were diluent drinks, small doses of calomel, nitrate of potash, &c."

Dr. Yonge, Plymouth :—

"I know of no remedies in particular for re-exciting the function of the kidneys, or any treatment, except such as restore the secretions generally."

Dr. Gwynne Bird, Swansea :—

"When the functions of the kidneys were restored, I could not observe that any remedial agent was specially productive of the result."

Dr. Roupell :—

"I cannot say that any of the means which I have tried have been successful. Cupping on the loins gives great relief, but turpentine and other remedies do not seem to avail in this condition."

Dr. Paul, Bermondsey :—

"I have not seen any good from medicines given for the restoration of the urinary secretion. As the system recovers itself, the flow of urine is re-established. I doubt of its being much influenced by treatment."

Dr. Dickinson and Dr. Burgess, Liverpool :—

"As the biliary and cutaneous secretions were restored, and the general state of congestion disappeared, the kidneys gradually resumed their functions without any special treatment."

Mr. Tebay, Westminster:—

"I am not satisfied that any particular remedy was of use in re-exciting the renal secretion."

Dr. White, Winchester:—

"In the cases which I have had under my care, the function of the kidneys has always been spontaneously re-established."

Dr. Rae, Plymouth:—

"The secretion of bile and of urine gradually returns with return-ing health, without the aid of any specific means."

Dr. Taylor, Fever Hospital, Liverpool:—

"The function of the kidneys was restored as the temperature returned, and the secretion of bile was re-established. Artificial means were not used for the purpose of exciting the flow of urine."

Muco-enterite.   During the consecutive fever, the intestinal tract is frequently in different parts the seat of persistent con-gestion with diptheritic inflammation and ulceration. The termina-tion of the ileum is most commonly thus affected, and is the fre-quent source of the bloody stools observed during reaction. In some rare instances, limited sloughs of the mucous membrane re-sult from effusion of blood into the submucous tissue. Such have been observed in the large intestine and in the stomach. The character of the local actions indicates a want of reparative power.

The treatment adapted to these lesions is probably that generally employed with success in other forms of gastro-enterite, such as gentle support, ammonia, serpentaria, and a moderate allowance of wine.

Woodfall and Kinder, Printers, Angel-court, Skinner-street, London.

March, 1854.

MR. CHURCHILL'S

𝔓𝔲𝔟𝔩𝔦𝔠𝔞𝔱𝔦𝔬𝔫𝔰

IN

MEDICINE, SURGERY,

AND

SCIENCE.

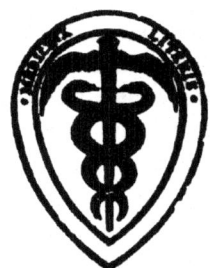

THE BRITISH AND FOREIGN MEDICO-CHIRURGICAL REVIEW;

OR,

QUARTERLY JOURNAL OF PRACTICAL MEDICINE.

Price Six Shillings. Nos. 1 to 25.

THE MEDICAL TIMES AND GAZETTE.

Published Weekly, price Sevenpence, or Stamped, Eightpence.
Annual Subscription, £1. 16s., or Stamped, £1. 14s. 8d., and regularly forwarded to all of the Kingdom.

The MEDICAL TIMES AND GAZETTE is favoured with an amount of Literary and Scientific support which enables it to reflect fully the progress of Medical Science, and insure the character, an influence, and a circulation possessed at the present time by no Medical odical.

THE HALF-YEARLY ABSTRACT OF THE MEDICAL SCIENCES.

Being a Digest of the Contents of the principal British and Continental Medical Journals, together with a Critical Report of the Progress of Medicine and the Collateral Sciences. Edited by W. H. RANKING, M.D., Cantab., and C. B. RADCLIFFE, M.D., Lond. Post cloth, 6s. 8d. Vols. 1 to 18.

THE JOURNAL OF PSYCHOLOGICAL MEDICINE AND MENTAL PATHOLOGY.

Being a Quarterly Review of Medical Jurisprudence and Insanity. Edited by For WINSLOW, M.D. Price 3s. 6d. Nos. 1 to 25.

THE PHARMACEUTICAL JOURNAL.

EDITED BY JACOB BELL, F.L.S., M.R.I.
Published Monthly, price One Shilling.
Under the sanction of the PHARMACEUTICAL SOCIETY, whose TRANSACTIONS form distinct portion of each Number.

. Vols. 1 to 12, bound in cloth, price 12s. 6d. each.

THE DUBLIN MEDICAL PRESS.

Published Weekly, Stamped, price Sixpence, free to any part of the Empire.

THE LONDON AND PROVINCIAL MEDICAL DIRECTO

Published Annually. 12mo. cloth, 7s. 6d.

Complete in Nine Fasciculi: imperial 4to., 20s. each;
half-bound morocco, gilt tops, 9l. 15s.;
whole bound morocco, 10l. 10s.

PATHOLOGY OF THE HUMAN EYE.

ILLUSTRATED IN A SERIES OF COLOURED PLATES,
FROM ORIGINAL DRAWINGS.

By JOHN DALRYMPLE, F.R.S., F.R.C.S.

The Publisher has the high satisfaction of announcing the completion of this beautiful work. Mr. Dalrymple had revised the last proof sheet, and the Artist had finished the last plate, a few days only previous to the lamented death of the Author, who thus leaves a monument to his scientific reputation, and of his ardent devotion to his Profession.

"A work reflecting credit on the profession has been brought to a successful conclusion. Had Mr. Dalrymple's life been spared but a few short months longer, the chorus of praise which now greets the completion of this great work would have fallen gratefully on his ear. The Publisher may well be proud of having issued such a work."—*London Journal of Medicine.*

"The satisfaction with which we should have announced the completion of this unrivalled work is overclouded by the regret which we feel, in common with all who were acquainted with its distinguished and estimable author, at his early decease. The value of this work can scarcely be over-estimated: it realises all that we believe it possible for art to effect in the imitation of nature."—*British and Foreign Medico-Chirurgical Review.*

SURGICAL ANATOMY.

A Series of Dissections, illustrating the Principal Regions of the Human Body.

By JOSEPH MACLISE, F.R.C.S.

The singular success of this Work exhausted the First Edition of 1000 Copies within six months of its completion.

The Second Edition, now in course of publication, Fasciculi I. to III. Imperial Folio, 5s. each.

PORTRAITS OF SKIN DISEASES.

By ERASMUS WILSON, F.R.S.

Fasciculi I. to XI., 20s. each. *To be completed in Twelve Numbers.*

" May be truly designated a splendid performance. We can scarcely speak too strongly of the merits of this work."—*British and Foreign Medico-Chirurgical Review.*

" We have never before seen a work more beautifully got up—they excel all other plates of diseases of the skin that have ever been published."—*Lancet.*

MR. ACTON, M.R.C.S.

A PRACTICAL TREATISE ON DISEASES OF THE URINARY
AND GENERATIVE ORGANS OF BOTH SEXES, INCLUDING SYPHILIS. Second Edition. 8vo. cloth, 20s.; or with Plates, 30s.

"Mr. Acton's work must be diligently studied by every practitioner who would desire to benefit instead of injuring his patient; it has a distinctive and pre-eminently diagnostic value."—*Med. Gazette*.

"The present edition of Mr. Acton's work is very much enlarged, and contains a most valuable collection of matter."—*The Lancet*.

"We cannot too highly recommend this treatise; it should be found wherever Surgery is practised throughout the British Empire."—*Provincial Medical Journal*.

DR. WILLIAM ADDISON, F.R.S., F.L.S.

ON HEALTHY AND DISEASED STRUCTURE, AND THE TRUE
PRINCIPLES OF TREATMENT FOR THE CURE OF DISEASE, ESPECIALLY CONSUMPTION AND SCROFULA, founded on MICROSCOPICAL ANALYSIS. 8vo. cloth, 12s.

"A work deserving the perusal of every one interested in the late rapid advance of physiology and pathology."—*Medico-Chirurgical Review*.

MR. ANDERSON, F.R.C.S.

L.

HYSTERICAL, HYPOCHONDRIACAL, EPILEPTIC, AND
OTHER NERVOUS AFFECTIONS; their Causes, Symptoms, and Treatment. 8vo. cloth, 5s.

II.

THE SYMPTOMS AND TREATMENT OF THE DISEASES OF
PREGNANCY. Post 8vo. 4s. 6d.

DR. ARMITAGE.

HYDROPATHY AS APPLIED TO ACUTE DISEASE.
Post 8vo. cloth, 3s.

DR. JAMES ARNOTT.

I.

ON THE REMEDIAL AGENCY OF A LOCAL ANÆSTHENIC
OR BENUMBING TEMPERATURE, in various painful and inflammatory Diseases. 8vo. cloth, 4s. 6d.

II.

ON INDIGESTION; its Pathology and its Treatment, by the Local
Application of Uniform and Continuous Heat and Moisture. With an Account of an improved Mode of applying Heat and Moisture in Irritative and Inflammatory Diseases. With a Plate. 8vo. 5s.

III.

PRACTICAL ILLUSTRATIONS OF THE TREATMENT OF
OBSTRUCTIONS IN THE URETHRA, AND OTHER CANALS, BY THE DILATATION OF FLUID PRESSURE. 8vo. boards, 3s.

F. A. ABEL, F.C.S.,
PROFESSOR OF CHEMISTRY AT THE ROYAL MILITARY ACADEMY, WOOLWICH; AND
O. L. BLOXAM,
FORMERLY FIRST ASSISTANT AT THE ROYAL COLLEGE OF CHEMISTRY.

HANDBOOK OF CHEMISTRY: THEORETICAL, PRACTICAL,
AND TECHNICAL. 8vo. cloth, 15s.

DR. G. C. CHILD.

ON INDIGESTION, AND CERTAIN BILIOUS DISORDERS

OFTEN CONJOINED WITH IT. Second Edition. 8vo. cloth, 6s.

SIR JAMES CLARK, M.D., BART.,
PHYSICIAN TO THE QUEEN.

THE SANATIVE INFLUENCE OF CLIMATE. With an Account

of the Principal Places resorted to by Invalids in England, South of Europe, the Colonies, &c. Fourth Edition, revised. Post 8vo. cloth, 10s. 6d.

MR. J. PATERSON CLARK, M.A.,
DENTIST EXTRAORDINARY TO HIS ROYAL HIGHNESS PRINCE ALBERT.

THE ODONTALGIST; OR, HOW TO PRESERVE THE TEETH,

CURE TOOTHACHE, AND REGULATE DENTITION FROM INFANCY TO AGE. With plates. Post 8vo. cloth, 5s.

DR. CONOLLY.

THE CONSTRUCTION AND GOVERNMENT OF LUNATIC

ASYLUMS AND HOSPITALS FOR THE INSANE. With Plans. Post 8vo. cloth, 6s.

MR. BRANSBY B. COOPER, F.R.S.,
SENIOR SURGEON TO GUY'S HOSPITAL.

LECTURES ON THE PRINCIPLES AND PRACTICE OF SUR-

GERY. 8vo. cloth, 21s.

"Mr. Cooper's book has reminded us, in its easy style and copious detail, more of Watson's Lectures, and we should not be surprised to see it occupy a similar position to that well-known work in professional estimation."—*Medical Times.*

MR. W. WHITE COOPER,
OPHTHALMIC SURGEON TO ST. MARY'S HOSPITAL.

ON NEAR SIGHT, AGED SIGHT, IMPAIRED VISION,

AND THE MEANS OF ASSISTING SIGHT. With 31 Illustrations on Wood. Second Edition. Fcap. 8vo. cloth, 7s. 6d.

MR. COOPER,
LATE PROFESSOR OF SURGERY IN THE UNIVERSITY COLLEGE, LONDON.

A DICTIONARY OF PRACTICAL SURGERY; comprehending all

the most interesting Improvements, from the Earliest Times down to the Present Period. Seventh Edition. One very thick volume, 8vo., 1l. 10s.

MR. COOLEY.
COMPREHENSIVE SUPPLEMENT TO THE PHARMACOPŒIAS.

THE CYCLOPÆDIA OF PRACTICAL RECEIPTS, AND COL-

LATERAL INFORMATION IN THE ARTS, MANUFACTURES, AND TRADES, INCLUDING MEDICINE, PHARMACY, AND DOMESTIC ECONOMY; designed as a Compendious Book of Reference for the Manufacturer, Tradesman, Amateur, and Heads of Families. Third Edition. *In the Press.*

DR. GAIRDNER.

ON GOUT; its History, its Causes, and its Cure. Second Edition. Post 8vo. cloth, 7s. 6d.

"No one can rise from the perusal of Dr. Gairdner's treatise without the conviction that it contains a trustworthy history of the disease,—that it conveys sound directions for treatment,—and that it is the work of a physician who, amid the wearying toil of a large and successful practice, keeps himself thoroughly conversant with all the recent advances in physiological science, both at home and abroad."—*Medical Times.*

MR. GALLOWAY,

I.

THE FIRST STEP IN CHEMISTRY. Post 8vo. cloth, 3s.

"We heartily commend this unpretending and useful work to the heads of scholastic establishments, and to others who are anxious to initiate their pupils into the principles of a most fascinating and most useful branch of human knowledge."—*London Journal of Medicine.*

II.

A MANUAL OF QUALITATIVE ANALYSIS. Post 8vo. cloth, 4s.

"This is really a valuable little book. We have not for a long time met with an introductory Manual which so completely fulfils its intention."—*Athenæum.*

DR. GAVIN.

ON FEIGNED AND FICTITIOUS DISEASES, chiefly of Soldiers and Seamen; on the means used to simulate or produce them, and on the best Modes of discovering Impostors; being the Prize Essay in the Class of Military Surgery in the University of Edinburgh. 8vo. cloth, 9s.

DR. GLOVER.

ON THE PATHOLOGY AND TREATMENT OF SCROFULA; being the Forthergillian Prize Essay for 1846. With Plates. 8vo. cloth, 10s. 6d.

MR. GRAY, M.R.C.S.

PRESERVATION OF THE TEETH indispensable to Comfort and Appearance, Health, and Longevity. 18mo. cloth, 3s.

"This small volume will be found interesting and useful to every medical practitioner, the heads of families, and those who have the care of children; while persons who have lost teeth will be made aware of the cause, and enabled to judge for themselves of the rationale of the principles pointed out for their replacement, and preservation of the remainder."

MR. GRIFFITHS.

CHEMISTRY OF THE FOUR SEASONS — Spring, Summer, Autumn, Winter. Illustrated with Engravings on Wood. Second Edition. Foolscap 8vo. cloth, 7s. 6d.

"This volume combines, in an eminent degree, amusement with instruction. The laws and properties of those wonderful and mysterious agents—heat, light, electricity, galvanism, and magnetism, are appropriately discussed, and their influence on vegetation noticed. We would especially recommend it to those commencing the study of medicine, both as an incentive to their natural curiosity, and an introduction to several of those branches of science which will necessarily soon occupy their attention."—*British and Foreign Medical Review.*

DR. GULLY.

I.

THE WATER CURE IN CHRONIC DISEASE: an Expositio.
the Causes, Progress, and Terminations of various Chronic Diseases of the Viscera, Nervous System, and Limbs, and of their Treatment by Water and other Hygienic M
Fourth Edition. Foolscap 8vo. sewed, 2s. 6d.

II.

THE SIMPLE TREATMENT OF DISEASE; deduced from
Methods of Expectancy and Revulsion. 18mo. cloth, 4s.

MR. GUTHRIE, F.R.S.

I.

THE ANATOMY OF THE BLADDER AND OF THE URETH
Third Edition. 8vo. cloth, 5s.

II.

ON INJURIES OF THE HEAD AFFECTING THE BRA
AND ON HERNIA. 4to. boards, 7s.

III.

ON WOUNDS AND INJURIES OF THE CHEST. 8vo. c
4s. 6d.

DR. GUY,
PHYSICIAN TO KING'S COLLEGE HOSPITAL.

HOOPER'S PHYSICIAN'S VADE-MECUM; OR, MANUAL
THE PRINCIPLES AND PRACTICE OF PHYSIC. New Edition, conside
enlarged, and re-written. Foolscap 8vo. cloth, 12s. 6d.

GUY'S HOSPITAL REPORTS. Vol. VIII. Part II., 7s., with Pl

CONTENTS.

1. On the Treatment to be adopted in Wounds in Arteries and Traumatic Aneu
   By the late BRANSBY B. COOPER, F.R.S.
2. Cases of Bright's Disease, with Remarks. By SAMUEL WILKS, M.D.
3. Case of Foreign Body introduced into the Bladder. By C. Syrum. With a Pl
4. Saccharine Matter; its Physiological Relations in the Animal Economy. By 1
   WILLIAM PAVY, M.B. With Plate.
5. On Dentine of Repair, and the Laws which Regulate its Formation. By S. J
   A. SALTER, M.B., F.L.S. With Plates.
6. Notes on the Development and Design of Portions of the Cranium; being a
   from the Lectures on Anatomy by JOHN HILTON, F.R.S. With Plates.
7. Cases of Laceration of the Perinaeum and Procidentia of the Uterus and
   remedied by Operation. By JOHN C. W. LEVER, M.D.
8. Half Yearly Report of all the Cases admitted into Guy's Hospital, from the C
   mencement of April to October, 1853. Medical Report by SAMUEL WILKS, M
   Surgical Report by A. POLAND, Esq.
9. Conclusion of a Case of Intestinal Obstruction treated by Operation. By J. Hn
   F.R.S.

DR. JAMES HOPE, F.R.S.

ON DISEASES OF THE HEART AND GREAT VESSE

Fourth Edition. Post 8vo. cloth, 10s. 6d.

"This is a new edition of the late Dr. Hope's well-known treatise, reduced in size and price; those who are desirous of possessing this truly standard work, we would strongly recommend the edition."—*Provincial Medical Journal.*

MR. THOMAS HUNT, M.R.C.S.

THE PATHOLOGY AND TREATMENT OF CERTAIN I

EASES OF THE SKIN, generally pronounced Intractable. Illustrated by up of Forty Cases. 8vo. cloth, 6s.

"We have found Mr. Hunt's practice exceedingly successful in severe obstinate cases."—*B waite's Retrospect of Medicine.*

"The facts and views he brings forward eminently merit attention."—*British and Foreign M Review.*

DR. ARTHUR JACOB, F.R.C.S.

PROFESSOR OF ANATOMY AND PHYSIOLOGY IN THE ROYAL COLLEGE OF SURGEONS IN IREL

A TREATISE ON THE INFLAMMATIONS OF THE EYE-BA

Foolscap 8vo. cloth, 5s.

It includes the Description and Treatment of the Idiopathic, Scrofulous, Rheum Arthritic, Syphilitic, Gonorrhœal, Post-febrile, and Neuralgic Species; as well as circumscribed Inflammations of the Cornea, Membrane of the Aqueous Humour, Cho Crystalline Lens and Retina; and also Inflammation from Injury, with the Sympathetic Phlebitic varieties.

MR. WHARTON JONES, F.R.S.

PROFESSOR OF OPHTHALMIC MEDICINE AND SURGERY IN UNIVERSITY COLLEGE

A MANUAL OF THE PRINCIPLES AND PRACTICE

OPHTHALMIC MEDICINE AND SURGERY; illustrated with 102 Engrav plain and coloured. Foolscap 8vo. cloth, 12s. 6d.

"We can assure students that they cannot meet with a hand-book on this subject that is more or more carefully written."—*Medical Gazette.*

"We entertain little doubt that this work will become a manual for daily reference and consult by the student and general practitioner."—*British and Foreign Medical Review.*

II.

THE WISDOM AND BENEFICENCE OF THE ALMIGHT

AS DISPLAYED IN THE SENSE OF VISION; being the Actonian Prize E for 1851. With Illustrations on Steel and Wood. Foolscap 8vo. cloth, 4s. 6d.

"A fit sequel to the Bridgewater Treatises: it is philosophically and admirably written."—*Lit Gazette.*

"This treatise resembles in style of treatment the famous Bridgewater Treatises."—*Athenæum.*

DR. BENCE JONES, F.R.S.

ON ANIMAL CHEMISTRY, in its relation to STOMACH and KEN

DISEASES. 8vo. cloth, 6s.

"The work of Dr. Bence Jones is one of the most philosophical and practical which has issued the press for many years past."—*Lancet.*

"Dr. Bence Jones is already favourably known as the author of works and papers on animal chemi and this contribution to his favourite science is calculated to extend his reputation as an able the and sound physician."—*Monthly Medical Journal.*

MR. NASMYTH, F.L.S., F.G.S., F.R.C.S.

RESEARCHES ON THE DEVELOPMENT, STRUCTURE, AND
DISEASES OF THE TEETH. With Ten finely-engraved Plates, and Forty Illustrations on Wood. 8vo. cloth, 1*l.* 1*s.*

DR. NOBLE.

I.

ELEMENTS OF PSYCHOLOGICAL MEDICINE: AN INTRO-
DUCTION TO THE PRACTICAL STUDY OF INSANITY. Post 8vo. cloth, 7*s.* 6*d.*

II.

THE BRAIN AND ITS PHYSIOLOGY. Post 8vo. cloth, 6*s.*

MR. NOURSE, M.R.C.S.

TABLES FOR STUDENTS. Price One Shilling.

1. Divisions and Classes of the Animal Kingdom.
2. Classes and Orders of the Vertebrate Sub-kingdom.
3. Classes of the Vegetable Kingdom, according to the Natural and Artificial Systems.
4. Table of the Elements, with their Chemical Equivalents and Symbols.

MR. NUNNELEY.

A TREATISE ON THE NATURE, CAUSES, AND TREATMENT
OF ERYSIPELAS. 8vo. cloth, 10*s.* 6*d.*

𝔒𝔵𝔣𝔬𝔯𝔡 𝔈𝔡𝔦𝔱𝔦𝔬𝔫𝔰.—Edited by Dr. GREENHILL.

I. ADDRESS TO A MEDICAL STUDENT. Second Edition, 18mo. cloth, 2*s.* 6*d.*

II. PRAYERS FOR THE USE OF THE MEDICAL PROFESSION. Second Edition, cloth, 1*s.* 6*d.*

III. LIFE OF SIR JAMES STONHOUSE, BART., M.D. Cloth, 4*s.* 6*d.*

IV. ANECDOTA SYDENHAMIANA. Second Edition, 18mo. 2*s.*

V. LIFE OF THOMAS HARRISON BURDER, M.D. 18mo. cloth, 4*s.*

VI. BURDER'S LETTERS FROM A SENIOR TO A JUNIOR PHYSICIAN, ON PROMOTING THE RELIGIOUS WELFARE OF HIS PATIENTS. 18mo. sewed, 6*d.*

VII. LIFE OF GEORGE CHEYNE, M.D. 18mo. sewed, 2*s.* 6*d.*

VIII. HUFELAND ON THE RELATIONS OF THE PHYSICIAN TO THE SICK, TO THE PUBLIC, AND TO HIS COLLEAGUES. 18mo. sewed, 9*d.*

IX. GISBORNE ON THE DUTIES OF PHYSICIANS. 18mo. sewed, 1*s.*

X. LIFE OF CHARLES BRANDON TRYE. 18mo. sewed, 1*s.*

XI. PERCIVAL'S MEDICAL ETHICS. Third Edition, 18mo. cloth, 3*s.*

XII. CODE OF ETHICS OF THE AMERICAN MEDICAL ASSOCIATION. 8*d.*

XIII. WARE ON THE DUTIES AND QUALIFICATIONS OF PHYSICIANS. 8*d.*

XIV. MAURICE ON THE RESPONSIBILITIES OF MEDICAL STUDENTS. 9*d.*

XV. FRASER'S QUERIES IN MEDICAL ETHICS. 9*d.*

PHARMACOPŒIA COLLEGII REGALIS MEDICORUM LON-
DINENSIS. 8vo. cloth, 9s.; or 24mo. 5s.

IMPRIMATUR.
Hic liber, cui titulus, PHARMACOPŒIA COLLEGII REGALIS MEDICORUM LONDINENSIS.
Datum ex Ædibus Collegii in comitiis censoriis, Novembris Mensis 14° 1850.

JOHANNES AYRTON PARIS. *Præses.*

THE PRESCRIBER'S PHARMACOPŒIA; containing all the Medi-
cines in the London Pharmacopœia, arranged in Classes according to their Action, with
their Composition and Doses. By a Practising Physician. Fourth Edition. 32mo.
cloth, 2s. 6d.; roan tuck (for the pocket), 3s. 6d.

" Never was half-a-crown better spent than in the purchase of this ' *Thesaurus Medicaminum.*' This
little work, with our visiting-book and stethoscope, are our daily companions in the carriage."—
Dr. Johnson's Review.

DR. PROUT, F.R.S.

ON THE NATURE AND TREATMENT OF STOMACH AND
RENAL DISEASES; being an Inquiry into the Connection of Diabetes, Calculus, and
other Affections of the Kidney and Bladder with Indigestion. Fifth Edition. With
Seven Engravings on Steel. 8vo. cloth, 20s.

SIR WM. PYM, K.C.H.,
INSPECTOR-GENERAL OF ARMY HOSPITALS.

OBSERVATIONS UPON YELLOW FEVER, with a Review of
"A Report upon the Diseases of the African Coast, by Sir WM. BURNETT and
Dr. BRYSON," proving its highly Contagious Powers. Post 8vo. 6s.

DR. RADCLIFFE.
I.

PROTEUS; OR, THE LAW OF NATURE. 8vo. cloth, 6s.

" We can truly commend Dr. Radcliffe's essay as full of interest, sound in its inferences, and calculated to enlarge our ideas of the vastness and simplicity of the scheme of creation, while, at the same
time, it tends to increase our reverent admiration of the Omnipotence and Omniscience which, amidst
such apparent incongruity, has established harmony, and has so marvellously combined unity of plan
with endless variety of detail."—*Medical Gazette.*

II.

THE PHILOSOPHY OF VITAL MOTION. 8vo. cloth, 6

*** The chief object of this work is to demonstrate the existence of a common law of motion in
the organic and inorganic world, by showing that the real operation of nervous and other vital
agencies, and of electricity and other physical forces, is not to excite or stimulate contraction in
muscle and other organic tissues, but to counteract this state and induce relaxation or expansion.
By this means vital contraction is shown to be a purely physical phenomenon, perfectly analogous
to that which takes place in a bar of metal when heat is withdrawn; and in addition to this, a
new and intelligible explanation is afforded of capillary action and the rhythmical action of the
heart.*

DR. ROYLE, F.R.S.
A MANUAL OF MATERIA MEDICA AND THERAPEUTICS.
With numerous Engravings on Wood. Second Edition. Fcap. 8vo. cloth, 12s. 6d.

"This is another of that beautiful and cheap series of Manuals published by Mr. Churchill. The execution of the wood-cuts of plants, flowers, and fruits is admirable. The work is indeed a most valuable one."—*British and Foreign Medical Review.*

MR. SAVORY,
MEMBER OF THE SOCIETY OF APOTHECARIES.
A COMPENDIUM OF DOMESTIC MEDICINE, AND COMPA-
NION TO THE MEDICINE CHEST; comprising Plain Directions for the Employment of Medicines, with their Properties and Doses, and Brief Descriptions of the Symptoms and Treatment of Diseases, and of the Disorders incidental to Infants and Children, with a Selection of the most efficacious Prescriptions. Intended as a Source of Easy Reference for Clergymen, and for Families residing at a Distance from Professional Assistance. Fourth Edition. 12mo. cloth, 5s.

DR. SHAPTER.
I.
THE CLIMATE OF THE SOUTH OF DEVON, AND ITS IN-
FLUENCE UPON HEALTH. With short Accounts of Exeter, Torquay, Teignmouth, Dawlish, Exmouth, Sidmouth, &c. Illustrated with a Map geologically coloured. Post 8vo. cloth, 7s. 6d.

"This volume is far more than a guide-book. It contains much statistical information, with very minute local details, that may be advantageously consulted by the medical man before he recommends any specific residence in Devonshire to his patient."—*Athenæum.*

II.
THE HISTORY OF THE CHOLERA IN EXETER IN 1832.
Illustrated with Map and Woodcuts. 8vo. cloth, 12s.

MR. SHAW.
THE MEDICAL REMEMBRANCER; OR, BOOK OF EMER-
GENCIES: in which are concisely pointed out the Immediate Remedies to be adopted in the First Moments of Danger from Poisoning, Drowning, Apoplexy, Burns, and other Accidents; with the Tests for the Principal Poisons, and other useful Information. Third Edition. 32mo. cloth, 2s. 6d.

"The plan of this little book is well conceived, and the execution corresponds thereunto. It costs little money, and will occupy little room; and we think no practitioner will regret being the possessor of what cannot fail, sooner or later, to be useful to him."—*British and Foreign Medical Review.*

MR. SKEY, F.R.S.
OPERATIVE SURGERY; with Illustrations engraved on Wood. 8vo. cloth, 18s.

"Mr. Skey's work is a perfect model for the operating surgeon, who will learn from it not only when and how to operate, but some more noble and exalted lessons, which cannot fail to improve him as a moral and social agent."—*Edinburgh Medical and Surgical Journal.*

"We pronounce Mr. Skey's 'Operative Surgery' to be a work of the very highest importance—a work by itself. The correctness of our opinion we trustfully leave to the judgment of the profession."—*Medical Gazette.*

DR. SPURGIN.
LECTURES ON MATERIA MEDICA, AND ITS RELATIONS
TO THE ANIMAL ECONOMY. Delivered before the Royal College of Physicians. 8vo. cloth, 5s. 6d.

"Dr. Spurgin has evidently devoted much time and labour to the composition of these lectures; and the result is, that he has produced one of the most philosophical essays on the subject of "Materia Medica" existing in the English language."—*Psychological Journal.*

VESTIGES OF THE NATURAL HISTORY OF CREATION.

Tenth Edition. Illustrated with 100 Engravings on Wood. 8vo. cloth, 12s. 6d.

BY THE SAME AUTHOR.

EXPLANATIONS: A SEQUEL TO "VESTIGES."

Second Edition. Post 8vo. cloth, 5s.

DR. VAN OVEN.

ON THE DECLINE OF LIFE IN HEALTH AND DISEASE;

being an Attempt to Investigate the Causes of LONGEVITY, and the Best Means of Attaining a Healthful Old Age. 8vo. cloth, 10s. 6d.

MR. WADE, F.R.C.S.,
SENIOR SURGEON TO THE WESTMINSTER DISPENSARY.

STRICTURE OF THE URETHRA; its Complications and Effects.

With Practical Observations on its Causes, Symptoms, and Treatment; and on a Safe and Efficient Mode of Treating its more Intractable Forms. 8vo. cloth, 5s.

" Mr. Wade is well known to have paid great attention to the subject of stricture for many years past, and is deservedly looked upon as an authority on this matter."—*Medical Times and Gazette.*

DR. WAGSTAFF.

ON DISEASES OF THE MUCOUS MEMBRANE OF THE

THROAT, and their Treatment by Topical Medication. Post 8vo. cloth, 4s. 6d.

DR. WALLER,
LECTURER ON MIDWIFERY AT ST. THOMAS'S HOSPITAL.

I.

ELEMENTS OF PRACTICAL MIDWIFERY; OR, COMPANION

TO THE LYING-IN ROOM. With Plates. Third Edition. 18mo. cloth, 3s. 6d.

" Students and practitioners in midwifery will find it an invaluable pocket companion."—*Medical Times and Gazette.*

II.

A PRACTICAL TREATISE ON THE FUNCTION AND DIS-

EASES OF THE UNIMPREGNATED WOMB. 8vo. cloth, 9s.

MR. HAYNES WALTON, F.R.C.S.,
SURGEON TO THE CENTRAL LONDON OPHTHALMIC HOSPITAL.

OPERATIVE OPHTHALMIC SURGERY. With Engravings on

Wood. 8vo. cloth, 18s.

" We have carefully examined the book, and can consistently say, that it is eminently a practical work, evincing in its author great research, a thorough knowledge of his subject, and an accurate and most observing mind."—*Dublin Quarterly Journal.*

DR. WARDROP.

ON DISEASES OF THE HEART. 8vo. cloth, 12s.

DR. WEGG.

OBSERVATIONS RELATING TO THE SCIENCE AND ART
OF MEDICINE. 8vo. cloth, 8s.

'We have much pleasure in stating, that the work is highly instructive, and proclaims its author to be a sober, sound, and able physician."—*London Journal of Medicine.*

DR. WHITEHEAD, F.R.C.S.,
SURGEON TO THE MANCHESTER AND SALFORD LYING-IN HOSPITAL.

I.

ON THE TRANSMISSION FROM PARENT TO OFFSPRING
OF SOME FORMS OF DISEASE, AND OF MORBID TAINTS AND TENDENCIES. 8vo. cloth, 10s. 6d.

II.

THE CAUSES AND TREATMENT OF ABORTION AND
STERILITY: being the result of an extended Practical Inquiry into the Physiological and Morbid Conditions of the Uterus, with reference especially to Leucorrhœal Affections, and the Diseases of Menstruation. 8vo. cloth, 12s.

"The work is valuable and instructive, and one that reflects much credit plus on the industry and practical skill of the author."—*Medico-Chirurgical Review.*

MR. WILLIAM R. WILDE, F.R.C.S.I.

AURAL SURGERY, AND THE NATURE AND TREATMENT
OF DISEASES OF THE EAR. 8vo. cloth, 12s. 6d.

"We have no hesitation in expressing our opinion that the book is by far the best treatise on Aural Surgery which has yet appeared in any language."—*Medical Times and Gazette.*

DR. JOHN CALTHROP WILLIAMS,
LATE PHYSICIAN TO THE GENERAL HOSPITAL, NOTTINGHAM.

PRACTICAL OBSERVATIONS ON NERVOUS AND SYM-
PATHETIC PALPITATION OF THE HEART, as well as on Palpitation the Result of Organic Disease. Second Edition, 8vo. cloth, 6s.

"From the extracts we have given, our readers will see that Dr. Williams's treatise is both able and practical."—*Medical Times.*
"The work is calculated to add to the author's reputation, and it is creditable to the provincial practitioners of England that so useful a treatise should have emanated from one of their body."—*Dublin Medical Press.*

DR. J. WILLIAMS.

I.

INSANITY: its Causes, Prevention, and Cure; including Apoplexy,
Epilepsy, and Congestion of the Brain. Second Edition. Post 8vo. cloth, 10s. 6d.

II.

ON THE ANATOMY, PHYSIOLOGY, AND PATHOLOGY OF
THE EAR; being the Prize Essay in the University of Edinburgh. With Plates. 8vo. cloth, 10s. 6d.

DR. G. C. WITTSTEIN.

PRACTICAL PHARMACEUTICAL CHEMISTRY: An Explanation
of Chemical and Pharmaceutical Processes, with the Methods of Testing the Purity of the Preparations, deduced from Original Experiments. Translated from the Second German Edition, by STEPHEN DARBY. 18mo. cloth, 6s.

Lightning Source UK Ltd.
Milton Keynes UK
UKOW05f1845050217
293666UK00008B/169/P

9 781334 646591